Surgery at a Glance

This new book is also available as an ebook.
For more details, please see www.wiley.com/buy/9781118272206
or scan this QR code:

<table>
<tr><td>Includes a companion website at:</td><td>**Companion website**</td></tr>
</table>

	Companion website
Includes a companion website at:	
	www.testgeneralsurgery.com
Featuring:	
– MCQs	
– Short answer questions.	

Surgery at a Glance

Pierce A. Grace

MA, MCh, FRCSI, FRCS
Professor of Surgical Science
Graduate Entry Medical School
University Hospital Limerick
Limerick, Ireland

Neil R. Borley

FRCS, FRCS (Ed), MS
Consultant Colorectal Surgeon
Cheltenham General Hospital
Cheltenham, UK

Fifth edition

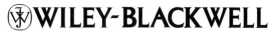
WILEY-BLACKWELL

A John Wiley & Sons, Ltd., Publication

This edition first published 2013 © 2013 by John Wiley & Sons, Ltd.
Previous editions 1999, 2002, 2006, 2009

Wiley-Blackwell is an imprint of John Wiley & Sons, formed by the merger of Wiley's global Scientific, Technical and Medical business with Blackwell Publishing.

Registered office: John Wiley & Sons, Ltd, The Atrium, Southern Gate, Chichester, West Sussex, PO19 8SQ, UK

Editorial offices: 9600 Garsington Road, Oxford, OX4 2DQ, UK
The Atrium, Southern Gate, Chichester, West Sussex, PO19 8SQ, UK
111 River Street, Hoboken, NJ 07030-5774, USA

For details of our global editorial offices, for customer services and for information about how to apply for permission to reuse the copyright material in this book please see our website at www.wiley.com/wiley-blackwell.

The right of the author to be identified as the author of this work has been asserted in accordance with the UK Copyright, Designs and Patents Act 1988.

Library of Congress Cataloging-in-Publication Data
Grace, P.A. (Pierce A.)
Surgery at a glance / Pierce Grace, Neil R.Borley. – 5ᵗʰ ed.
p. ; cm.
Includes bibliographical references and index.
ISBN 978-1-118-27220-6 (pbk.: alk.paper)
1. Borley, Neil R. 11. Title. [DNLM. 1. Surgical Procedures, Operative–Handbooks.
2. Diagnostic
Techniques and Procedures – Handbooks. WO 39]

617'.9—dc23

2012032718

Cover image: SCIENCE PHOTO LIBRARY © MAURO FERMARIELLO
Cover design by Meaden Creative

A catalogue record for this book is available from the British Library.

Set in Times 9/11.5 pt by Toppan Best-set Premedia Limited
Printed and bound in Malaysia by Vivar Printing Sdn Bhd

1   2013

Contents

Companion website

Includes a companion website at:

www.testgeneralsurgery.com

Featuring:
- MCQs
- Short answer questions.

Preface

Surgery at a Glance continues to be a very popular text with medical students and others who study surgery. In full colour, the book, in keeping with the *At a Glance* series in general, has a very user-friendly layout and is easy to read. A key feature of *Surgery at a Glance* is its division into clinical presentations and surgical diseases. Thus, in one volume is combined the ways that patients present with surgical problems and the surgical diseases that underlie those presentations. Fourteen years on we are delighted to present the revised and updated fifth edition of *Surgery at a Glance*. The new edition contains some additions. In response to feedback from medical students we have added four new chapters on orthopaedics as well as updating the text and illustrations throughout the book. The book retains its colour profile and beautiful illustrations. We have had lots of help and suggestions from several people in putting this book together. We would like to thank the many medical students and colleagues who have read the book and given us good advice. Students seem to like this book particularly for revision in preparation for exams. We especially thank the publishing team and illustrators at Wiley-Blackwell for their hard work in bringing this beautifully presented book to completion. We believe that the fifth edition of *Surgery at a Glance* is an excellent book and we hope that this text will continue to help students understand surgery.

Pierce A. Grace
Neil R. Borley
2013

List of abbreviations

AAA	abdominal aortic aneurysm	CEA	carcinoembryonic antigen
AAT	aspartate amino transferase	CEA	carotid endarterectomy
ABI	ankle–brachial pressure index	cfu	colony forming units
Abs	antibiotics	CgA	chromogranin A
ACE	angiotensin converting enzyme	CK	creatinine kinase
Ach	acetylcholine	CLO	*Campylobacter*-like organism
ACN	acute cortical necrosis	CMV	cisplatin, methotrexate, vinblastine
ACS	acute coronary syndrome	CMV	cytomegalovirus
ACTH	adrenocorticotrophic hormone	CNS	central nervous system
ADH	antidiuretic hormone	COCP	combined oral contraceptive pill
AF	atrial fibrillation	COPD	chronic obstructive pulmonary disease
AFP	α-fetoprotein	COX	cyclo-oxygenase
Ag	antigen	CPK-MB	creatine phosphokinase (cardiac type)
AJCC	American Joint Committee on Cancer	CRC	colorectal carcinoma
AKI	acute kidney injury	CRF	chronic renal failure
Alb	albumin	CRP	C-reactive protein
ALI	acute lung injury	CSF	cerebrospinal fluid
ALND	axillary lymph node dissection	CT	computed tomography
ANCA	antineutrophil cytoplasmic antibody	CTA	computed tomographic angiogram
ANDI	abnormalities of the normal development and involution (of the breast)	CTCV	congenital talipes calcaneo valgus
		CVA	cerebrovascular accident
AP	angina pectoris	CVI	chronic venous insufficiency
AP	anteroposterior	CVP	central venous pressure
APACHE	acute physiology and chronic health evaluation	CVS	cardiovascular system
APTT	activated partial thromboplastin time	CXR	chest X-ray
ARB	angiotensin receptor blocker	D_2	type 2 dopaminergic receptors
ARDS	adult/acute respiratory distress syndrome	DCIS	ductal carcinoma in situ
ARF	acute renal failure	DDAVP	1-desamino-8-arginine vasopressin (desmopressin)
ASA	American Society of Anesthesiologists	DDH	developmental dysplaia of the hip
ASCA	anti-*Saccharomyces cerevisiae* antibodies	DHEA	dihydroepiandrosterone
ATN	acute tubular necrosis	DIC	disseminated intravascular coagulation
AV	arteriovenous	DM	diabetes mellitus
BCC	basal cell carcinoma	DMARDs	disease-modifying antirheumatic drugs
BCG	bacillus Calmette–Guérin	DMSA	dimercaptosuccinic acid
b.d.	twice daily	DU	duodenal ulcer
BDM	bone mineral density	DVT	deep venous thrombosis
BE	base excess	Dx	diagnosis
BEP	bleomycin, etoposide, cisplatin	DXA	dual energy X-ray absorptiometry
BMI	body mass index	DXT	deep X-ray therapy
BP	blood pressure	EAS	external anal sphincter
BPH	benign prostatic hypertrophy	EBV	Epstein–Barr virus
BS	breath sounds	ECG	electrocardiogram
bx	biopsy	EMLA	Eutetic Mixture of Local Anaesthetic
C&S	culture and sensitivity	ER	oestrogen receptor
CABG	coronary artery bypass graft	ERCP	endoscopic retrograde cholangio-pancreatograph
CAD	coronary artery disease	ESR	erythrocyte sedimentation rate
cAMP	cyclic adenosine monophosphate	ESWL	extracorporeal shock-wave lithotripsy
CA-MRSA	community-associated methicillin-resistant *Staphylococcus aureus*	EUA	examination under anaesthesia
		EUS	endoscopic ultrasound
CAS	carotid angioplasty and stent	FAP	familial polyposis coli
CBD	common bile duct	FBC	full blood count
CCF	congestive cardiac failure	FCD	fibrocystic disease
CD	*Clostridium difficile*	FFP	fresh frozen plasma
CDH	congenital dysplaia of the hip	FHx	family history
CDI	central diabetes insipidus		

FNAC	fine-needle aspiration cytology
FSH	follicle-stimulating hormone
5-FU	5-fluorouracil
gFOBT	guaiac faecal occult blood test
γ-GT	gamma glutamyl transpeptidase
GA	general anaesthetic
GC	gemcitabine, cisplatin
GCS	Glasgow Coma Scale
GFR	glomerular filtration rate
GH	growth hormone
GI	gastrointestinal
GIST	gastrointestinal stromal tumour
Gm+, Gm−	Gram-positive, Gram-negative
GORD	gastro-oesophageal reflux disease
GSF	greater sciatica foramen
GTN	glyceryl trinitrate
GU	gastric ulcer
GU	genito-urinary
GVHD	graft-versus-host disease
HALO	haemorrhoidal artery ligation operation
Hb	haemoglobin
HCG	human chorionic gonadotrophin
β-HCG	beta-human chorionic gonadotrophin
Hct	haematocrit
HCT	hematopoietic cell transplantation
HDL	high density lipoprotein
HDU	high-dependency unit
HER2/neu	human epidermal growth factor receptor 2
HIDA	hepatabiliary imido-diacetic acid
HLA	human leucocyte antigen
HNPCC	hereditary non-polyposis colorectal cancer (Lynch syndrome)
HoLEP	holium laser enucleation of prostate
hPTH	human parathyroid hormone
HRT	hormone replacement therapy
HVA	homovanillic acid
Hx	history
I&D	incision and drainage
IBS	irritable bowel syndrome
ICP	intracranial pressure
ICS	intercostal space
ICU	intensive care unit
IFN-γ	interferon gamma
Ig	immunoglobulin
IGF	insulin-like growth factor
IL	interleukin
iNOS	inducible nitric oxide synthetase
INR	international normalized ratio
IPPV	intermittent positive pressure ventilation
IV	intravenous
IVC	inferior vena cava
IVU	intravenous urogram
JGA	juxtaglomerular apparatus
JVP	jugular venous pulse
KUB	kidney, ureter, bladder
LA	local anaesthetic
LAD	left anterior descending
LATS	long-acting thyroid stimulating (factor)
LBO	large bowel obstruction
LCA	left coronary artery
LDH	lactate dehydrogenase
LDL	low density lipoprotein
LDUH	low dose unfractionated heparin
LFT	liver function test
LH	luteinizing hormone
LHRH	LH-releasing hormone
LIF	left iliac fossa
LMWH	low molecular weight heparin
LOC	loss of consciousness
LOS	lower oesophageal sphincter
LPS	lipopolysaccharide
LRD	living related donor
LSE	left sternal edge
LSF	lesser sciatica foramen
LSV	long saphenous vein
LUQ	left upper quadrant
LURD	living unrelated donor
LUTS	lower urinary tract symptoms
LV	left ventricle
LVF	left ventricular failure
MAG3	mercapto acetyl triglycine
MAP	mean arterial pressure
MCP	metacarpophalangeal
MC+S	microscopy cultures and sensitivity
MDRO	multidrug-resistant organisms
MDT	multidisciplinary team
MEAC	minimum effective analgesic concentration
MEN	multiple endocrine neoplasia
MI	myocardial infarction
MIBG	*meta*-iodo-benzyl guanidine
MM	malignant melanoma
MND	motor neurone disease
MODS	multiple organ dysfunction syndrome
MRA	magnetic resonance angiography
MRCP	magnetic resonance cholangio-pancreatography
MRI	magnetic resonance imaging
MRSA	methicillin-resistant *Staphylococcus aureus*
MS	multiple sclerosis
MSH	melanocyte-stimulating hormone
MSU	mid-stream urine
MT	major trauma
mTOR	mammalian target of rapamycin
MTP	metatarsophalangeal
MUGA	multiple uptake gated analysis
MVAC	methotrexate, vinblastine, doxorubicin (Adriamycin), cisplatin
N&V	nausea and vomiting
NAdr	noradrenaline/norepinephrine
NDI	nephrogenic diabetes insipidus
NF-κB	nuclear factor-κB
NG	nasogastric
NK	natural killer
NPO	nil *per oram* (nil by mouth)
NSAID	non-steroidal anti-inflammatory drug
NSGCT	non-seminomatous germ cell tumour
NSTEMI	non-ST elevation myocardial infarction
NSU	non-specific urethritis
OA	osteoarthritis

OAB	overactive bladder	SGCT	seminomatous germ cell tumour
o/e	on examination	SIADH	syndrome of inappropriate antidiuretic hormone
OGD	oesophago-gastro-duodenoscopy	SIRS	systemic inflammatory response syndrome
OGJ	oesophago-gastric junction	SLE	systemic lupus erythematosus
PA	posteroanterior	SLN	superior laryngeal nerve
PAD	peripheral arterial disease	SPECT	sestamibi-single photon emission computed tomography
PAF	platelet activating factor		
PAI-1	plasminogen activator inhibitor	SRS	somatostatin receptor scintigraphy
pANCA	perinuclear antineutrophil cytoplasmic antibody	SSV	short saphenous vein
PCA	patient-controlled analgesia	STEMI	ST elevation myocardial infarction
PCI	percutaneous coronary intervention	SVC	superior vena cava
PCV	packed cell volume	T_3	tri-iodothyronine
PE	pulmonary embolism	T_4	thyroxine
PEEP	positive end expiratory pressure	TAA	thoracic aortic aneurysm
PEG	percutaneous endoscopic gastrostomy	TB	tuberculosis
PET	positron emission tomography	TCC	transitional cell carcinoma
PHPT	primary hyperparathyroidism	TED	thrombo-embolic deterrent
PID	pelvic inflammatory disease	TENS	transcutaneous electrical nerve stimulation
PIP	proximal inter phalangeal	tLOSR	transient lower esophageal relaxation
PL	prolactin	TIA	transient ischaemic attack
POP	plaster of Paris	TKI	tyrosine kinase inhibitor
POVD	peripheral occlusive vascular disease	TNF	tumour necrosis factor
PPI	proton pump inhibitor	TNM	tumour, node, metastasis (UICC)
PR	per rectum	tPA	tissue plasminogen activator
PSA	prostate-specific antigen	TPHA	treponema pallidum haemagglutination (test)
PT	prothrombin time	TPR	temperature, pulse, respiration
PTH	parathyroid hormone	TRUS	transrectal ultrasound
PUD	peptic ulcer disease	TSH	thyroid-stimulating hormone
PUO	pyrexia of unknown origin	TURP	transurethral resection of the prostate
PV	*per vaginum*	TURT	transurethral resection of tumour
PVD	peripheral vascular disease	TxP	transplantation
QoL	quality of life	UC	ulcerative colitis
RA	rheumatoid arthritis	UDT	undescended testis
RBC	red blood cell	U+E	urea and electrolytes
RCC	renal cell carcinoma	UI	urinary incontinence
RD	respiratory depression	uPA	urokinase plasminogen activator
rhAPC	recombinant human activated protein C	U/S	ultrasound
RIA	radioimmunoassay	UTI	urinary tract infection
RIF	right iliac fossa	VEGF	vascular endothelial growth factor
RLN	recurrent laryngeal nerve	VEGFR	vascular endothelial growth factor receptor
RPLND	retroperitoneal lymph node dissection	VF	ventricular fibrillation
RS	respiratory system	VHL	von Hippel–Lindau
RT	radiotherapy	VIP	vasoactive intestinal peptide
RTA	road traffic accident	VMA	vanillyl mandelic acid
RUQ	right upper quadrant	V/Q	ventilation–perfusion
RV	right ventricle	VRE	vancomycin-resistant enterococcus
RVF	right ventricular failure	VSD	ventricular septal defect
Rx	treatment	VV	varicose veins
SCC	squamous cell carcinoma	WBC	white blood cell
SCFE	slipped capital femoral epiphysis	WCC	white cell count
SERM	selective oestrogen receptor modulators	ZE	Zollinger Ellison

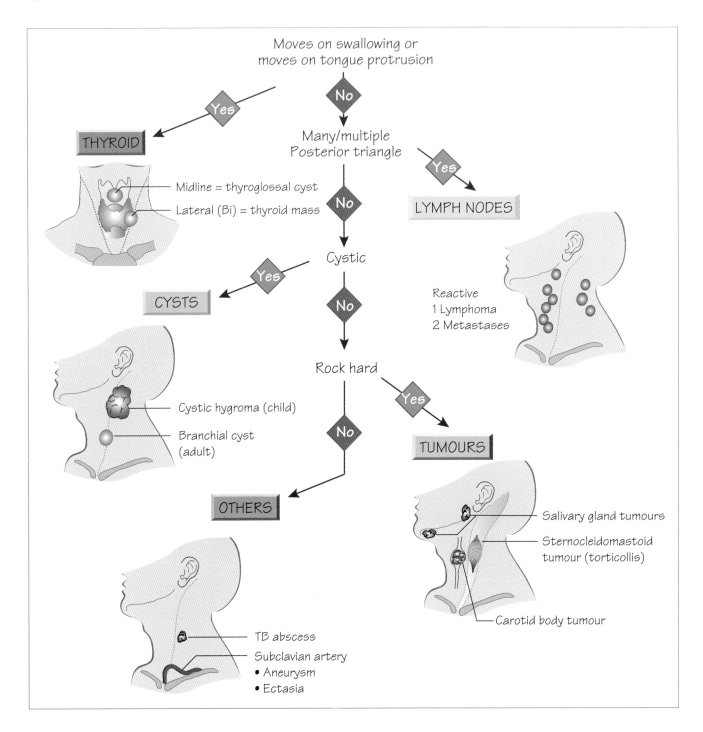

Moves on swallowing or
moves on tongue protrusion

Yes → **THYROID**

Midline = thyroglossal cyst
Lateral (Bi) = thyroid mass

No

Many/multiple
Posterior triangle

Yes → **LYMPH NODES**

Reactive
1 Lymphoma
2 Metastases

No

Cystic

Yes → **CYSTS**

Cystic hygroma (child)
Branchial cyst (adult)

No

Rock hard

Yes → **TUMOURS**

Salivary gland tumours
Sternocleidomastoid tumour (torticollis)
Carotid body tumour

No → **OTHERS**

TB abscess
Subclavian artery
• Aneurysm
• Ectasia

Definition

A *neck lump* is any congenital or acquired mass arising in the anterior or posterior triangles of the neck between the clavicles inferiorly and the mandible and base of the skull superiorly.

> ## Key points
>
> - Thyroid swellings move upwards (with the trachea) on swallowing.
> - Most abnormalities of the neck are visible as swellings.
> - Ventral lumps attached to the hyoid bone, such as thyroglossal cysts, move upwards with both swallowing and protrusion of the tongue.
> - Multiple lumps are almost always lymph nodes.
> - In all cases of lymphadenopathy a full head and neck examination, including the oral cavity is mandatory.

Differential diagnosis

- 50% of neck lumps are thyroid in origin.
- 40% of neck lumps are caused by malignancy (80% metastatic usually from primary lesion above the clavicle; 20% primary neoplasms: lymphomas, salivary gland tumours).
- 10% of neck lumps are inflammatory or congenital in origin.

Thyroid
- Goitre, cyst, neoplasm.

Neoplasm
- Metastatic carcinoma.
- Primary lymphoma.
- Salivary gland tumour.
- Sternocleidomastoid tumour.
- Carotid body tumour (rare).

Inflammatory
- Acute infective adenopathy.
- Collar stud abscess.
- Parotitis.

Congenital
- Thyroglossal duct cyst.
- Dermoid cyst.
- Torticollis.
- Branchial cyst.
- Cystic hygroma.

Vascular
- Subclavian or brachiocephalic ectasia (common).
- Subclavian aneurysm (rare).

Important diagnostic features
Children
- Congenital and inflammatory lesions are common.
- Cystic hygroma: in infants, base of the neck, brilliant transillumination, 'come and go'.

- Thyroglossal or dermoid cyst: midline, discrete, elevates with tongue protrusion.
- Torticollis: rock hard mass, more prominent with head flexed, associated with fixed rotation (a fibrous mass in the sternocleidomastoid muscle).
- Branchial cyst (also fistulae or sinus): anterior to the upper third of the sternocleidomastoid.
- Viral/bacterial adenitis: usually affects jugular nodes, multiple, tender masses.
- Neoplasms are unusual in children (lymphoma most common).

Young adults
Inflammatory neck masses and thyroid malignancy are common.
- Viral (e.g. infectious mononucleosis) or bacterial (tonsillitis/pharyngitis) adenitis.
- Papillary thyroid cancer: isolated, non-tender, thyroid mass, possible lymphadenopathy.

Over-40s
Neck lumps are malignant until proven otherwise.
- Metastatic lymphadenopathy: multiple, rock hard, non-tender, tendency to be fixed.
- 75% in primary head and neck (thyroid, nasopharynx, tonsils, larynx, pharynx), 25% from infraclavicular primary (stomach, pancreas, lung).
- Primary lymphadenopathy (thyroid, lymphoma): fleshy, matted, rubbery, large size.
- Primary neoplasm (thyroid, salivary tumour): firm, non-tender, fixed to tissue of origin.

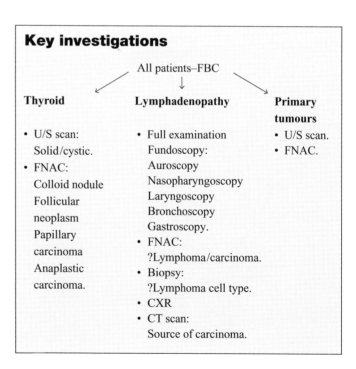

> ## Key investigations
>
> All patients–FBC
>
> ### Thyroid
> - U/S scan:
>   Solid/cystic.
> - FNAC:
>   Colloid nodule
>   Follicular
>   neoplasm
>   Papillary
>   carcinoma
>   Anaplastic
>   carcinoma.
>
> ### Lymphadenopathy
> - Full examination
>   Fundoscopy:
>   Auroscopy
>   Nasopharyngoscopy
>   Laryngoscopy
>   Bronchoscopy
>   Gastroscopy.
> - FNAC:
>   ?Lymphoma/carcinoma.
> - Biopsy:
>   ?Lymphoma cell type.
> - CXR
> - CT scan:
>   Source of carcinoma.
>
> ### Primary tumours
> - U/S scan.
> - FNAC.

2 Dysphagia

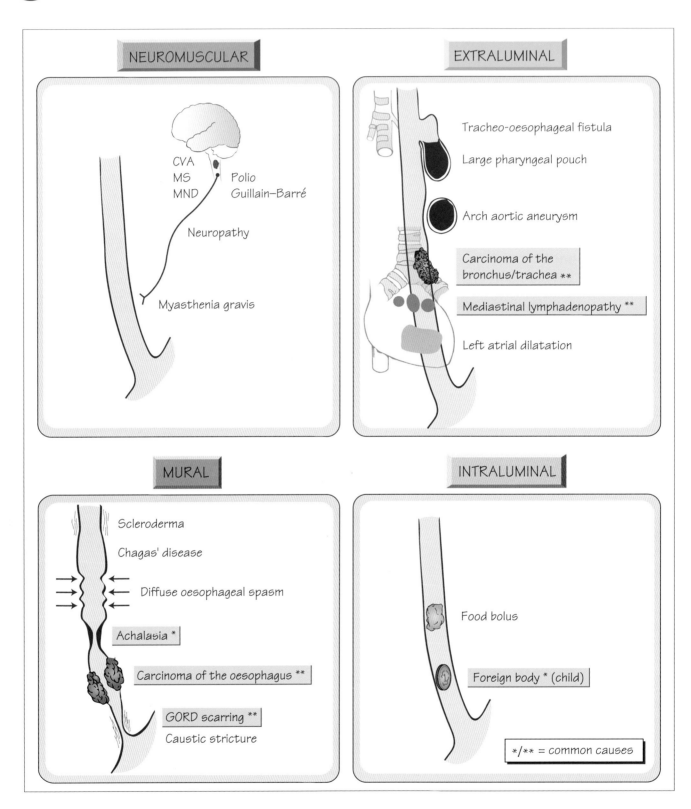

NEUROMUSCULAR

CVA
MS   Polio
MND   Guillain–Barré

Neuropathy

Myasthenia gravis

EXTRALUMINAL

Tracheo-oesophageal fistula

Large pharyngeal pouch

Arch aortic aneurysm

Carcinoma of the bronchus/trachea **

Mediastinal lymphadenopathy **

Left atrial dilatation

MURAL

Scleroderma

Chagas' disease

Diffuse oesophageal spasm

Achalasia *

Carcinoma of the oesophagus **

GORD scarring **
Caustic stricture

INTRALUMINAL

Food bolus

Foreign body * (child)

*/** = common causes

Definition

Dysphagia literally means difficulty with swallowing, which may be associated with ingestion of solids or liquids or both.

Key points

- Most causes of dysphagia are oesophageal in origin.
- In children, foreign bodies and corrosive liquids are common causes.
- In young adults, reflux stricture and achalasia are common.
- In the middle aged and elderly, carcinoma and reflux are common.
- Because the segmental nerve supply of the oesophagus corresponds to the intercostal dermatomes, a patient with dysphagia can accurately pinpoint the level of obstruction.
- Any new symptoms of progressive dysphagia should be assumed to be malignant until proven otherwise. All need endoscopic ± radiological investigation.
- Tumour and achalasia may mimic each other. Endoscopy and biopsy are advisable unless the diagnosis is clear.

Important diagnostic features

Mural causes

- Carcinoma of the oesophagus: progressive course, associated weight loss and anorexia, low-grade anaemia, possible small haematemesis.
- Reflux oesophagitis and stricture: preceded by heartburn, progressive course, nocturnal regurgitation (24-hour oesophageal pH monitoring may be indicated).
- Achalasia: onset in young adulthood or old age, liquids disproportionately difficult to swallow, frequent regurgitation, recurrent chest infections, long history.
- Tracheo-oesophageal fistula: recurrent chest infections, coughing after drinking. Present in infants (congenital) or late adulthood (post trauma, deep X-ray therapy (DXT) or malignant).
- Chagas' disease (*Trypanosoma cruzi*): South American prevalence, associated with dysrhythmias and colonic dysmotility.

- Caustic stricture: examination shows corrosive ingestion, chronic dysphagia, onset may be months after ingestion of caustic agent. Long term risk of developing SCC (1–4%).
- Scleroderma: slow onset, associated with skin changes, Raynaud's phenomenon and mild arthritis.

Intraluminal causes

Foreign body: acute onset, marked retrosternal discomfort, dysphagia even to saliva is characteristic.

Extramural causes

- Pulsion diverticulum (proximal: pharyngo-oesophageal [Zenker's]; distal: epiphrenic): intermittent symptoms, unexpected regurgitation, halitosis.
- External compression: mediastinal lymph nodes, left atrial hypertrophy, bronchial malignancy.

Key investigations

All
FBC: anaemia (tumours much more commonly cause this than reflux).
LFTs: (hepatic disease).
↓
OGD
(moderate risk, specialist, good for differentiating tumour vs. achalasia vs. reflux stricture, allows biopsy for tissue diagnosis, allows possible treatment).
Video contrast swallow
(low risk, easy, good for possible fistula, high tumour, diverticulum, reflux).
↓

If ?dysmotility
- achalasia
- neurogenic causes
↓
Video contrast swallow
Oesophageal manometry

If ?extrinsic compression
↓
CXR (AP and lateral)
CT scan: low risk, good for extrinsic compression, allows tumour staging

3 Haemoptysis

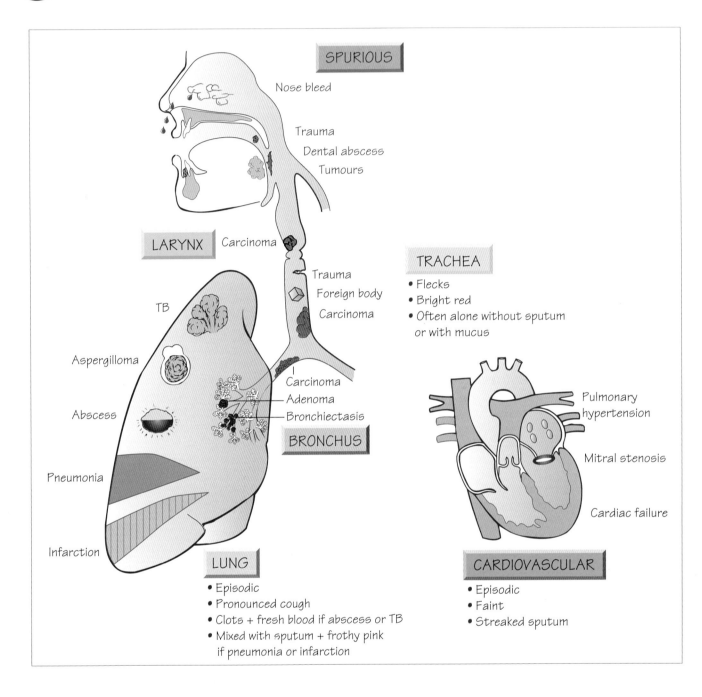

SPURIOUS
Nose bleed
Trauma
Dental abscess
Tumours

LARYNX   Carcinoma

TRACHEA
• Flecks
• Bright red
• Often alone without sputum or with mucus

Trauma
Foreign body
Carcinoma

TB
Aspergilloma
Abscess
Pneumonia
Infarction

Carcinoma
Adenoma
Bronchiectasis
BRONCHUS

Pulmonary hypertension
Mitral stenosis
Cardiac failure

LUNG
• Episodic
• Pronounced cough
• Clots + fresh blood if abscess or TB
• Mixed with sputum + frothy pink if pneumonia or infarction

CARDIOVASCULAR
• Episodic
• Faint
• Streaked sputum

Definition

Haemoptysis (blood spitting) is the symptom of coughing up blood from the lungs. Blood from the nose, mouth or pharynx that may also be spat out is termed 'spurious haemoptysis'.

Key points

- Blood from the proximal bronchi or trachea is usually bright red. It may be frank blood or mixed with mucus and debris, particularly from a tumour.
- Blood from the distal bronchioles and alveoli is often pink and mixed with frothy sputum (e.g. pulmonary oedema).

Important diagnostic features

The sources, causes and features are listed below.

Spurious haemoptysis

Mouth and nose
- Blood dyscrasias: associated nose bleeds, spontaneous bruising.
- Scurvy (vitamin C deficiency): poor hair/teeth, skin bruising.
- Dental caries, trauma, gingivitis.
- Oral tumours: painful intraoral mass, discharge, fetor.
- Hypertensive/spontaneous: no warning, brief bleed, often recurrent.
- Nasal tumours (common in South-East Asia).

True haemoptysis

Larynx and trachea
- Foreign body: choking, stridor, pain.
- Carcinoma: hoarse voice, bovine cough.

Bronchus
- Carcinoma: spontaneous haemoptysis, chest infections, weight loss, monophonic wheezing.
- Adenoma (e.g. carcinoid): recurrent chest infections, carcinoid syndrome.
- Bronchiectasis: chronic chest infections, fetor, blood mixed with copious purulent sputum; physical examination may show TB or severe chest infections.
- Foreign body: recurrent chest infections, sudden-onset inexplicable 'asthma'.

Lung
- TB: weight loss, fevers, night sweats, dry or productive cough.
- Pneumonia: fever, rigors, cough, myalgia, headache, chest pain, dyspnoea.
- Lung abscess: fever, cough, foul-smelling sputum, night sweats, anorexia, gingival disease, clubbing of fingers.
- Pulmonary infarct (secondary to PE): pleuritic chest pain, tachypnoea, pleural rub.
- Aspergilloma.

Cardiac
- Mitral stenosis: frothy pink sputum, recurrent chest infections.
- LVF: frothy pink sputum, pulmonary oedema.

Key investigations

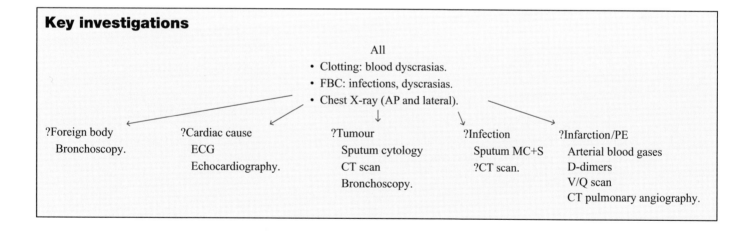

All
- Clotting: blood dyscrasias.
- FBC: infections, dyscrasias.
- Chest X-ray (AP and lateral).

?Foreign body	?Cardiac cause	?Tumour	?Infection	?Infarction/PE
Bronchoscopy.	ECG	Sputum cytology	Sputum MC+S	Arterial blood gases
	Echocardiography.	CT scan	?CT scan.	D-dimers
		Bronchoscopy.		V/Q scan
				CT pulmonary angiography.

4 Breast lump

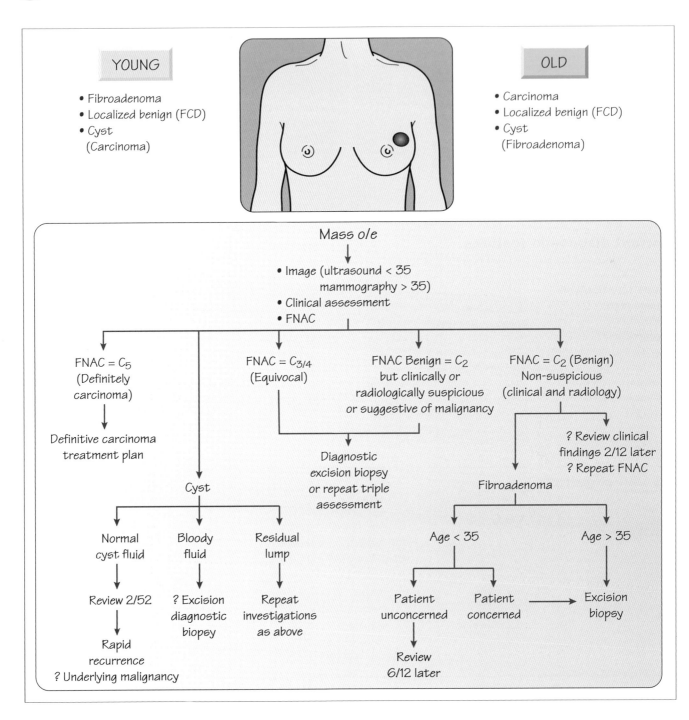

Mass o/e

↓

- Image (ultrasound < 35
  mammography > 35)
- Clinical assessment
- FNAC

FNAC = C_5 (Definitely carcinoma)

↓

Definitive carcinoma treatment plan

FNAC = $C_{3/4}$ (Equivocal)

↓

Cyst

FNAC Benign = C_2 but clinically or radiologically suspicious or suggestive of malignancy

↓

Diagnostic excision biopsy or repeat triple assessment

FNAC = C_2 (Benign) Non-suspicious (clinical and radiology)

↓

Fibroadenoma

? Review clinical findings 2/12 later ? Repeat FNAC

Normal cyst fluid

↓

Review 2/52

↓

Rapid recurrence ? Underlying malignancy

Bloody fluid

↓

? Excision diagnostic biopsy

Residual lump

↓

Repeat investigations as above

Age < 35

Patient unconcerned

↓

Review 6/12 later

Patient concerned →

Age > 35

Excision biopsy

Definition

A *breast lump* is defined as any palpable mass in the breast. A breast lump is the most common presentation of both benign and malignant breast disease. Enlargement of the whole breast can occur either uni- or bilaterally, but this is not strictly a breast lump.

Key points

- The most common breast lumps occurring under the age of 35 years are fibroadenomas and fibrocystic disease.
- The most common breast lumps occurring over the age of 50 years are carcinomas and cysts.
- Pain is more characteristic of infection/inflammation than tumours.
- Skin/chest wall tethering is more characteristic of tumours than benign disease.
- Multiple lesions are usually benign (cysts or fibrocystic disease).

Differential diagnosis

Swelling of the whole breast (mammoplasia)

Bilateral
- Pregnancy, lactation.
- Idiopathic hypertrophy.
- Drug induced (e.g. diethylstilbestrol, antidepressants).
- Gynaecomastia in males.

Unilateral
- Enlargement in the newborn.
- Puberty.
- Gynaecomastia in males.

Localized swellings in the breast

Mastitis/breast abscess
- During lactation: red, hot, tender lump, systemic upset.
- Tuberculous abscess: chronic, 'cold', recurrent, discharging sinus.

Cysts
- Galactocele: more common postpartum, tender but not inflamed, milky contents.
- Fibrocystic disease: irregular, ill defined, often tender.

Solid lumps
Benign include:
- Fibroadenoma: discrete, firm, well defined, regular, highly mobile.
- Fat necrosis: irregular, ill defined, hard, ?skin tethering.
- Lipoma: well defined, soft, non-tender, fairly mobile.
- Cystosarcoma phylloides: usually large tumour (5 cm), firm, mobile, well circumscribed, non-tender breast mass. (rare, 1% of breast tumours, 10% are malignant).

Malignant include:
- Carcinoma
  early: ill defined, hard, irregular, skin tethering
  late: spreading fixity, ulceration, fungation, '*peau d'orange*'.

Swellings behind the breast
- Rib deformities, chondroma, costochondritis (Tietze's disease).

Key investigations

All lumps should have triple assessment – clinical examination, FNAC, imaging (ultrasound or mammography).
- FNAC: tumours, fibroadenoma, fibrocystic disease, fat necrosis, mastitis.
- Ultrasound (better in young women with denser breasts): fibroadenoma, cysts, tumours.
- Mammography (better in older women with less dense breasts): tumours, cysts, fibrocystic disease, fat necrosis.
- Biopsy ('Trucut'/core, rarely open surgical): usually provides definitive histology (may be radiologically guided if lump is small or impalpable, e.g. detected by mammography as part of breast screening programme).

5 Breast pain

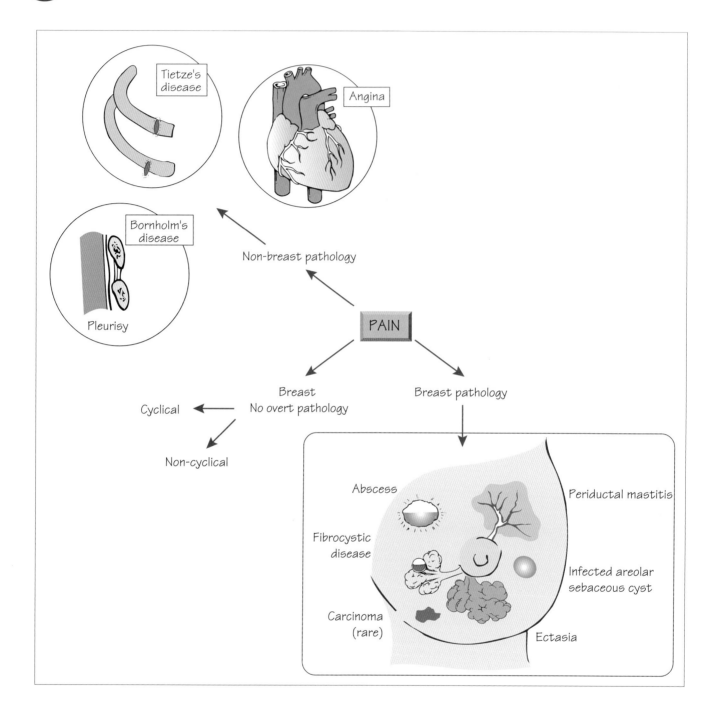

Surgery at a Glance, Fifth Edition. Pierce A. Grace and Neil R. Borley. © 2013 John Wiley & Sons, Ltd. Published 2013 by John Wiley & Sons, Ltd.

Definition

Mastalgia is any pain felt in the breast. *Cyclical mastalgia* is pain in the breast that varies in association with the menstrual cycle. *Non-cyclical mastalgia* is pain in the breast that follows no pattern or is intermittent.

Key points

- Mastalgia is commonly due to disorders of the breast or nipple tissue but may also be due to problems in the underlying chest wall or overlying skin.
- Pain is an uncommon presenting feature of tumours but any underlying lump should be investigated as for a lump (see Chapter 4).
- Always look for an associated infection in the breast.
- Mammography should be routine in women presenting over the age of 45 years to help exclude occult carcinoma.

Important diagnostic features

Non-breast conditions

- Tietze's disease (costochondritis): tenderness over medial ends of ribs (typically 2nd/3rd/4th), not limited to the breast area of the chest wall, typically unilateral, relieved by NSAIDs.
- Bornholm's disease (epidemic pleurodynia caused by coxsackie A virus): marked pain with no physical signs in the breast, worse with inspiration, no underlying respiratory disease, relieved with NSAIDs.
- Pleurisy: associated respiratory infection, pleural rub, may be bilateral.
- Angina: usually atypical angina, may be hard to diagnose, previous history of associated vascular disease.

Mastalgia due to breast pathology

Mastitis/breast abscess

- During lactation: red hot tender lump, systemic upset.
Treatment: aspirate abscess (may need to be repeated), do not stop breastfeeding, oral antibiotics.
- Non-lactational abscesses: recurrent, associated with smoking, associated with underlying ductal ectasia:

treatment: outpatient aspiration, give oral antibiotics, stop smoking, prophylactic metronidazole for recurrent sepsis, repeat aspiration if necessary.

Infected sebaceous cyst

- Single lump superficially in the skin of the periareolar region, previous history of painless cystic lump:
    treatment: excise infected cyst ± antibiotics.

Fibrocystic disease

- Common condition. Breast discomfort, dull heavy pain and tenderness. Variable symptoms and intensity, worse premenstrually. Cobblestone consistency to breast on palpation—upper outer quadrants:
    treatment: as for mastalgia without breast pathology.

Mastalgia without breast pathology

- Pain often felt throughout the breast, often worse in the axillary tail, moderately tender to examination:
    general treatment: restrict dietary fat and avoid caffeine, possibly vitamin E, well-fitting bra to provide good breast support
    treatment for cyclical mastalgia: paracetamol, danazol, tamoxifen, bromocriptine, γ linoleic acid (evening primrose oil)
    treatment for non-cyclical mastalgia: paracetamol, NSAIDs.

Key investigations

Non-breast origin
Chest X-ray, ECG, stress test.

Breast pathology
- FNAC (MC+S): associated palpable lump, ?fibrocystic disease, ?mastitis/abscess.
- Ultrasound (young women/dense breasts) or mammography (older women/small breasts).

Mastalgia without breast pathology
Mammography in women over 45 years.

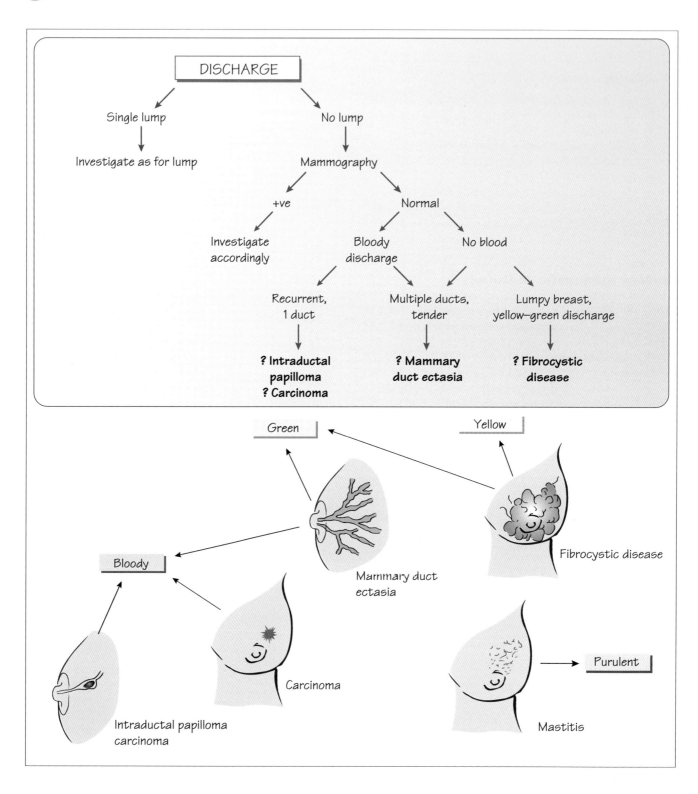

Definition

Any fluid (which may be physiological or pathological) emanating from the nipple.

Differential diagnosis

Physiological discharges

Milky or clear

- Lactation.
- Lactorrhoea in the newborn ('witches' milk').
- Lactorrhoea at puberty (may be in either sex).

Pathological discharges

Serous yellow-green

- Fibrocystic disease: cyclical, tender, lumpy breasts.
- Mammary duct ectasia: usually multiple ducts, intermittent, may be associated with low-grade mastitis.

Bloody

- Duct papilloma: single duct, ?retro-areolar, 'pea-sized' lump.
- Carcinoma: ?palpable lump.
- Mammary duct ectasia: usually multiple ducts, intermittent, may be associated with low-grade mastitis.

Pus ± milk

- Acute suppurative mastitis: tender, swollen, hot breast, multiple ducts discharging.
- Tuberculous (rare): chronic discharge, periareolar fistulae, 'sterile' cultures on normal media.

Key investigations

- MC+S: acute mastitis, TB (Lowenstein–Jensen medium, Ziehl–Neelsen stains).
- Discharge cytology: carcinoma.
- Mammography: tumours, fibrocystic disease, ?ectasia.
- Ductal excision: may be needed for exclusion of neoplasia.

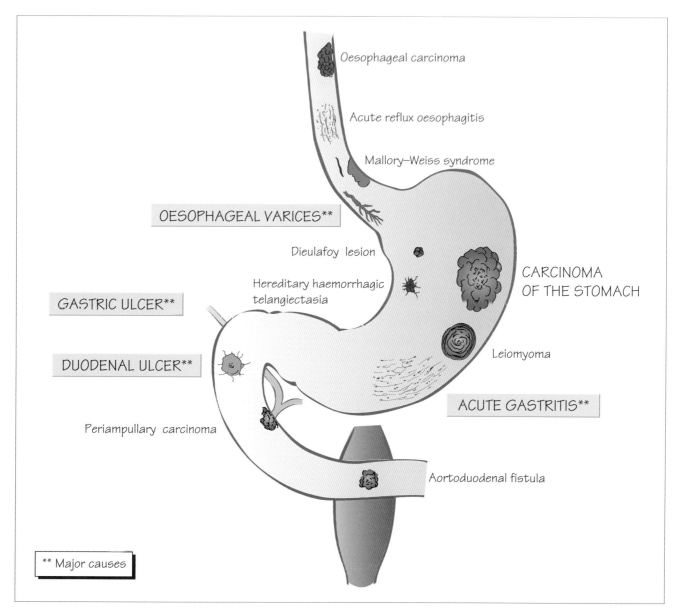

Oesophageal carcinoma

Acute reflux oesophagitis

Mallory–Weiss syndrome

OESOPHAGEAL VARICES**

Dieulafoy lesion

Hereditary haemorrhagic telangiectasia

GASTRIC ULCER**

CARCINOMA OF THE STOMACH

Leiomyoma

DUODENAL ULCER**

ACUTE GASTRITIS**

Periampullary carcinoma

Aortoduodenal fistula

** Major causes

Definitions

GI bleeding is any blood loss from the GI tract (anywhere from the mouth to the anus), which may present with haematemesis, melaena, rectal bleeding or anaemia. *Haematemesis* is defined as vomiting blood and is usually caused by upper GI disease. *Melaena* is the passage PR of a black treacle-like stool that contains altered blood, usually as a result of proximal bowel bleeding. *Haematochesia* is the presence of undigested blood in the stool usually from lower GI causes.

Upper GI bleeding

Key points

- Haematemesis is usually caused by lesions proximal to the duodeno-jejunal junction.

- Melaena may be caused by lesions anywhere from oesophagus to colon.
- Haematochesia is usually caused by lower GI pathology (colorectal tumours, haemorrhoids, diverticulitis, angiodysplasia), brisk acute upper GI bleeding may also present in this way.
- Most tumours more commonly cause anaemia than frank haematemesis.
- In young adults, PUD, congenital lesions and varices are common causes.
- In the elderly, tumours, PUD and angiodysplasia are common causes.

Important diagnostic features

Oesophagus

- Reflux oesophagitis: small volumes, bright red, associated with regurgitation.
- Oesophageal carcinoma: scanty, blood-stained debris, rarely significant volume, associated with weight loss, anergia, dysphagia.
- Bleeding varices (oesophageal or gastric): sudden onset, painless, large volumes, dark or bright red blood, history of (alcoholic) liver disease, other features of portal hypertension (ascites, dilated abdominal veins, encephalopathy, reduced platelets or white cells).
- Trauma during vomiting (Mallory–Weiss syndrome): bright red bloody vomit usually preceded by several normal but forceful vomiting episodes.

Stomach

- Erosive gastritis: small volumes, bright red, may follow alcohol or NSAID intake, history of dyspepsia.
- Gastric ulcer: often larger sized bleed, painless, possible preceding (herald) smaller bleeds, accompanied by altered blood ('coffee grounds'), history of PUD.
- Gastric cancer: rarely large bleed, anaemia more common, associated weight loss, anorexia, dyspeptic symptoms.
- Gastric leiomyoma (rare): spontaneous-onset moderate-sized bleed.
- Dieulafoy's disease (rare): younger patients, spontaneous large bleed, difficult to diagnose.

Duodenum

- Duodenitis: small volumes, bright red, may follow alcohol or NSAID use, history of dyspepsia.
- Duodenal ulcer: past history of duodenal ulcer, melaena often also prominent, symptoms of back pain, hunger pains, NSAID use.
- Aortoduodenal fistula (rare): usually infected graft post AAA repair, massive haematemesis and PR bleed, usually fatal.

Key investigations

- FBC: iron deficiency anaemia: carcinoma, reflux oesophagitis.
- LFTs: liver disease (varices).
- Clotting: alcohol, bleeding diatheses.
- OGD: investigation of choice. High diagnostic accuracy, allows therapeutic manoeuvres (varices: injection or banding; ulcers: injection/cautery). Test for *H. pylori* infection.
- Angiography (or CT angiography) : rare duodenal causes, obscure recurrent bleeds.
- Barium meal and follow through: limited use in patients who are unfit for OGD (respiratory disease) and ?proximal jejunal lesions.

Essential management of upper GI bleeding

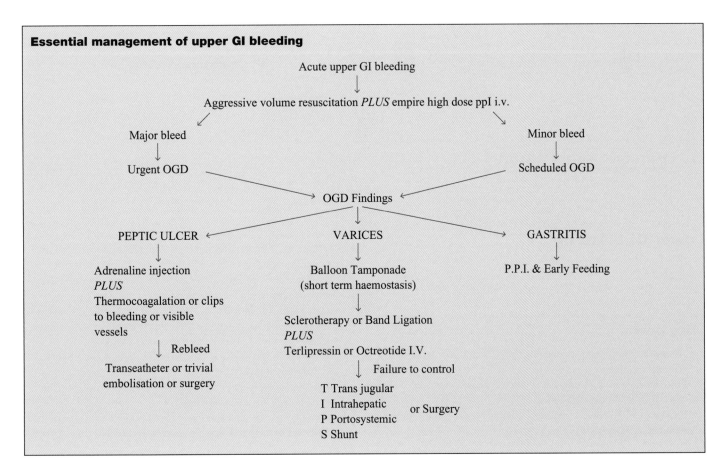

Gastrointestinal bleeding/2

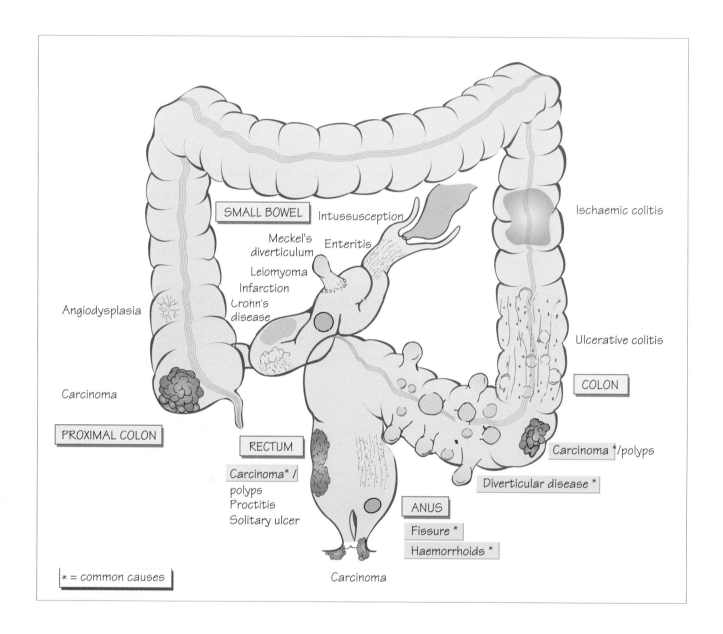

SMALL BOWEL Intussusception

Meckel's diverticulum Enteritis

Leiomyoma
Infarction
Crohn's disease

Ischaemic colitis

Angiodysplasia

Ulcerative colitis

COLON

Carcinoma

PROXIMAL COLON

RECTUM

Carcinoma* / polyps
Proctitis
Solitary ulcer

Carcinoma */polyps

Diverticular disease *

ANUS

Fissure *
Haemorrhoids *

* = common causes

Carcinoma

Lower GI bleeding

Key points

- Anorectal bleeding is characteristically bright red, associated with defaecation.
- Left-sided/sigmoid bleeding is characteristically dark red, with clots, may be mixed with the stool.
- Proximal colonic/ileal bleeding is usually dark red, fully mixed with the stool or occult.

- Always do a rectal examination and proctoscopy ± flexible sigmoidoscopy.
- New rectal bleeding age >55 always deserves colonic investigation– never assume it is a simple anal cause.
- Acute major PR bleeding is usually due to diverticular disease or angiodysplasia; colonic ischaemia, Meckel's diverticulum, ulcerative colitis or haemorrhoids are less likely.
- In children – anal fissure, Meckel's diverticulum and intussusception should be considered
- In young adults – anal causes (haemorrhoids, fissure, proctitis), colitis polyps are common causes
- In the elderly – colorectal tumours, diverticular disease, angiodysplasia and colonic ischaemia should be considered

Important diagnostic features

Small intestine
- Meckel's diverticulum: children and young adults, painless bleeding, darker red/melaena common.
- Intussusception: young children (3–12 months), colicky abdominal pain, retching, bright red/mucus stool.
- Enteritis (infective/radiation/Crohn's).
- Ischaemic: severe abdominal pain, physical examination shows mesenteric ischaemia or AF, few signs, later collapse and shock.
- Tumours (leiomyoma/lymphoma): rare, intermittent history, often modest volumes lost.

Colon
- Angiodysplasia: proximal colon, common in the elderly, painless, no warning, often large volume, fresh and clots mixed.
- Diverticular disease: spontaneous onset, painless, large volume, mostly fresh blood, previous history of constipation.
- Polyps/carcinoma: may be large volume or small, possible associated change in bowel habit, blood often mixed with stool. Caecal carcinoma commonly causes anaemia rather than PR bleeding.
- Ulcerative colitis: blood mixed with mucus, associated with systemic upset, long history, intermittent course, diarrhoea prominent.
- Ischaemic colitis: elderly, severe abdominal pain, AF, bloody diarrhoea, collapse and shock later.

Rectum
- Carcinoma of the rectum: change in bowel habit common, rarely large volumes.
- Proctitis: bloody mucus, purulent diarrhoea in infected, perianal irritation common.
- Solitary rectal ulcer: bleeding post-defaecation, small volumes, feeling of 'lump in anus', mucus discharge.

Anus
- Haemorrhoids: bright red bleeding post-defaecation, stops spontaneously, perianal irritation.
- Fissure-*in-ano*: children and young adults, extreme pain on defaecation, small volumes bright red blood on stool and toilet paper.
- Carcinoma of the anus: elderly, mass in anus, small volumes bloody discharge, anal pain, unhealing ulcers.
- Perianal Crohn's disease.

Key investigations

- FBC: iron deficiency anaemia–tumours/chronic colitis.
- Clotting: bleeding diatheses.
- FOB: testing.
- PR/proctoscopy/flexible sigmoidoscopy: anorectal tumours, prolapse, haemorrhoids, distal colitis.
- Abdominal X-ray, ultrasound: intussusception.
- Flexible sigmoidoscopy: suspected colitis, sigmoid tumours or diverticular disease.
- Colonoscopy: diverticular disease, colon tumours, angiodysplasia.
- Angiography: angiodysplasia, small bowel causes (especially Meckel's). (Needs active bleeding 0.5 ml/min, highly accurate when positive, invasive, allows embolization therapy.)
- Technetium-99m-pertechnate labelled RBC scan: angiodysplasia, small bowel causes including Meckel's diverticulum, obscure colonic causes. (Needs active bleeding 1ml/min, less accurate placement of source, non-invasive, non-therapeutic.)
- Small bowel enema: small bowel tumours.

Essential management of acute lower GI bleeding

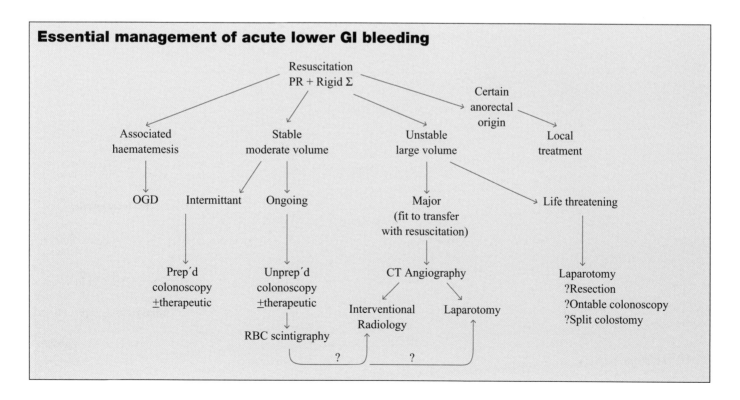

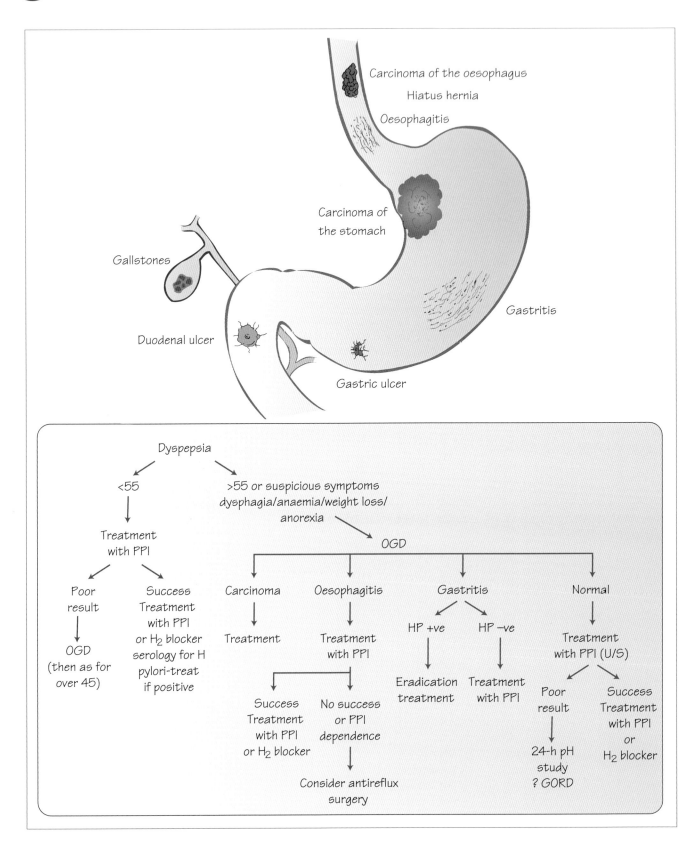

Definition

Dyspepsia is the feeling of discomfort or pain in the upper abdomen or lower chest. *Indigestion* may be used by the patient to mean dyspepsia, regurgitation symptoms or flatulence.

Key points

- Dyspepsia may be the only presenting symptom of upper GI malignancy. All older patients and patients with alarm symptoms (dysphagia, vomiting, anorexia and weight loss, GI bleeding) should have endoscopy.
- Dyspepsia in young people without alarm symptoms is very unlikely to be due to malignancy.
- In young adults, gastro-oesophageal reflux and *Helicobacter pylori*-positive gastritis are common causes.
- Dyspepsia is rarely the only symptom of gallstones – they are more often incidental findings.

Differential diagnosis

Oesophagus

- Reflux oesophagitis: retrosternal dyspepsia, worse after large meal/lying down, associated symptoms of regurgitation, pain on swallowing.
- Oesophageal carcinoma: new-onset dyspepsia in older patient, associated symptoms of dysphagia/weight loss/haematemesis, failure to respond to acid suppression treatment.

Stomach

- Gastritis: recurrent episodes of epigastric pain, transient or short-lived symptoms, may be associated with diet, responds well to antacids/acid suppression.
- Gastric ulcer: typically chronic epigastric pain, worse with food, 'food fear' may lead to weight loss, exacerbated by smoking/alcohol, occasionally relieved by vomiting.
- Carcinoma of the stomach: progressive symptoms, associated weight loss/anorexia, iron-deficient anaemia common, early satiety, epigastric mass.
- Hiatus hernia: recurrent epigastric and retrosternal discomfort, may be associated with diet, symptoms of reflux, may respond to acid suppression.

Duodenum

- Duodenal ulcer: epigastric and back pain, chronic exacerbations lasting several weeks, relieved by food especially milky drinks, relieved by bed rest, more common in younger men, associated with *H. pylori* infection.
- Duodenitis: often transient, mild symptoms only, associated with alcohol and smoking.

Gallstones

Dyspepsia is rarely the only symptom, associated RUQ pain, needs normal OGD and positive ultrasound to be considered as cause for dyspeptic symptoms.

Key investigations

- FBC: anaemia suggests malignancy.
- Tests for *H. pylori*: breath test (C14 or C13 urea), blood (antibodies to *H. pylori*) or endoscopic biopsy urease test (CLO test).
- OGD: tumours, PUD, assessment of oesophagitis.
- 24-hour pH monitoring: ?GORD.
- Oesophageal manometry: ?dysmotility.
- Ultrasound: ?gallstones.

9 Vomiting

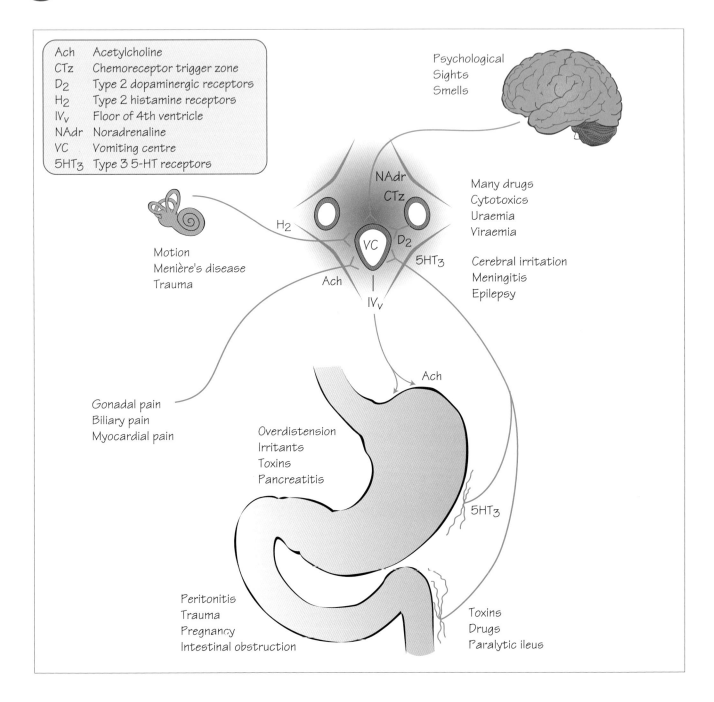

Ach   Acetylcholine
CTz   Chemoreceptor trigger zone
D_2 Type 2 dopaminergic receptors
H_2 Type 2 histamine receptors
IV_v Floor of 4th ventricle
NAdr   Noradrenaline
VC   Vomiting centre
$5HT_3$ Type 3 5-HT receptors

Psychological
Sights
Smells

NAdr
CTz

Many drugs
Cytotoxics
Uraemia
Viraemia

H_2

VC D_2

$5HT_3$

Cerebral irritation
Meningitis
Epilepsy

Motion
Menière's disease
Trauma

Ach

IV_v

Ach

Gonadal pain
Biliary pain
Myocardial pain

Overdistension
Irritants
Toxins
Pancreatitis

$5HT_3$

Peritonitis
Trauma
Pregnancy
Intestinal obstruction

Toxins
Drugs
Paralytic ileus

 Surgery at a Glance, Fifth Edition. Pierce A. Grace and Neil R. Borley. © 2013 John Wiley & Sons, Ltd. Published 2013 by John Wiley & Sons, Ltd.

Definitions

Vomiting is defined as the involuntary return to, and forceful expulsion from, the mouth of all or part of the contents of the stomach. *Water-brash* is the sudden secretion and accumulation of saliva in the mouth as a reflex associated with dyspepsia. *Retching* is the process whereby forceful contractions of the diaphragm and abdominal muscles occur without evacuation of the stomach contents.

Key points

- Vomiting is initiated when the vomiting centre in the medulla oblongata is stimulated, either directly (central vomiting) or via various afferent fibres (reflex vomiting).
- Vomiting of different origins is mediated by different pathways and transmitters. Therapy is best directed according to cause.
- Consider mechanical causes (e.g. gastric outflow or intestinal obstruction) before starting therapy.

Important diagnostic features

Central vomiting
- Drugs, e.g. morphine sulphate, chemotherapeutic agents.
- Uraemia.
- Viral hepatitis.
- Hypercalcaemia of any cause.
- Acute infections, especially in children.
- Pregnancy.

Reflex vomiting

Gastrointestinal causes ($5\text{-}HT_3$ and Ach mediated – treatment: promotilants, $5\text{-}HT_3$ antagonists)
- Ingestion of irritants:
  bacteria, e.g. salmonella (gastroenteritis)
  emetics, e.g. zinc sulphate, ipecacuanha
  drugs, e.g. alcohol, salicylates (gastritis)
  poisons, e.g. salt, arsenic, phosphorus.
- PUD: especially gastric ulcer; vomiting relieves the pain.
- Intestinal obstruction:
  hour-glass stomach (carcinoma of the stomach)
  pyloric stenosis – infant: hypertrophic pyloric stenosis, projectile vomiting; adult: pyloric outlet obstruction secondary to PUD or malignant disease
  small bowel obstruction: adhesions, hernia, neoplasm, Crohn's disease
  large bowel obstruction: malignancy, volvulus, diverticular disease.
- Inflammation: appendicitis, peritonitis, pancreatitis, cholecystitis, biliary colic.

General causes (Ach and D_2 mediated – treatment: anticholinergics, antidopaminergics)
- Myocardial infarction.
- Ovarian disease, ectopic pregnancy.
- Severe pain (e.g. kick to the testis, gonadal torsion, blow to the epigastrium).
- Severe coughing (e.g. pulmonary TB, pertussis).

CNS causes (NAdr and Ach mediated – treatment: anticholinergics, sedatives)
- Raised intracranial pressure:
  head injury
  cerebral tumour or abscess
  hydrocephalus
  meningitis
  cerebral haemorrhage.
- Migraine.
- Epilepsy.
- Offensive sights, tastes and smells.
- Hysteria.
- Middle ear disorders (H_2 mediated – treatment: antihistamines): Menière's disease, travel/motion sickness.

10 Acute abdominal pain

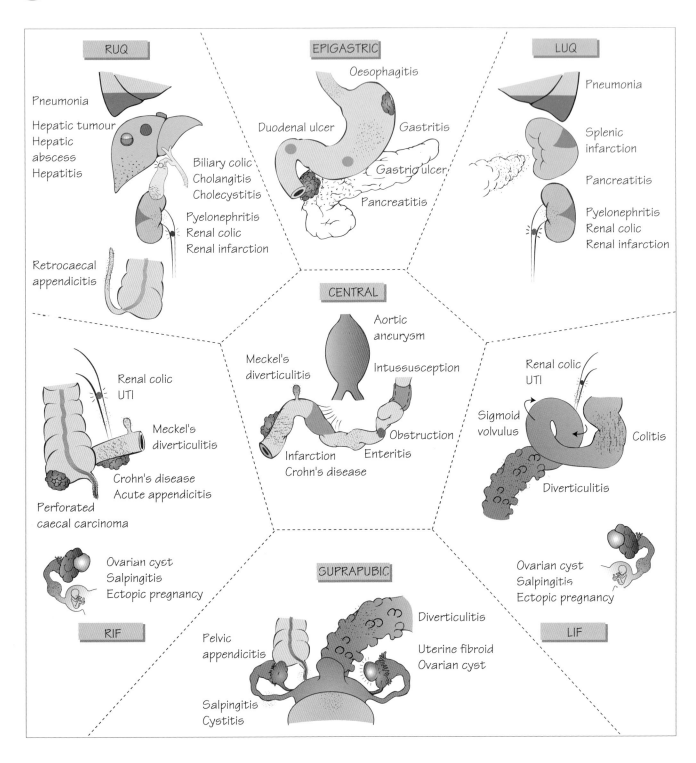

Definitions

Abdominal pain is a subjective unpleasant sensation felt in any of the abdominal regions. *Acute abdominal pain* is usually used to refer to pain of sudden onset, and/or short duration. *Referred pain* is the perception of pain in an area remote from the site of origin of the pain.

Surgery at a Glance, Fifth Edition. Pierce A. Grace and Neil R. Borley. © 2013 John Wiley & Sons, Ltd. Published 2013 by John Wiley & Sons, Ltd.

Important diagnostic features

History of the pain

- The site of pain relates to its origin: foregut – upper; midgut – middle, hindgut – lower.
- Colicky (visceral) pain is caused by stretching or contracting a hollow viscus (e.g. gallbladder, ureter, ileum).
- Constant localized (somatic) pain is due to peritoneal irritation and indicates the presence of inflammation/infection (e.g. pancreatitis, cholecystitis, appendicitis).
- Associated back pain suggests retroperitoneal pathology (aortic aneurysm, pancreatitis, posterior DU, pyelonephritis).
- Associated sacral or perineal pain suggests pelvic pathology (ovarian cyst, PID, pelvic abscess).
- Pain out of proportion to the physical signs suggests ischaemia with or without perforation.
- Remember referred causes of pain: pneumonia (right lower lobe), myocardial infarction, lumbar nerve root pathology.

Abdominal examination

Inspection: Scaphoid or distended, movement on respiration, swellings, scars, lesions, bruising.

Palpation: Superficial and deep.

- Tenderness: pain or discomfort when affected area is touched.
- Rebound tenderness: pain or discomfort on removing one's hand from the affected area.
- Guarding (*défense musculaire*): involuntary spasm of the anterior abdominal wall muscles over inflamed abdominal vicera, e.g. in RIF in patients with appendicitis.
- Rigidity: stiff, hard, unyielding abdominal wall due to abdominal wall muscle spasm; indicates extensive peritonitis.
- Palpate for organs and masses: liver, spleen, bladder, gallbladder, appendix mass, AAA.

Percussion: May detect distended bladder or enlarged liver/spleen.

Auscultation: Listen for bowel sounds. Absent or deceased in peritonitis, increased with intestinal obstruction.

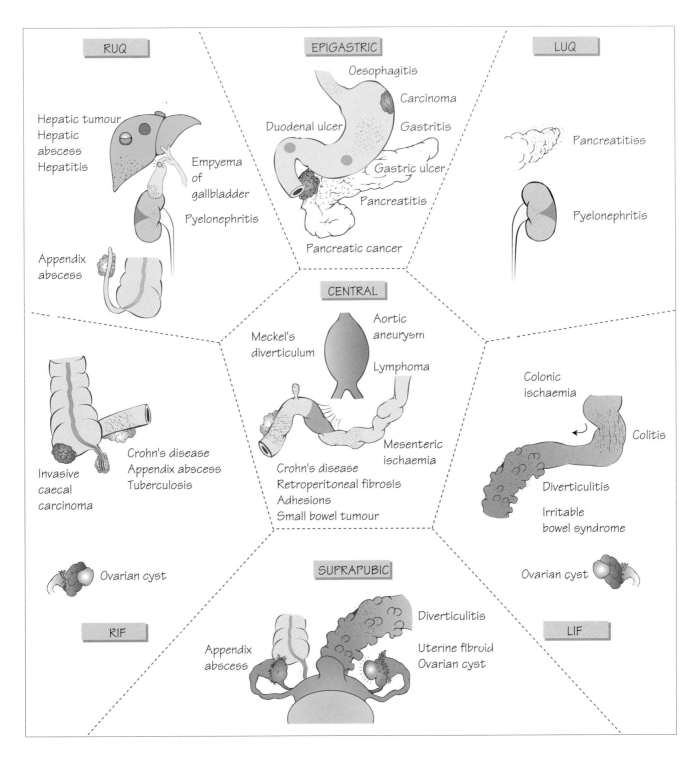

Definition

Chronic abdominal pain is usually used to refer to pain that is either long-standing, of prolonged duration or of recurrent/intermittent nature. Chronic pain may be associated with acute exacerbations.

Key points

- Chronic abdominal pain of prolonged duration requires investigation.
- Adhesions as a cause of chronic abdominal pain should be a diagnosis of exclusion.
- IBS is less common than supposed – any atypical bowel symptoms should be investigated fully before diagnosing IBS.
- Back pain suggests a retroperitoneal origin (e.g. pancreas, duodenum, upper urinary tract, aorta).
- Sacral pain suggests a pelvic origin.
- Relationship to food strongly suggests a physical pathology and always requires investigation.

Important diagnostic features

Irritable bowel syndrome

- Syndrome of colicky abdominal pain, bloating, hard pellety or watery stools, sensation of incomplete evacuation, often associated with frequency and urgency.
- Blood with stools, mucus, abdominal physical findings, weight loss, recent onset of symptoms or onset in old age should suggest an organic cause and require thorough investigation.

Adhesions

Associated with several syndromes of chronic or recurrent abdominal symptoms.

Adhesional abdominal pain

Difficult to diagnose with any confidence, usually a diagnosis of exclusion, may be suggested by small bowel enema showing evidence of delayed transit or fixed strictures, uncertain response to surgical (laparoscopic) adhesiolysis.

Recurrent incomplete small bowel obstruction

Transient episodes of obstructive symptoms, often do not have all classic signs or symptoms present, abdominal signs may be unremarkable, self-limiting. Obstruction due to adhesions often settles with conservative treatment (IV fluids, NPO, NG tube). Non-resolution or development of physical signs (e.g. abdominal tenderness) are indica-

tions for laparotomy/laparoscopy. Best investigation – contrast follow through.

Mesenteric angina

Classically occurs shortly after eating in elderly patients, colicky central abdominal pain, vomiting, food fear and weight loss. Usually associated with other occlusive vascular disease. Difficult to diagnose. Best investigation – CT angiography.

Meckel's diverticulum

May cause undiagnosed central abdominal pain in young adults. Occasionally associated with obscure PR bleeding, anaemia. Best investigation – radionuclide scanning (technetium-99m-pertechnate).

Key investigations

- FBC: leucocytosis – chronic infective/inflammatory diseases; anaemia – occult malignancy, PUD; lymphocytosis – lymphoma.
- LFTs: common bile duct gallstones, hepatitis, liver tumours (primary/secondary).
- MSU: urinary tract infection (++ve nitrites, blood, protein), renal stone (++ve blood).
- Faecal occult blood: may be positive in any cause of GI bleeding (see Chapter 7).
- ECG: ischaemic heart disease.
- Abdominal X-ray: chronic pancreatitis (small calcification throughout gland).
- Ultrasound:
  intra-abdominal abscesses (diverticular, appendicular, pelvic, hepatic)
  'gallstones', 'chronic cholecystitis'
  ovarian pathology (cyst)
  aortic aneurysm, renal tumours.
- OGD: PUD, gastritis, gastric or oesophageal carcinoma.
- Colonoscopy: diverticular disease, chronic colonic ischaemia, colonic polyps and tumours.
- CT scan: chronic pancreatitis, pancreatic carcinoma, aortic aneurysm, retroperitoneal pathologies (fibrosis, lymphadenopathy, tumours), bowel tumours.
- IVU: renal stones, renal tract tumours, renal tract obstruction.
- Visceral angiography/CT angiogram/mesenteric MRA: mesenteric vascular disease.
- ERCP: chronic pancreatitis, pancreatic carcinoma.
- Small bowel enema: Crohn's disease, small bowel tumours, Meckel's diverticulum.
- Barium enema: ischaemic strictures, chronic colitis.

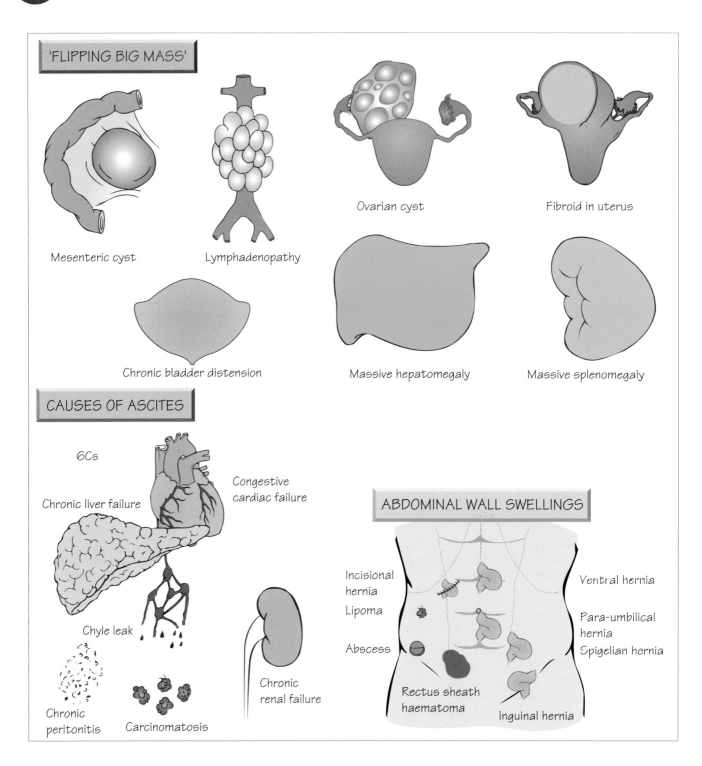

'FLIPPING BIG MASS'

Mesenteric cyst

Lymphadenopathy

Ovarian cyst

Fibroid in uterus

Chronic bladder distension

Massive hepatomegaly

Massive splenomegaly

CAUSES OF ASCITES

6Cs

Chronic liver failure

Congestive cardiac failure

Chyle leak

Chronic renal failure

Chronic peritonitis

Carcinomatosis

ABDOMINAL WALL SWELLINGS

Incisional hernia
Lipoma

Abscess

Rectus sheath haematoma

Inguinal hernia

Ventral hernia

Para-umbilical hernia

Spigelian hernia

Definition

An abdominal swelling is an abnormal protuberance that arises from the abdominal cavity or the abdominal wall and may be general or localized, acute or chronic, cystic or solid.

Key points

- Generalized abdominal swellings affect the entire abdominal cavity.
- Localized swellings can be located in the various regions of the abdomen.
- Abdominal wall swellings can be differentiated from intra-abdominal swellings by asking the patient to raise his or her head from the couch (intraperitoneal swellings disappear while abdominal wall swellings persist).
- Giant masses, other than ovarian cystadenocarcinoma or lymphomatous lymphadenopathy, are rarely malignant.

Important diagnostic features

'Fat'

Obesity: deposition of fat in the abdominal wall and intra-abdominally (extraperitoneal layer, omentum and mesentery). Commoner in males than females (where hip and thigh obesity is more common). Clinical obesity = body weight 120% greater than that recommended for their height, age and sex (BMI = weight (kg)/height (m)^2). A BMI of >25 is overweight, >30 obese.

'Flatus'

Intestinal obstruction: swallowed air accumulates in the bowel causing distension. This gives a tympanic note on percussion and produces the characteristic air–fluid levels and 'ladder' pattern on an abdominal radiograph. Sigmoid or caecal volvulus produces gross distension with characteristic features of distended loops on abdominal X-ray.

'Fluid'

- Intestinal obstruction: as well as air, fluid accumulates in the obstructed intestine.
- Ascites: fluid accumulates in the peritoneal cavity due to the '7 Cs':
  chronic peritonitis (e.g. tuberculosis)
  carcinomatosis (malignant deposits, especially ovary and stomach)
  chronic liver disease (cirrhosis, secondary deposits, portal or hepatic vein obstruction, parasitic infections)
  chronic pancreatitis (ascites only in 4% of patients)
  congestive heart failure (RVF)
  chronic renal failure (nephrotic syndrome)
  chyle (lymphatic duct disruption e.g. post AAA surgery).

'Faeces'

Chronic constipation: faeces accumulate in the colon producing abdominal distension. Congenital causes include spina bifida and Hirschsprung's disease. Acquired causes include chronic dehydration, drugs (opiates, anticholinergics, phenothiazines), hypothyroidism and emotional disorders,.

'Fetus'

Pregnancy: swelling arises out of the pelvis.

'Flipping big mass'

Usually cystic lesions: giant ovarian cystadenoma, mesenteric cyst, retroperitoneal lymphadenopathy (lymphoma), giant uterine fibroid, giant splenomegaly, giant hepatomegaly, giant renal tumour, desmoid tumour. Occasionally, very distended bladder.

Key investigations – abdominal masses

- FBC: lymphomas, infections.
- LFT: liver disease.
- U+E: renal disease.
- Abdominal X-ray:
  ascites ('ground glass' appearance, loss of visceral outlines)
  large mass (bowel gas pattern eccentric, paucity of gas in one quadrant)
  fibroid ('popcorn' calcification).
- Ultrasound: ascites, may show cystic masses.
- CT scan: investigation of choice, differentiates origin and relationships.
- Paracentesis: MC+S (infections), cytology (tumours), amylase (pancreatic ascites).
- Biopsy: liver – undiagnosed hepatomegaly, omental 'cake' – ovarian carcinoma.

Key investigations – abdominal wall swellings

- Ultrasound: subcutaneous lumps.
- CT scan: abscesses, hernias.
- Laparoscopy: diagnosis and possible treatment of hernia.
- Herniography: rarely used for possible hernias with negative other investigations.

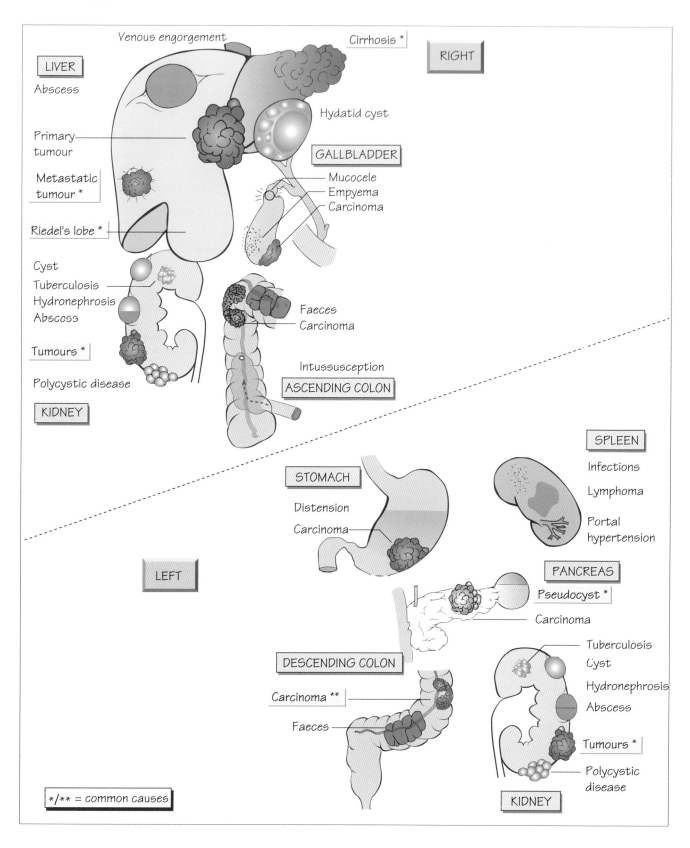

Venous engorgement

Cirrhosis *

RIGHT

LIVER

Abscess

Hydatid cyst

Primary tumour

GALLBLADDER

Mucocele
Empyema
Carcinoma

Metastatic tumour *

Riedel's lobe *

Cyst
Tuberculosis
Hydronephrosis
Abscess

Faeces
Carcinoma

Tumours *

Intussusception

ASCENDING COLON

Polycystic disease

KIDNEY

SPLEEN

Infections

Lymphoma

STOMACH

Portal hypertension

Distension

Carcinoma

LEFT

PANCREAS

Pseudocyst *

Carcinoma

Tuberculosis
Cyst
Hydronephrosis

DESCENDING COLON

Abscess

Carcinoma **

Tumours *

Faeces

Polycystic disease

KIDNEY

*/** = common causes

Liver

- Riedel's lobe: normal anatomical variant, smooth, non-tender, lateral/right lobe, 'tongue-like', women > men.
- Infective hepatitis: smooth, tender, global enlargement.
- Liver abscess: usually one large abscess, ?amoebic, very tender, systemically unwell.
- Hydatid cyst: smooth, may be loculated, ?history of tropical travel.
- Venous congestion: smooth, tender, pulsatile (slightly irregular (cirrhotic) if chronic).
- Cirrhosis: irregular, firm, 'knobbly'.
- Tumours:
  primary: solitary, large, non-tender, ?lobulated
  secondary: often multiple, irregular, rock hard, centrally umbilicated.

Gallbladder

- Generally: oval, smooth, projects towards RIF, beneath the tip of the ninth rib, moves with respiration.
- Mucocele: large gallbladder, moderately tender, smooth walled.
- Empyema: tender mass in RUQ, difficult to delineate clearly because of pain and omentum surrounding GB.
- Carcinoma of gallbladder: nodular, hard, irregular.

- Malignant obstruction of the lower end of the bile duct: palpable, painless, smooth gallbladder with jaundice. (Courvoisier's law: a palpable gallbladder in the presence of jaundice is unlikely to be due to gallstones.)

Renal masses

- Perinephric abscess/pyonephrosis: acutely tender, systemic signs, rarely large.
- Hydronephrosis: large, smooth, tense kidney. May be massive.
- Solitary cyst: smooth, non-tender, may be massive.
- Polycystic disease: frequently very large, lobulated, smooth.
- Renal carcinoma: irregular, nodular, often hard, ?fixed.
- Nephroblastoma: large mass in children.

Suprarenal gland

- Generally: only palpable when large, moves with respiration, difficult to define borders.
- Adenomas: usually cystic if palpable.
- Infections: ?chronic fungal infections, may be tender, systemic features.
- Congenital hyperplasia: young children, endocrine disorders associated, smooth, non-tender.

Abdominal swellings (localized) – upper abdominal/2

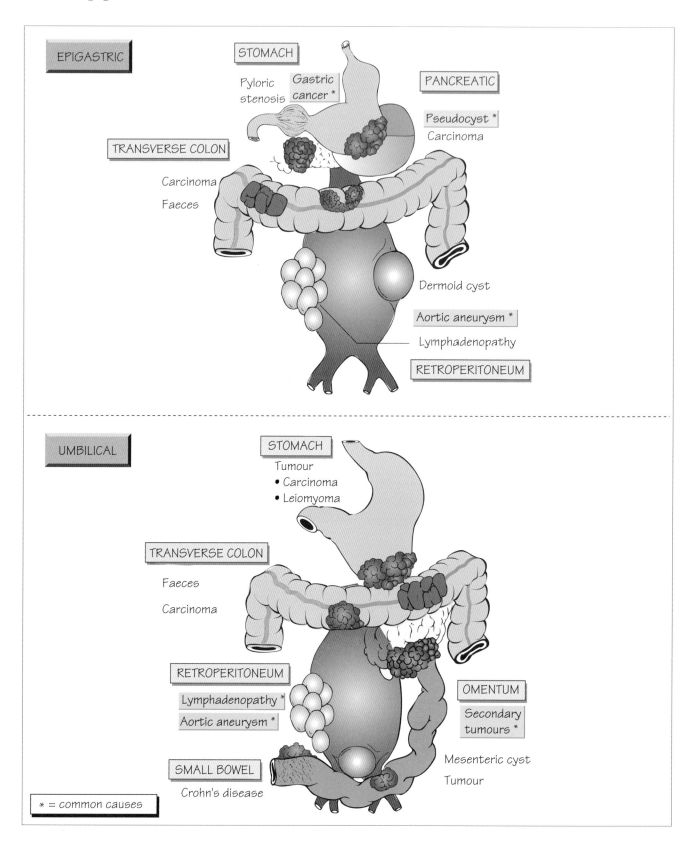

EPIGASTRIC

STOMACH

Pyloric stenosis

Gastric cancer *

PANCREATIC

Pseudocyst *

Carcinoma

TRANSVERSE COLON

Carcinoma

Faeces

Dermoid cyst

Aortic aneurysm *

Lymphadenopathy

RETROPERITONEUM

UMBILICAL

STOMACH

Tumour
• Carcinoma
• Leiomyoma

TRANSVERSE COLON

Faeces

Carcinoma

RETROPERITONEUM

Lymphadenopathy *

Aortic aneurysm *

OMENTUM

Secondary tumours *

Mesenteric cyst

Tumour

SMALL BOWEL

Crohn's disease

* = common causes

Colon

• Faeces: soft, putty-like mass, mobile, non-tender, can be indented.
• Carcinoma: firm-hard, irregular, non-tender, may be mobile (fixity strongly suggests carcinoma).
• Intussusception: mobile, smooth, sausage-shaped mass usually in RUQ.

Stomach

• Gastric distension: soft, fluctuant, succussion splash present.
• Neoplasm: irregular, hard, craggy, immobile, does not descend on inspiration.

Pancreas

• Generally: does not move with respiration, fixed to retroperitoneum, poorly defined.
• Pseudocyst/cyst: mildly tender (worse if infected), symptoms of gastric obstruction.
• Carcinoma: hard, irregular, non-tender, fixed.

Retroperitoneum

• Lymphadenopathy: solid, immobile, irregular, 'rubbery', may be massive, particularly if lymphomatous.

• Aortic aneurysm: smooth, fusiform, pulsatile, expansile, may be tender.
• Dermoid cysts (rare): deep seated, smooth, recurrent after surgery.

Omentum

Secondary carcinoma: hard, irregular, mobile, 'pancake-like', often ovarian carcinoma.

Key investigations

• FBC: anaemia, tumours.
• WCC: lymphomas, Crohn's disease, appendicitis/diverticulitis.
• LFTs: liver lesions.
• Ultrasound: pancreatic (pseudo)cysts, aortic aneurysm.
• CT scan: pancreatic tumours, lymphadenopathy, retroperitoneal/mesenteric cysts, aortic aneurysm, omental deposits.
• Gastroscopy: stomach tumours.
• Colonoscopy: colonic tumours.
• Small bowel enema: small intestinal tumours.
• Barium enema: colonic tumours.

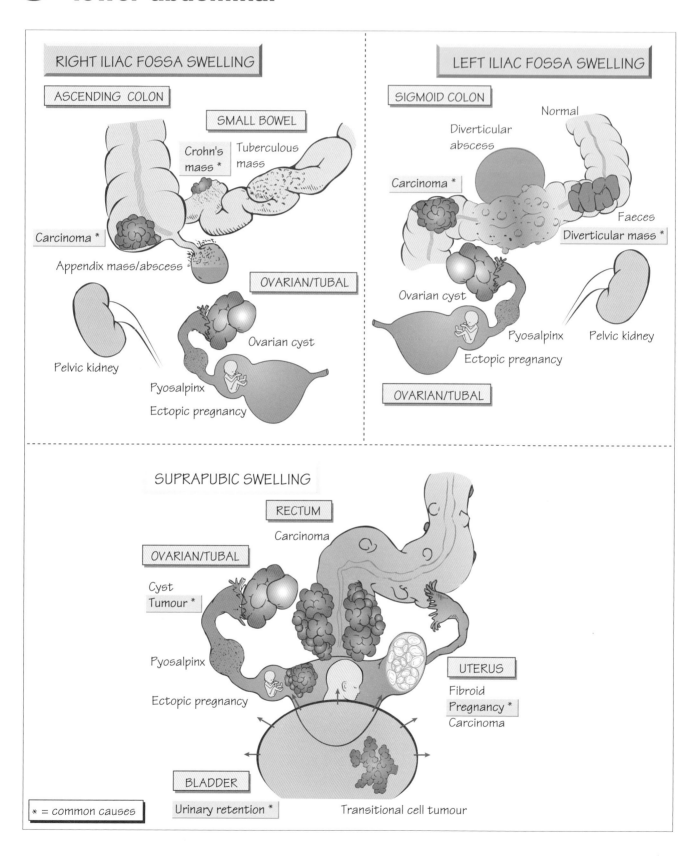

RIGHT ILIAC FOSSA SWELLING

ASCENDING COLON

SMALL BOWEL

Crohn's mass *   Tuberculous mass

Carcinoma *

Appendix mass/abscess

OVARIAN/TUBAL

Pelvic kidney

Ovarian cyst

Pyosalpinx

Ectopic pregnancy

LEFT ILIAC FOSSA SWELLING

SIGMOID COLON

Normal

Diverticular abscess

Carcinoma *

Faeces

Diverticular mass *

Ovarian cyst

Pyosalpinx   Pelvic kidney

Ectopic pregnancy

OVARIAN/TUBAL

SUPRAPUBIC SWELLING

RECTUM

Carcinoma

OVARIAN/TUBAL

Cyst
Tumour *

Pyosalpinx

Ectopic pregnancy

UTERUS

Fibroid
Pregnancy *
Carcinoma

BLADDER

* = common causes

Urinary retention *   Transitional cell tumour

Sigmoid colon

- Diverticular mass: tender, ill defined, rubbery hard, non-mobile.
- Paracolic abscess: acutely tender, ill defined, ?fluctuant, features of systemic sepsis.
- Carcinoma: hard, craggy, non-tender unless perforated, immobile, associated with altered bowel habit/obstructive symptoms.
- Faeces: firm, indentable/'malleable', mobile with colon.
- Normal: only in a thin person, non-tender, chord-like.
- Volvulus: usually generalized distension and signs of obstruction rather than localized swelling.

Caecum/ascending colon

- Appendix mass/abscess: acutely tender, ill defined, ?fluctuant, features of systemic sepsis.
- Carcinoma: hard, craggy, non-tender unless perforated, immobile, associated with anaemia/weight loss and anergia.

Terminal ileum

- Crohn's mass: tender, ill defined, rubbery hard, non-mobile, may have features of systemic sepsis is secondary complications such as abscess or localized perforation.
- Tuberculous mass: mildly tender, ill defined, firm, associated with cutaneous sinuses, ?systemic TB.

Ovary/fallopian tube

- Cyst: may be massive, usually mobile, ?bimanually palpable on PV examination.
- Neoplasm.
- Ectopic pregnancy: very tender, associated with PV bleeding/intra-abdominal bleeding and collapse.
- Salpingo-oophoritis: very tender, bimanually palpable, associated with PV discharge.

Bladder

- Generally: midline swelling, extends up towards umbilicus, dull to percussion, non-mobile, cannot 'get below' it.

- Retention of urine: stony dull to percussion, associated with desire to pass urine, disappears on voiding/catheterization. May be no desire to pass urine with chronic retention.
- Transitional cell carcinoma: hard, irregular, fixed, may be associated with dysuria, haematuria and desire to pass urine on examination.

Uterus

- Pregnancy: smooth, regular, fetal heart sounds heard/movements.
- Leiomyoma ('fibroids'): usually smooth, may be pedunculated and mobile, non-tender, associated menorrhagia.
- Uterine carcinoma: firm uterus, may be tender, irregular only if tumour is extrauterine, associated PV bloody discharge.

Rectum

Carcinoma: firm, irregular, non-tender, relatively immobile, associated alteration in bowel habit/PR bleeding.

Urachus (rare)

Cyst: small swelling in midline, ?associated umbilical discharge.

Other

Pelvic kidney: smooth, regular, non-tender, non-mobile.

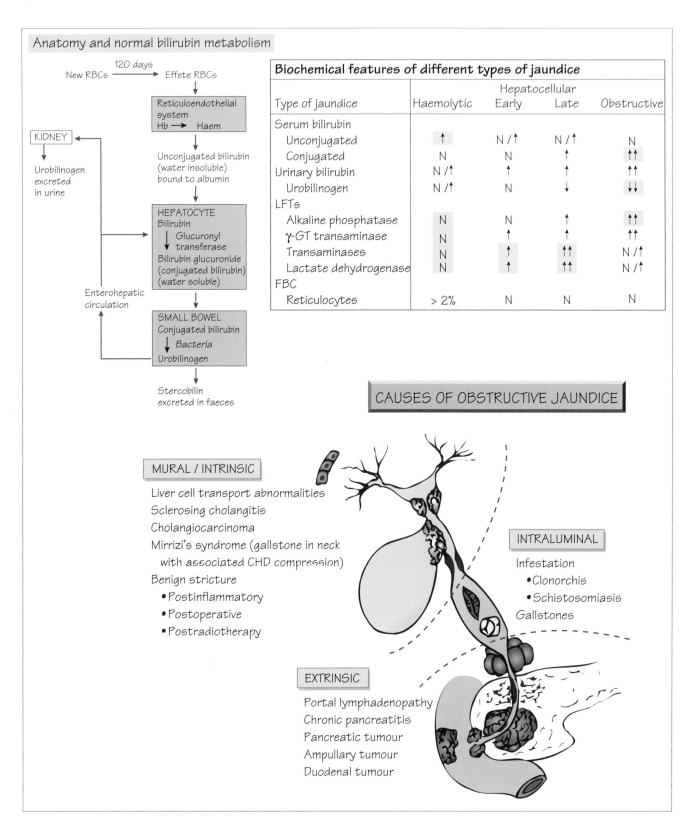

Anatomy and normal bilirubin metabolism

New RBCs —120 days→ Effete RBCs

Reticuloendothelial system
Hb → Haem

Unconjugated bilirubin (water insoluble) bound to albumin

KIDNEY

Urobilinogen excreted in urine

HEPATOCYTE
Bilirubin
↓ Glucuronyl transferase
Bilirubin glucuronide (conjugated bilirubin) (water soluble)

Enterohepatic circulation

SMALL BOWEL
Conjugated bilirubin
↓ Bacteria
Urobilinogen

Stercobilin excreted in faeces

Biochemical features of different types of jaundice

Type of jaundice	Haemolytic	Hepatocellular Early	Hepatocellular Late	Obstructive
Serum bilirubin				
Unconjugated	↑	N/↑	N/↑	N
Conjugated	N	N	↑	↑↑
Urinary bilirubin	N/↑	↑	↑	↑↑
Urobilinogen	N/↑	N	↓	↓↓
LFTs				
Alkaline phosphatase	N	N	↑	↑↑
γ-GT transaminase	N	↑	↑	↑↑
Transaminases	N	↑	↑↑	N/↑
Lactate dehydrogenase	N	↑	↑↑	N/↑
FBC				
Reticulocytes	> 2%	N	N	N

CAUSES OF OBSTRUCTIVE JAUNDICE

MURAL / INTRINSIC

Liver cell transport abnormalities
Sclerosing cholangitis
Cholangiocarcinoma
Mirrizi's syndrome (gallstone in neck with associated CHD compression)
Benign stricture
• Postinflammatory
• Postoperative
• Postradiotherapy

INTRALUMINAL

Infestation
• Clonorchis
• Schistosomiasis
Gallstones

EXTRINSIC

Portal lymphadenopathy
Chronic pancreatitis
Pancreatic tumour
Ampullary tumour
Duodenal tumour

Definition

Jaundice (also called *icterus*) is defined as yellowing of the skin and sclera from accumulation of the pigment bilirubin in the blood and tissues. The bilirubin level has to exceed 35–40 mmol/L before jaundice is clinically apparent.

Key points

- Jaundice can be classified simply as pre-hepatic (haemolytic), hepatic (hepatocellular) and post-hepatic (obstructive).
- Most of the surgically treatable causes of jaundice are post-hepatic (obstructive).
- Painless progressive jaundice is highly likely to be due to malignancy.

Differential diagnosis

The following list explains the mechanisms behind the causes of jaundice.

Pre-hepatic/haemolytic jaundice

Haemolytic/congenital hyperbilirubinaemias

Excess production of unconjugated bilirubin exhausts the capacity of the liver to conjugate the extra load, such as in haemolytic anaemias (e.g. hereditary spherocytosis, sickle cell disease, hypersplenism, thalassaemia).

Hepatic/hepatocellular jaundice

Hepatic unconjugated hyperbilirubinaemia

- Failure of transport of unconjugated bilirubin into the cell, e.g. Gilbert's syndrome.
- Failure of glucuronyl transferase activity, e.g. Crigler–Najjar syndrome.

Hepatic conjugated hyperbilirubinaemia

Hepatocellular injury. Hepatocyte injury results in failure of excretion of bilirubin:

- Infections: viral hepatitis.
- Poisons: CCl$_4$, aflatoxin.
- Drugs: paracetamol, halothane.

Post-hepatic/obstructive jaundice

Post-hepatic conjugated hyperbilirubinaemia

Anything that blocks the release of conjugated bilirubin from the hepatocyte or prevents its delivery to the duodenum.

Courvoisier's law

'A palpable gallbladder in the presence of jaundice is unlikely to be due to gallstones.' It usually indicates the presence of a neoplastic (tumour of pancreas, ampulla, duodenum, CBD) or chronic pancreatitic stricture.

Key investigations

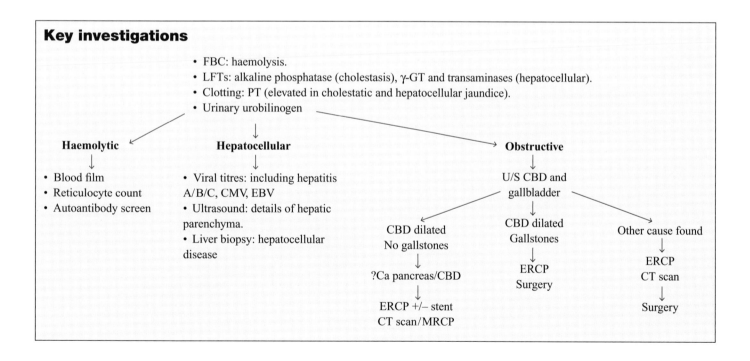

- FBC: haemolysis.
- LFTs: alkaline phosphatase (cholestasis), γ-GT and transaminases (hepatocellular).
- Clotting: PT (elevated in cholestatic and hepatocellular jaundice).
- Urinary urobilinogen

Haemolytic
- Blood film
- Reticulocyte count
- Autoantibody screen

Hepatocellular
- Viral titres: including hepatitis A/B/C, CMV, EBV
- Ultrasound: details of hepatic parenchyma.
- Liver biopsy: hepatocellular disease

Obstructive
U/S CBD and gallbladder

CBD dilated
No gallstones
↓
?Ca pancreas/CBD
↓
ERCP +/− stent
CT scan/MRCP

CBD dilated
Gallstones
↓
ERCP
Surgery

Other cause found
↓
ERCP
CT scan
↓
Surgery

16 Diarrhoea

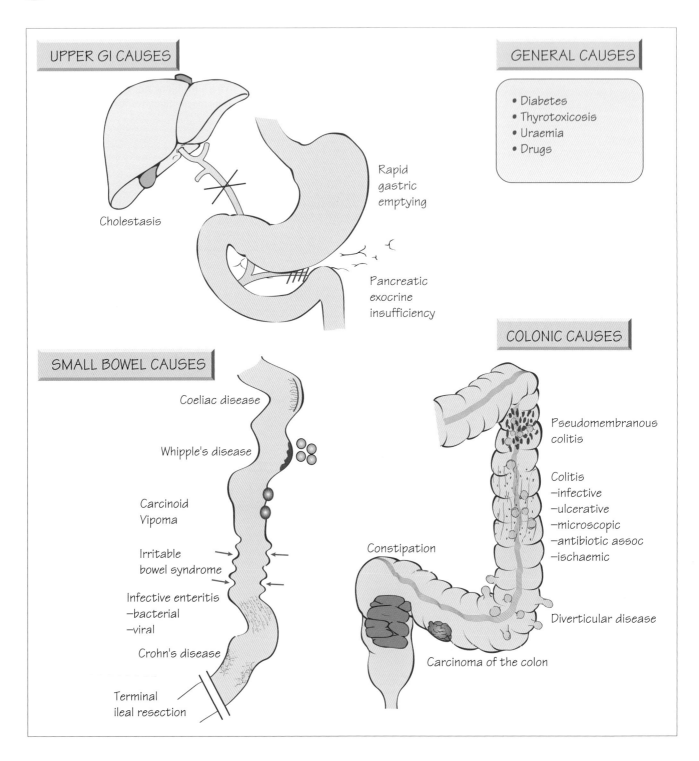

UPPER GI CAUSES

Cholestasis

Rapid gastric emptying

Pancreatic exocrine insufficiency

GENERAL CAUSES

- Diabetes
- Thyrotoxicosis
- Uraemia
- Drugs

SMALL BOWEL CAUSES

Coeliac disease

Whipple's disease

Carcinoid
Vipoma

Irritable bowel syndrome

Infective enteritis
–bacterial
–viral

Crohn's disease

Terminal ileal resection

COLONIC CAUSES

Pseudomembranous colitis

Colitis
–infective
–ulcerative
–microscopic
–antibiotic assoc
–ischaemic

Constipation

Diverticular disease

Carcinoma of the colon

 Surgery at a Glance, Fifth Edition. Pierce A. Grace and Neil R. Borley. © 2013 John Wiley & Sons, Ltd. Published 2013 by John Wiley & Sons, Ltd.

Definitions

Diarrhoea is defined as the passage of loose, liquid stool. *Urgency* is the sensation of the need to defaecate without being able to delay. It may indicate rectal irritability but also occurs where the volume of liquid stool is too large, causing the rectum to be overwhelmed as a storage vessel. *Frequency* merely reflects the number of stools passed and may or may not be associated with urgency or diarrhoea. *Dysentery* is an infective, inflammatory disorder of the lower intestinal tract resulting in pain, severe diarrhoea and passage of blood and mucus per rectum.

Key points

- Bloody diarrhoea is always pathological and usually indicates colitis of one form or another.
- Infective causes are common in acute transient diarrhoea.
- In diarrhoea of uncertain origin, remember the endocrine causes.
- Consider parasitic/atypical bacterial infections in a history of foreign travel.
- Alternating morning diarrhoea and normal/pellety stools later in the day is rarely pathological.
- Diarrhoea developing in hospitalized patients may be due to *Clostridium difficile* infection – check for CD toxin in the stool.

Important diagnostic features

Acute diarrhoea

Infections

- Viral: rotavirus, enteric adenovirus, calicivirus, e.g. norovirus (acute watery diarrhoea).
- Bacteria: *Vibrio cholera* (severe diarrhoea, 'rice water' stool, dehydration, history of foreign travel), *Shigella/Salmonella*, *Campylobacter*, *Yersinia* (bacterial dysentery – diarrhoea + blood + mucus), *Clostridium difficile* (green, offensive diarrhoea).
- Protozoa: *Giardia intestinalis*, *Cryptosporidium parvum* (watery diarrhoea), *Entamoeba histolytica* (occasionally diarrhoea + blood + mucus – amoebic dysentery).

Antibiotic related

Due to disruption of the normal colonic flora. Usually short-lived, self-limiting, mild colicky abdominal pain. May be prolonged and slow to resolve (possibly associated with microscopic colitis on biopsy.

Pseudomembranous colitis

Most severe form of *Clostridium difficile* infection, characterized by severe diarrhoea which may be bloody but occasionally acute constipation may indicate severe disease. Characteristic features on colonoscopy ('baked bean'-like adherent mucopurulent pseudomembranes). Treatment is with oral metronidazole or vancomycin for 10 days.

Chronic diarrhoea

Small bowel disease

- Crohn's disease: diarrhoea, pain prominent, blood and mucus less common, young adults, long history, chronic malnourishment and weight loss. May be signs of perianal disease. May follow from surgical resection.
- Coeliac disease: history of wheat and cereals intolerance rarely clear, may present in adulthood with chronic diarrhoea and weight loss, abdominal pains, iron deficiency (anaemia).
- 'Blind loop' syndrome: frothy, foul-smelling liquid stool, due to bacterial overgrowth and fermentation, usually associated with previous surgery, may complicate Crohn's disease.
- Whipple's disease: malabsorption caused by bacterium *Tropheryma whipplei*, weight loss, arthritis, diarrhoea, lymphadenopathy. M : F = 10 : 1.

Large bowel disease

- Ulcerative colitis: intermittent, blood and mucus, colicky pains, young adults. May be a short history in first presentations. Rarely presents with acute fulminant colitis with acute abdominal signs.
- Colon cancer: older, occasional blood streaks and mucus, change in frequency may be the only feature, positive faecal occult blood, rectal mass.
- Ischaemic colitis: elderly, other evidence of cardiovascular disease; abdominal pain, fever, diarrhoea and rectal bleeding.
- Irritable bowel syndrome: diarrhoea and constipation mixed, bloating, colicky pain, small stool pellets, never blood.
- Spurious: impacted faeces in rectum, liquefied stool passes around faecal obstruction, elderly, mental illness, constipating drugs.
- Polyps (villous) (rare): watery, mucoid diarrhoea, K^+ loss, most common in rectum.
- Diverticular disease (rare).

Systemic disease

Thyrotoxicosis, anxiety, peptides from tumours (VIP, serotonin, substance P, calcitonin), laxative abuse.

Key investigations

- FBC: leucocytosis (infective causes, colitis), anaemia (colon cancer, ulcerative colitis, diverticular disease).
- Anti α-gliadin Abs TTG lutaminase: coeliac disease.
- Thyroid function tests: hyperthyroidism.
- Stool culture: infections (remember microscopy for parasites).
- Proctoscopy/sigmoidoscopy: cancer, colitis, polyps (simple, easy, cheap and safe; performed in outpatients).
- Flexible sigmoidoscopy: cancer, polyps, colitis, infections (relatively safe, well tolerated, high sensitivity).
- Colonoscopy: colitis (extent and severity), pseudomembranous colitis.
- Small bowel enema: Crohn's disease, coeliac disease, Whipple's disease.
- Faecal elastase, faecal fat estimation/ERCP: pancreatic insufficiency.

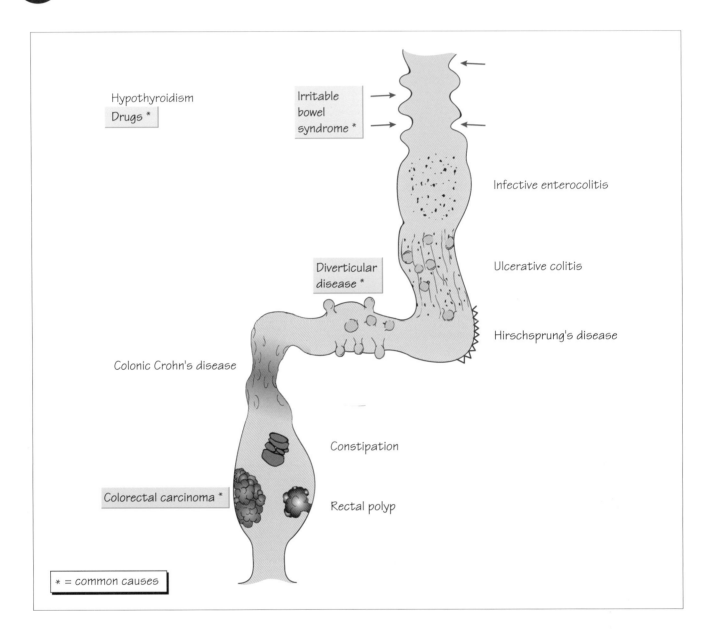

Hypothyroidism

Drugs *

Irritable bowel syndrome *

Infective enterocolitis

Ulcerative colitis

Diverticular disease *

Hirschsprung's disease

Colonic Crohn's disease

Constipation

Colorectal carcinoma *

Rectal polyp

* = common causes

Definitions

'Normal' bowel habit varies widely from person to person. Alterations in bowel habit are common manifestations of GI disease. *Constipation* is defined as infrequent or difficult evacuation of faeces and can be acute or chronic. *Absolute constipation* is defined as the inability to pass either faeces or flatus. *Diarrhoea* is an increase in the fluidity of stool. *Tenesmus* is the sensation of incomplete or unsatisfactory evacuation, often with rectal pain/discomfort.

Key points

- Acute constipation often indicates intestinal obstruction. The cardinal symptoms of obstruction are colicky abdominal pain, vomiting, absolute constipation and distension.
- Chronic constipation may be a lifelong problem or may develop slowly in later life.
- All alterations in bowel habit that persist must be investigated for an underlying cause – colorectal neoplasms are common causes, especially in the elderly.
- IBS is a diagnosis of exclusion and should rarely be considered for new symptoms age >55.
- Always do a PR examination and a rigid sigmoidoscopy – anorectal causes must be excluded.

Important diagnostic features

Chronic constipation

Bowel disease

- Colon cancer: gradual onset, colicky abdominal pain, associated weight loss, anergia, anaemia, positive faecal occult bloods, abdominal mass.
- Diverticular disease: associated LIF pains, inflammatory episodes, rectal bleeding.
- Perianal pain, e.g. fissure, perianal abscess – due to spasm of the internal anal sphincter, common in children.

Adynamic bowel

- Hirschsprung's disease: constipation from birth, gross abdominal distension. Short-segment Hirschsprung's disease (involving only the lower rectum) may present in adulthood with worsening chronic constipation and megarectum/megasigmoid.
- Drugs: opiates, anticholinergics, antipsychotics, secondary to chronic laxative abuse.
- Pregnancy: due to progesterone effects on smooth muscle of bowel wall.

Key investigations

- Digital rectal examination: rectal cancer, rectal adenoma.
- FBC: iron deficiency anaemia – colon cancer, ulcerative colitis, diverticular disease.
- Stool culture: infections (remember microscopy for parasites).
- Proctoscopy/sigmoidoscopy: cancer, colitis, polyps (simple, easy, cheap and safe; performed in outpatients).
- Flexible sigmoidoscopy: cancer, polyps, colitis, infections (relatively safe, well tolerated, high sensitivity).
- Barium enema: where colonoscopy contraindicated or colonic strictures present/suspected.
- Colonoscopy: colitis (extent and severity).
- Rectal biopsy (full thickness): Hirschprung's disease.

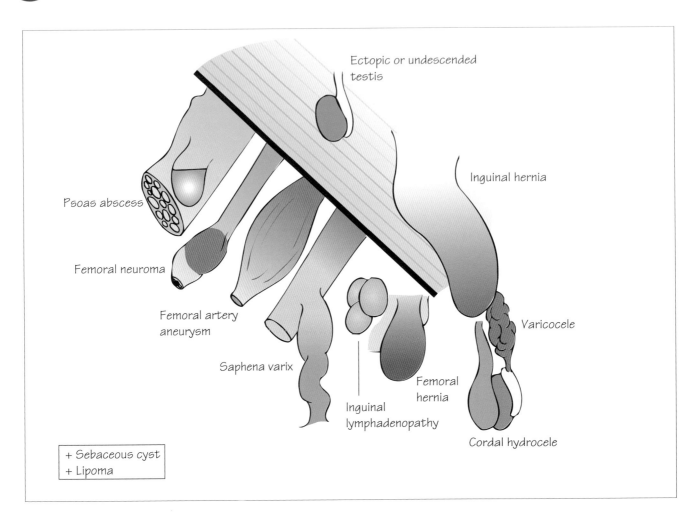

Ectopic or undescended testis

Inguinal hernia

Psoas abscess

Femoral neuroma

Femoral artery aneurysm

Saphena varix

Inguinal lymphadenopathy

Femoral hernia

Varicocele

Cordal hydrocele

+ Sebaceous cyst
+ Lipoma

 Surgery at a Glance, Fifth Edition. Pierce A. Grace and Neil R. Borley. © 2013 John Wiley & Sons, Ltd. Published 2013 by John Wiley & Sons, Ltd.

Definition

Any swelling in the inguinal area or upper medial thigh.

Key points

- The groin crease does not mark the inguinal ligament and is an unreliable landmark.
- Inguinal hernias are common, always start above and medial to the pubic tubercle, may be medial or lateral to it and usually emphasize the groin crease on that side.
- Femoral hernias always start below and lateral to the pubic tubercle, usually flatten the skin crease on that side and are often irreducible.
- Femoral hernias are more common in women, are high risk and need urgent attention.
- Masses in the groin and scrotum together are inguinal hernias.
- Inguinal lymphadenopathy may be isolated or may be part of systemic lymphadenopathy. A cause should always be sought.

Important diagnostic features

The types, causes and features are listed below.

Inguinal hernia

- Direct inguinal hernia: not controlled by pressure over internal ring, characteristically causes a 'forward' bulge in the groin, does not descend into the scrotum.
- Indirect inguinal hernia: controlled by pressure over internal ring, 'slides' through the inguinal canal, often descends into the scrotum.
- Undescended testis: often mass at the external ring or inguinal canal, associated with hypoplastic hemi-scrotum, frequently associated with indirect inguinal hernia.
- Spermatic cord: 'cordal' hydrocele, does not have a cough impulse, may be possible to define upper edge, fluctuates and transilluminates.
- Lipoma: soft, fleshy, does not transilluminate or fluctuate.

Femoral hernia

- Femoral hernia: elderly women (mostly), may be tender and non-expansile, not reducible, groin crease often lost, high risk of strangulation and obstruction.

- Saphena varix: expansile, cough impulse, thrill on percussion of distal saphenous vein.
- Lymphadenopathy: hard, discrete nodules, often multiple or an indistinct mass.
- Femoral artery aneurysm: expansile, pulsatile, thrill and bruit may be present.
- Psoas abscess (rare): soft, fluctuant and compressible, lateral to the femoral artery, may be 'cold' abscesses caused by TB.
- Femoral neuroma (very rare): hard, smooth, moves laterally but not vertically, pressure may cause pain in the distribution of the femoral nerve.
- Hydrocele of femoral sac (very very rare).

Key investigations

- FBC: causes of lymphadenopathy.
- Ultrasound: femoral aneurysm, saphena varix, psoas abscess, ectopic testicle. Also sometimes useful to identify small femoral hernias.
- CT scan: cause of psoas abscess.
- Herniography: rarely needed to confirm presence of hernia if operative indication not clear.
- Laparoscopy: may be used as both diagnostic and therapeutic manoeuvre.

Principles of hernia surgery

- Femoral hernia: close the canal only (usually sutured – may be mesh 'plug' if large defect).
- Infantile inguinal hernia: excise/close the sac/processus vaginalis only ('herniotomy'). No repair of the canal ('herniorraphy') is required. No mesh.
- Adult inguinal hernia – open or laparoscopic surgical approach:
  open (transcutaneous) under GA, LA or spinal + sedation – reduce the contents, excise or reduce the sac and reinforce the canal without tension (usually mesh) 'Lichtenstein' technique
  laparoscopic (Totally ExtraPeritoneal: TEPS; TransAbdominal Pre-peritoneal: TAPS) – always GA, reduce the sac and contents only, always mesh.

19 Claudication

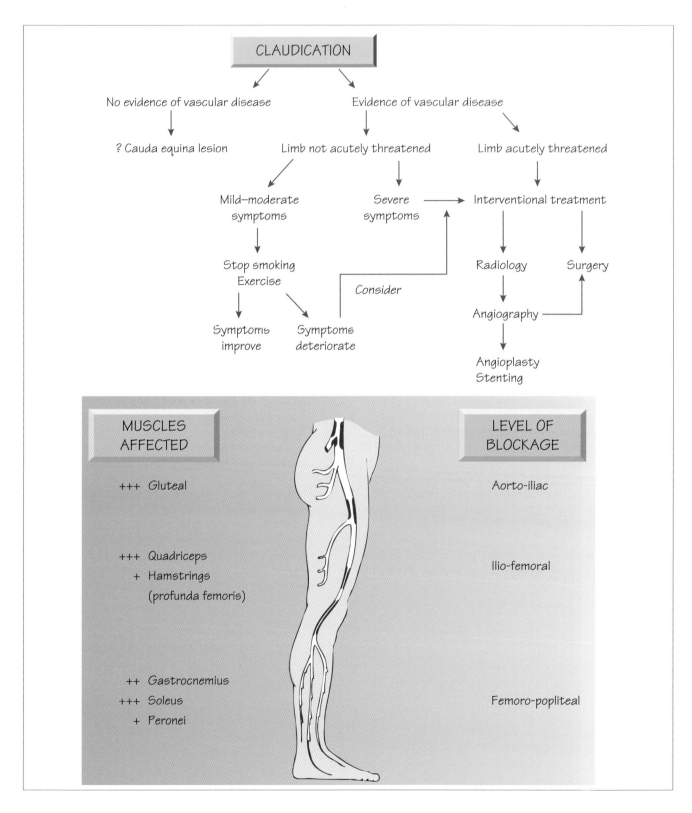

CLAUDICATION

No evidence of vascular disease → ? Cauda equina lesion

Evidence of vascular disease
- Limb not acutely threatened
- Limb acutely threatened

Limb not acutely threatened → Mild–moderate symptoms / Severe symptoms

Limb acutely threatened → Interventional treatment

Mild–moderate symptoms → Stop smoking / Exercise → Symptoms improve / Symptoms deteriorate

Consider → Interventional treatment

Interventional treatment → Radiology → Angiography → Angioplasty Stenting / Surgery

MUSCLES AFFECTED

+++ Gluteal

+++ Quadriceps
  + Hamstrings
    (profunda femoris)

 ++ Gastrocnemius
+++ Soleus
  + Peronei

LEVEL OF BLOCKAGE

Aorto-iliac

Ilio-femoral

Femoro-popliteal

 Surgery at a Glance, Fifth Edition. Pierce A. Grace and Neil R. Borley. © 2013 John Wiley & Sons, Ltd. Published 2013 by John Wiley & Sons, Ltd.

Definition

Intermittent claudication is defined as an aching pain in the leg muscles, usually the calf, that is precipitated by walking and is relieved by rest.

Key points

- Claudication pain is always reversible and relieved by rest.
- Claudication tends to improve with time and exercise due to the opening up of new collateral supply vessels and improved muscle function.
- The site of disease is one level higher than the highest level of affected muscles, e.g. disease in the superficial femoral artery (SFA) produces calf claudication.
- Most patients with claudication have associated vascular disease and investigation for occult coronary or cerebrovascular is mandatory.
- All patients with peripheral vascular disease should be commenced on an antiplatelet agent and a statin, and be encouraged to exercise and stop smoking.
- Cauda equina ischaemia caused by osteoarthritis of the spine can also cause intermittent claudication.

Differential diagnosis

Vascular

Atheroma

- Typical patient: male, over 45 years, ischaemic heart disease, smoker, diabetic, overweight.
- Aortic occlusion: buttock, thigh and possibly calf claudication, impotence in males, absent femoral pulses and below in both legs (Leriche's syndrome).
- Iliac or common femoral stenosis: thigh and calf claudication, absent/weak femoral pulses in affected limb.
- Femoro-popliteal stenosis: calf claudication only, absent popliteal and distal pulses.

Neurological

Cauda equina

Elderly patients, atypical history, history of chronic back pain or back injury, pain may be bilateral and in the distribution of the S1–S3 dermatomes, may be accompanied by paraesthesia in the feet and loss of ankle jerks, all peripheral pulses palpable and legs well perfused.

Key investigations

- FBC: exclude polycythaemia.
- Glucose: diabetes.
- Lipids: hyperlipidaemia.
- ABI: (pre and post exercise) estimate of disease severity.
- ECG: coronary artery disease.
- Angiography: precise location and extent of disease, pre-procedure planning.
  catheter angiography: a catheter is inserted into the artery and contrast given intra-arterially, standard or digital substraction X-ray images obtained – invasive
  CT angiography: IV contrast given and CT images obtained
  MRA: IV contrast given (gadolinium), MR images obtained – no radiation.
  Duplex ultrasound scanning sometimes used instead of angiography.

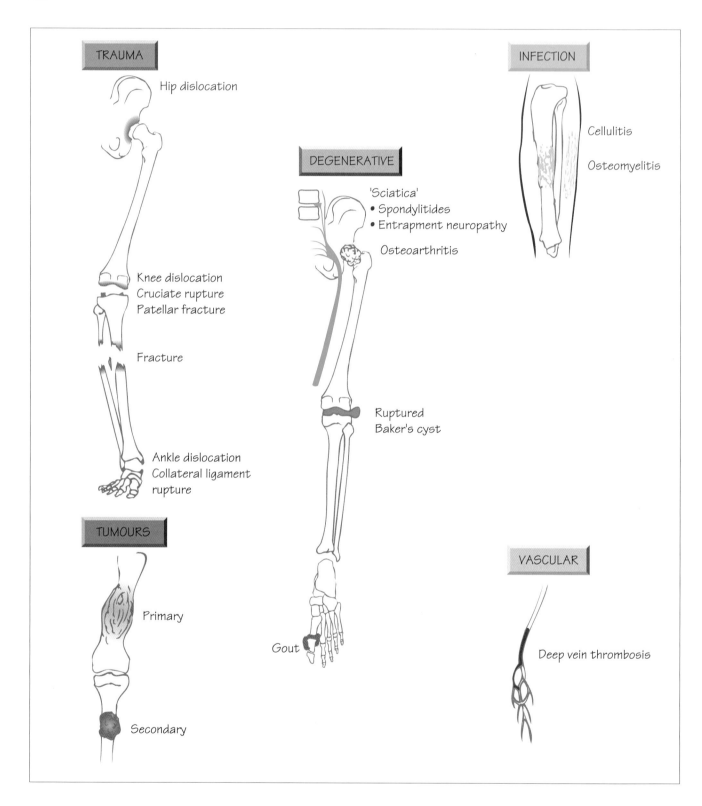

TRAUMA

Hip dislocation

Knee dislocation
Cruciate rupture
Patellar fracture

Fracture

Ankle dislocation
Collateral ligament
rupture

TUMOURS

Primary

Secondary

DEGENERATIVE

'Sciatica'
• Spondylitides
• Entrapment neuropathy

Osteoarthritis

Ruptured
Baker's cyst

Gout

INFECTION

Cellulitis

Osteomyelitis

VASCULAR

Deep vein thrombosis

Definitions

Acute leg pain is a subjective, unpleasant sensation felt somewhere in the lower limb. *Referred pain* is the perception of pain in an area remote from the site of origin of the pain, e.g. leg pain from lumbar disc herniation, knee pain from hip pathology. *Cramps* are involuntary, painful contractions of voluntary muscles. *Sciatica* is a nerve pain caused by irritation of the sciatic nerve roots characterized by lumbosacral pain radiating down the back of the thigh, lateral side of the calf and into the foot.

Key points

- May be due to pathology arising in any of the tissues of the leg.
- Constant or lasting pain suggests local pathology.
- Transient or intermittent pain suggests referred pathology.
- Systemic symptoms or upset suggests inflammation.

Important diagnostic features

Infection

- Infection of skin (cellulitis): painful, swollen, red, hot leg, associated systemic features – pyrexia, rigors, anorexia, commonly caused by *Streptococcus pyogenes*. May be associated lymphangitis (inflammation of lymphatics).
- Acute osteomyelitis: staphylococcal infection, affects metaphyses, acute pain, tenderness and oedema over the end of a long bone, common in children, may be history of skin infection or trauma.

Trauma

- Muscle: swollen, tender and painful, pain worse on attempted movement of the affected muscle.
- Bone: painful, tender. Swelling, deformity, discoloration, bruising and crepitus suggest fracture.

- Joints: painful, limited movement, deformity if dislocated, locking and instability with knee injury.

Degenerative

- Gout: first MTP joint (big toe), males, associated signs of joint inflammation.
- Disc herniation (sciatica): pain in distribution of one or two nerve roots, sudden onset, back pain and stiffness, lumbar scoliosis due to muscle spasm.
- Ruptured Baker's cyst: pain mostly behind the knee, previous history of knee arthritis, calf may be hot and swollen.

Tumours

Bone: deep pain, worse in morning and after exercise, overlying muscle tenderness, pathological fractures, primary (e.g. osteosarcoma, osteoclastoma) or secondary (e.g. breast, prostate, lung metastasis).

Vascular

DVT: calf pain, swelling, redness, prominent superficial veins, tender on calf compression, low-grade pyrexia.

Key investigations

- FBC: WCC in infection.
- D-Dimers: suspected DVT.
- Blood cultures: spreading cellulitis.
- Serum uric acid – gout.
- Clotting: DVT.
- Plain X-ray: trauma, osteomyelitis, bone tumours, gout.
- MRI: suspected disc herniation.
- Duplex ultrasound: DVT.
- Venography: rarely used now as duplex ultrasound is as good, non-invasive and widely available.

21 Acute 'cold' leg

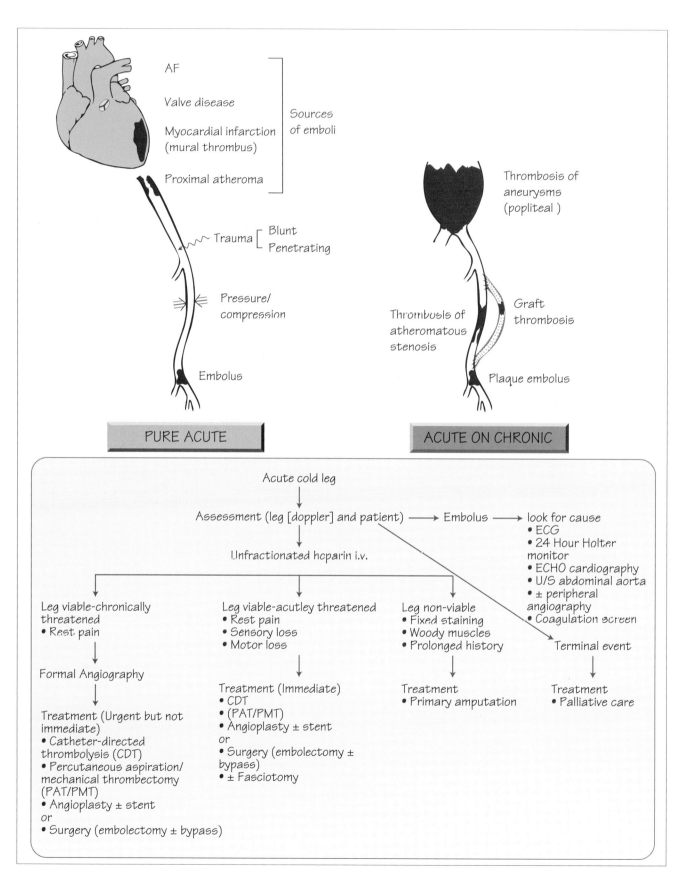

AF

Valve disease

Myocardial infarction (mural thrombus)

Proximal atheroma

Sources of emboli

Trauma — Blunt / Penetrating

Pressure/ compression

Embolus

PURE ACUTE

Thrombosis of aneurysms (popliteal)

Thrombosis of atheromatous stenosis

Graft thrombosis

Plaque embolus

ACUTE ON CHRONIC

Acute cold leg
↓
Assessment (leg [doppler] and patient) → Embolus → look for cause
• ECG
• 24 Hour Holter monitor
• ECHO cardiography
• U/S abdominal aorta
• ± peripheral angiography
• Coagulation screen

Unfractionated heparin i.v.

Leg viable-chronically threatened
• Rest pain

Formal Angiography
↓
Treatment (Urgent but not immediate)
• Catheter-directed thrombolysis (CDT)
• Percutaneous aspiration/ mechanical thrombectomy (PAT/PMT)
• Angioplasty ± stent
or
• Surgery (embolectomy ± bypass)

Leg viable-acutley threatened
• Rest pain
• Sensory loss
• Motor loss
↓
Treatment (Immediate)
• CDT
• (PAT/PMT)
• Angioplasty ± stent
or
• Surgery (embolectomy ± bypass)
• ± Fasciotomy

Leg non-viable
• Fixed staining
• Woody muscles
• Prolonged history
↓
Treatment
• Primary amputation

Terminal event
↓
Treatment
• Palliative care

 Surgery at a Glance, Fifth Edition. Pierce A. Grace and Neil R. Borley. © 2013 John Wiley & Sons, Ltd. Published 2013 by John Wiley & Sons, Ltd.

Definition

The 'acute cold leg' is a clinical syndrome comprising sudden onset of symptoms indicative of the presence of ischaemia sufficient to threaten the viability of the limb or part of it.

Key points

- Remember the '6 Ps' of acute ischaemia – pain, pallor, paraesthesia, paralysis, pulselessness, perishing cold.
- An acute cold leg is a surgical emergency and requires prompt diagnosis and treatment.
- 80% of acute cold legs presenting as an emergency have underlying chronic vascular pathology.
- Fasciotomies should always be considered as part of treatment if a leg is being revascularized.
- Despite appropriate treatment up to 25% of patients have a major amputation.

Important diagnostic features

Isolated arterial embolus

- Sudden-onset severe ischaemia, no previous symptoms of vascular disease, previous history of atrial fibrillation/recent myocardial infarction/valvular heart disease, all peripheral pulses on the unaffected limb normal (suggesting no underlying PVD).
- Limb usually acutely threatened due to complete occlusion with no collateral supply.
- Common sites of impaction are: popliteal bi(tri)furcation, distal superficial femoral artery (adductor canal), origin of the profunda femoris. 'Saddle' embolus at aortic bifurcation causes bilateral acute ischaemic limbs.

Trauma

- May be due to direct injury to the vessel or by secondary compression due to bone fragments or haematoma.

- Direct injuries may be due to complete division of the vessel, distraction injury, intimal damage and *in situ* thrombosis, foreign body, false aneurysm.

Thrombosis (in situ)

- Usually associated with underlying atheroma predisposing to thrombosis after minor trauma or immobility (after a fall or illness).
- May be subacute in onset, previous history of known vascular disease or intermittent claudication, associated risk factors for peripheral vascular disease, abnormal pulses in the unaffected limb.
- Paradoxically, the limb may not be as acutely threatened as in isolated arterial embolus because collateral vessels may already be present due to underlying disease.

Graft thrombosis

Often subacute in onset, limb not acutely threatened, progressive symptoms, loss of graft pulsation.

Aneurysm thrombosis

- Most common site – popliteal aneurysms.
- Sudden-onset limb ischaemia, acutely threatened, may be associated embolization as well, non-pulsatile mass in popliteal fossa, many have contralateral asymptomatic popliteal aneurysm.

Key investigations

- FBC: polycythaemia.
- U+E: renal impairment, myonecrosis.
- Clotting: thrombophilia.
- ECG, ECHO: atrial fibrillation, myocardial infarction, valve disease.
- Duplex scanning: graft patency, popliteal aneurysm.
- Angiography: wherever possible – facilitates treatment plan – arterial embolism, thrombosis, underlying PVD.

22 Leg ulceration

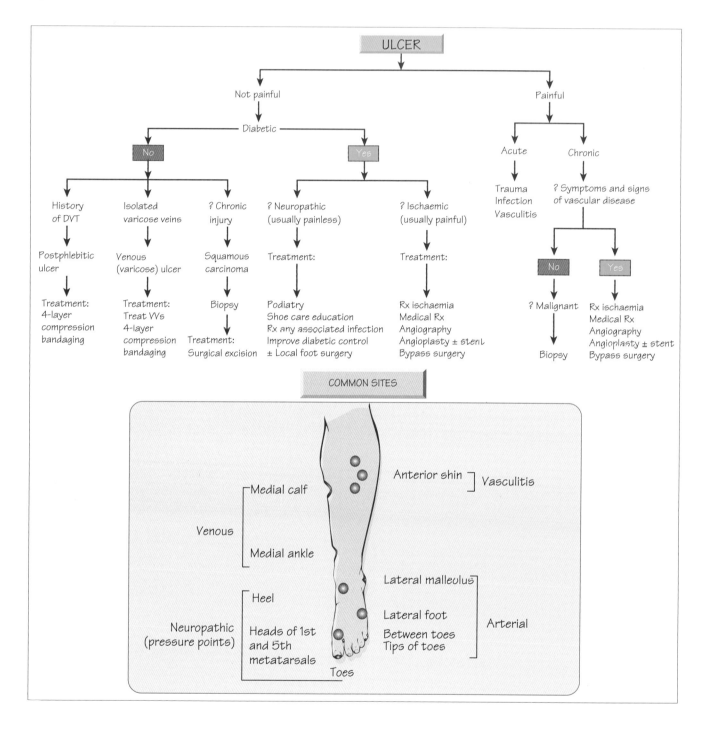

ULCER

- Not painful
  - Diabetic
    - **No**
      - History of DVT → Postphlebitic ulcer → Treatment: 4-layer compression bandaging
      - Isolated varicose veins → Venous (varicose) ulcer → Treatment: Treat VVs 4-layer compression bandaging
      - ? Chronic injury → Squamous carcinoma → Biopsy → Treatment: Surgical excision
    - **Yes**
      - ? Neuropathic (usually painless) → Treatment: Podiatry Shoe care education Rx any associated infection Improve diabetic control ± Local foot surgery
      - ? Ischaemic (usually painful) → Treatment: Rx ischaemia Medical Rx Angiography Angioplasty ± stent Bypass surgery
- Painful
  - Acute → Trauma Infection Vasculitis
  - Chronic → ? Symptoms and signs of vascular disease
    - **No** → ? Malignant → Biopsy
    - **Yes** → Rx ischaemia Medical Rx Angiography Angioplasty ± stent Bypass surgery

COMMON SITES

- Anterior shin] Vasculitis
- Venous { Medial calf / Medial ankle
- Neuropathic (pressure points) { Heel / Heads of 1st and 5th metatarsals / Toes
- Lateral malleolus / Lateral foot / Between toes / Tips of toes] Arterial

 Surgery at a Glance, Fifth Edition. Pierce A. Grace and Neil R. Borley. © 2013 John Wiley & Sons, Ltd. Published 2013 by John Wiley & Sons, Ltd.

Definition

An *ulcer* is defined as an area of discontinuity of the surface epithelium. A *leg ulcer* is an area of ulceration anywhere on the lower limb but usually sited below the knee or on the foot.

Key points

- Pain suggests ischaemia or infection.
- Neuropathic ulcers occur over points of pressure and trauma.
- Marked worsening of a chronic ulcer suggests malignant change.
- The underlying cause must be treated first or the ulcer will not heal.
- Several precipitating causes may coexist (e.g. diabetes, PVD and neuropathy).
- If underlying varicose veins are present with a venous ulcer they should be treated.

Important diagnostic features

Venous ulcers

- Venous hypertension secondary to DVT or varicose veins: ulceration on the medial side of the leg, above the ankle, any size, shallow with sloping edges, bleeds after minor trauma, weeps readily, associated dermato-liposclerosis.
- Duplex scanning of the veins is indicated to assess the functional status (patency and competence) of the superficial and deep venous systems.

Arterial ulcers

Occlusive arterial disease: painful ulcers, do not bleed, non-healing, lateral ankle, heel, metatarsal heads, tips of the toes, associated features of ischaemia, e.g. claudication, absent pulses, pallor. Elderly patients may present with 'blue toe' syndrome which is caused by microemboli.

Diabetic ulcers

- Ischaemic: same as arterial ulcers.
- Neuropathic: deep, painless ulcers, plantar aspect of foot or toes, associated with cellulitis, deep tissue abscesses, oedema, warm foot, pulses may be present.

Malignant ulcers

- Squamous cell carcinoma: may arise *de novo* or malignant change in a chronic ulcer or burn (Marjolin's ulcer). Large ulcer, heaped up, everted edges. Lymphadenopathy – highly suspicious.
- Basal cell carcinoma: uncommon on the leg, rolled edges, pearly white.
- Malignant melanoma: lower limb is a common site, consider malignant if increase in size or pigmentation, bleeding, itching or ulceration.

Miscellaneous ulcers

- Trauma: may be caused by minor trauma. Predisposing factors are poor circulation, malnutrition or steroid treatment.
- Vasculitis (rare): e.g. rheumatoid arthritis, SLE.
- Infections (rare): syphilis, TB, tropical infections.
- Pyoderma gangrenosum: multiple necrotic ulcers over the legs that start as nodules. Seen with ulcerative colitis and Crohn's disease.

Key investigations

- FBC: infections.
- Glucose: diabetes.
- Special blood tests: TPHA (syphilis), ANCA (SLE), Rh factor.
- ABI measurement to exclude underlying PVD. Toe pressures more accurate in diabetes.
- Biopsy: malignancy. Melanoma – always excision biopsy. Others may be incision/'punch'.
- Duplex ultrasound/angiography/(rarely venography)/: extent and severity of disease. Planning treatment.

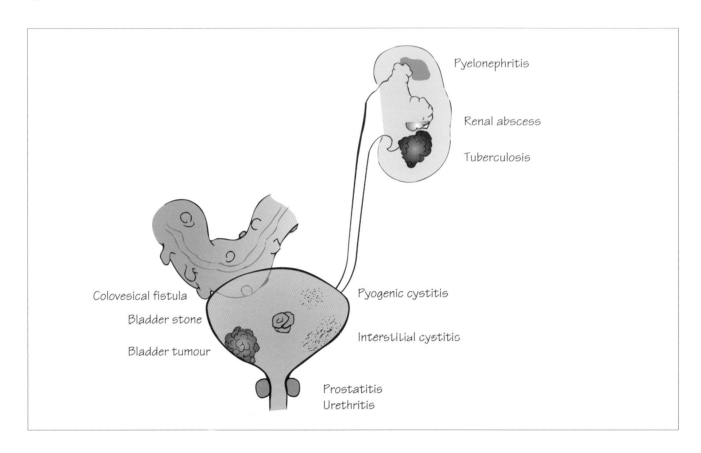

Definitions

Dysuria is defined as a pain that arises from an irritation of the urethra and is felt during micturition. *Frequency* indicates increased passage of urine during the daytime; *nocturia* indicates increased passage of urine during the night. *Urgency* is an uncontrollable desire to micturate and may be associated with *incontinence*, which is the involuntary loss of urine. *Pneumaturia* is the passage of gas (air) mixed with urine and may be described by patients as passing bubbles in the urine.

Key points

- UTI is the most common cause of dysuria in adults.
- Features of systemic sepsis and loin pain suggest an ascending UTI (pyelonephritis).
- Elderly men with recurrent UTIs often have an underlying problem of bladder emptying due to prostate disease.
- Recurrent infections require investigation to exclude an underlying cause.
- Pneumaturia, 'bits/debris' in the urine and coliform infections suggest a colovesical fistula.

Important diagnostic features

Urinary tract infection

Acute pyelonephritis

Cause: Upper tract infection.

Predisposing causes:

- Outflow tract obstruction.
- Vesicoureteric reflux (in children).
- Renal or bladder calculi.
- Diabetes mellitus.
- Neuropathic bladder dysfunction.

Features: Pyrexia, rigors, flank pain, dysuria, malaise, anorexia, leucocytosis, pyuria (>10 WBC/mm^3 urine), bacteriuria, microscopic haematuria, C&S >100000 organisms/ml. Sterile pyuria may be caused by perinephric abscess, urethral syndrome, chronic prostatitis, renal TB and fungal infections.

Acute cystitis

Causes:

- Lower tract infection.
- Usually coliform bacteria.

- Because of short urethra more common in females.
- *Proteus* infections may indicate stone disease.

Features: Dysuria, frequency, urgency, suprapubic pain, low back pain, incontinence and microscopic haematuria.

Urethritis

Causes:

- Sexually transmitted diseases.
- May be gonococcal, chlamydial or mycoplasmal.

Features: Dysuria and meatal pruritus, occurs 3–10 days after sexual contact, yellowish purulent urethral discharge suggests *Gonococcus*, thin mucoid discharge suggests *Chlamydia*.

Other causes of dysuria

Urethral syndrome

A condition characterized by frequency, urgency and dysuria in women with urine cultures showing no growth or low bacterial counts.

Vaginitis

A condition characterized by dysuria, pruritus and vaginal discharge. Urine cultures are negative, but vaginal cultures often reveal *Trichomonas vaginalis*, *Candida albicans* or *Haemophilus vaginalis*.

Bladder problems

- Bladder tumours are an uncommon cause of dysuria (10%), they usually present with haematuria.
- Interstitial cystitis: a chronic inflammatory condition of the bladder that causes frequent, urgent and painful urination with or without pelvic discomfort.
- Colovesical fistula: usually caused by diverticular disease, rarely by Crohn's disease, carcinoma of the colon or bladder and very rarely by gas-producing bacterial infection of the urinary tract.

Key investigations

- FBC: WCC – infection, normocytic anaemia – chronic infection.
- Ultrasound: renal abscess.
- CT scan (CT IVU) : renal abscess, diverticular disease.
- Cystoscopy: bladder tumours, stones, cystitis, prostatic disease.
- Transrectal ultrasound (TRUS): prostate disease (?carcinoma).

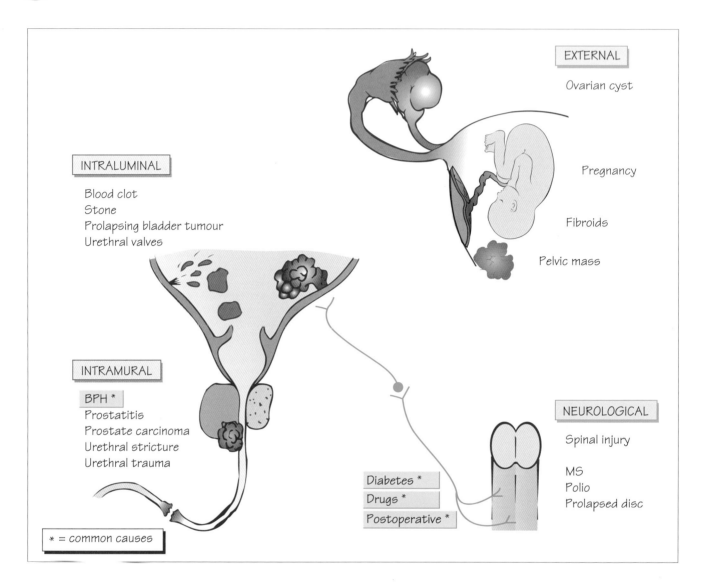

EXTERNAL
Ovarian cyst
Pregnancy
Fibroids
Pelvic mass

INTRALUMINAL
Blood clot
Stone
Prolapsing bladder tumour
Urethral valves

INTRAMURAL
BPH *
Prostatitis
Prostate carcinoma
Urethral stricture
Urethral trauma

NEUROLOGICAL
Spinal injury
MS
Polio
Prolapsed disc

Diabetes *
Drugs *
Postoperative *

* = common causes

Definitions

Urinary retention is defined as an inability to micturate (pass urine). *Acute urinary retention* is the sudden inability to micturate in the presence of a painful bladder. *Chronic urinary retention* is the presence of an enlarged, full, often painless bladder with or without difficulty in micturition. *Overflow incontinence* is an uncontrollable leakage and dribbling of urine from the urethra in the presence of a full bladder.

Key points

- Acute retention: characterized by pain, sensation of bladder fullness, bladder often only mildly distended or not clinically detectable unless superadded on chronic retention.
- Chronic retention: characterized by symptoms of bladder irritation (frequency, dysuria, small volume), or painless, marked distention, overflow incontinence (often associated with secondary UTI).
- Urinary retention is uncommon in young adults and always requires investigation to exclude underlying cause.
- Retention is common in elderly men – often due to prostate pathology.

Differential diagnosis

Age

Acute retention
- Children – abdominal pain, drugs.
- Young – postoperative, drugs, acute UTI, trauma, haematuria.
- Elderly – acute on chronic retention with BPH, tumours, postoperative.

Chronic retention
- Children – congenital abnormalities.
- Young – trauma, postoperative.
- Elderly – BPH, strictures, prostatic carcinoma.

Mechanical

In the lumen of the urethra
- Congenital valves (rare): neonates, males, recurrent UTIs.
- Foreign body (rare).
- Stones (rare): acute pain in penis and glans.

- Tumour (rare): TCC or squamous cell carcinoma, history of haematuria, working in dye or rubber industry.

In the wall of the urethra
- BPH: frequency, nocturia, hesitancy, poor stream, dribbling, urgency.
- Tumour: as above.
- Stricture: history of trauma or serious infection, gradual onset of poor stream.
- Trauma: blood at meatus.

Outside the wall of the urethra
- Pregnancy.
- Fibroids: palpable, bulky uterus, menorrhagia, dysmenorrhoea.
- Ovarian cyst: mobile iliac fossa mass.
- Faecal impaction: spurious diarrhoea.

Neurological
- Postoperative: pain, drugs, pelvic nerve disturbance.
- Drugs: narcotics, anticholinergics, antihistamines, antipsychotics.
- Upper motor neuron lesions produce chronic retention with reflex incontinence.
- Lower motor neuron lesions produce chronic retention with overflow incontinence.
- Spinal cord injuries: acute phase is lower motor neurone type, late phase is upper motor neurone type.
- Diabetes: progressive lower motor neuron pattern.
- Idiopathic: detrusor sphincter dyssynergia, ?bladder neurone degeneration.

Key investigations

- U+E and creatinine: renal function.
- MSU MC+S: associated infection, include cytology where tumour suspected.
- Ultrasound bladder scan.
- Cystography: urethral valves, strictures.
- IVU: renal/bladder stones.
- Urodynamics: allows identification and assessment of neurological problems, assesses BPH through uroflowmetry – average flow for an adult is 18 ml/s.
- Cystoscopy.

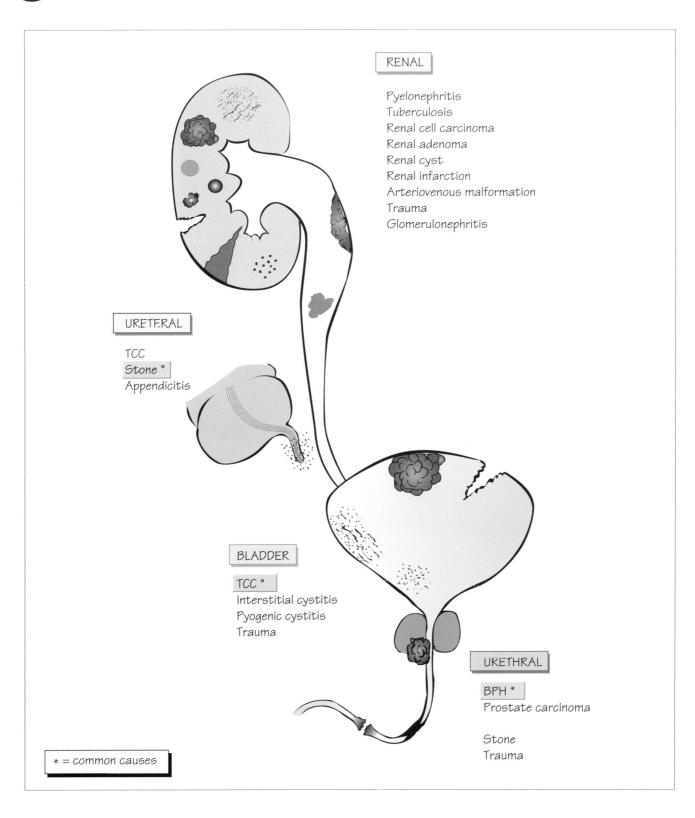

RENAL

Pyelonephritis
Tuberculosis
Renal cell carcinoma
Renal adenoma
Renal cyst
Renal infarction
Arteriovenous malformation
Trauma
Glomerulonephritis

URETERAL

TCC
Stone *
Appendicitis

BLADDER

TCC *
Interstitial cystitis
Pyogenic cystitis
Trauma

URETHRAL

BPH *
Prostate carcinoma

Stone
Trauma

* = common causes

Definitions

Haematuria is the passage of blood in the urine. *Frank haematuria* is the presence of blood on macroscopic examination, while *microscopic haematuria* indicates that RBCs are only seen on microscopy. *Haemoglobinuria* is defined as the presence of free Hb in the urine.

Key points

- Haematuria always requires investigation to exclude an underlying cause.
- Initial haematuria (blood on commencing urination) suggests a urethral cause.
- Terminal haematuria (blood after passing urine) suggests a bladder base or prostatic cause.
- Ribbon clots suggest a pelvi-ureteric cause.
- Renal bleeding can mimic colic due to clots passing down the ureter.

Important diagnostic features

Kidney

- Trauma: mild to moderate trauma commonly causes renal bleeding, severe injuries may not bleed (avulsed kidney – complete disruption).
- Tumours: may be profuse or intermittent.
- Renal cell carcinoma: associated mass, loin pain, clot, colic or fever, occasional polycythaemia, hypercalcaemia and hypertension.
- TCC: characteristically painless, intermittent haematuria.
- Calculus: severe loin/groin pain, gross or microscopic, associated infection.
- Glomerulonephritis: usually microscopic, associated systemic disease (e.g. SLE).
- Pyelonephritis (rare).
- Renal tuberculosis (rare): sterile pyuria, weight loss, anorexia, PUO, increased frequency of micturition day and night.
- Polycystic disease (rare): palpable kidneys, hypertension, chronic renal failure.

- Renal arteriovenous malformation or simple cyst (very rare): painless, no other symptoms.
- Renal infarction (very rare): may be caused by an arterial embolus, painful tender kidney.

Ureter

- Calculus: severe loin/groin pain, gross or microscopic, associated infection.
- TCC: see below.

Bladder

- Calculus: sudden cessation of micturition, pain in perineum and tip of penis.
- TCC: characteristically painless, intermittent haematuria, history of smoking, exposure to rubber or chemical dyes.
- Acute cystitis: suprapubic pain, dysuria, frequency and bacteriuria.
- Interstitial cystitis (rare): may be autoimmune, drug or radiation induced, frequency and dysuria common.
- Schistosomiasis (very rare): history of foreign travel, especially North Africa.

Prostate

- BPH: painless haematuria, associated obstructive symptoms, recurrent UTI.
- Carcinoma (rare).

Urethra

- Trauma: blood at meatus, history of direct blow to perineum, e.g. falling astride, acute retention.
- Calculus (rare).
- Urethritis (rare).

Key investigations

- FBC: WCC – infection, iron deficiency anaemia – renal tumours.
- Ultrasound: renal tumours, cysts, trauma.
- CT scan (CT IVU): renal tumours/stones/AVM, bladder tumours.
- Cystoscopy: bladder tumours, cystitis, prostatic disease.
- Transrectal ultrasound (TRUS): prostate disease (?carcinoma).
- Cystogram: bladder/urethral trauma.

26 Scrotal swellings

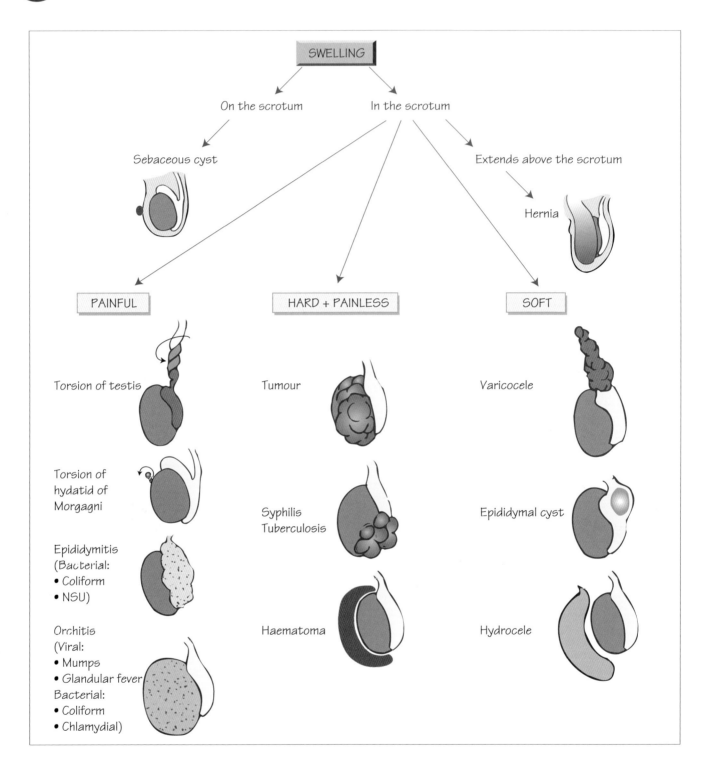

Definition

Any swelling in or on the scrotum or its contents.

Key points

- Always evaluate scrotal swellings for extension to the groin. If present they are almost always inguinoscrotal hernias.
- Torsion is most common in adolescence and in the early twenties. Whenever the diagnosis is suspected, urgent assessment and usually emergency surgery are required.
- Young adult men: tumours, trauma and acute infections are common.
- Older men: hydrocele and hernia are common.

Differential diagnosis

The causes and features are listed below.

Scrotum

- Sebaceous cyst: attached to the skin, just fluctuant, does not transilluminate, punctum.
- Infantile scrotal oedema: acute idiopathic scrotal swelling, hot, tender, bright red, testicle less tender than in torsion, most common in young boys.

Testis

Painful conditions

- Orchitis: confined to testis, young men (mumps, brucellosis).
- Epididymo-orchitis: painful and swollen, epididymis more than testis, associated erythema of scrotum, fever and pyuria, unusual below the age of 25 years, pain relieved by elevating the testis. May be related to sexually transmitted disease.
- Torsion of the testis: rapid onset, pubertal males, often high investment of tunica vaginalis on the cord – 'bellclapper testis', testis may lie high and transversely in the scrotum, 'knot' in the cord may be felt.
- Torsion of appendix testis (hydatid of Morgagni): mimics full torsion, early signs are a lump at the upper pole of the testis and a blue spot on transillumination, later the whole testis becomes swollen, may require explorative surgery to exclude full torsion.

Hard conditions

- Testicular tumour: painless swelling, younger adult men (20–50 years), may have lax secondary hydrocele, associated abdominal lymphadenopathy.
- Haematocele: firm, does not transilluminate, testis cannot usually be felt, history of trauma.
- Syphilitic gummata – firm, rubbery, usually associated with other features of secondary syphilis. TB – uncommon.

Soft conditions

- Hydrocele: soft, fluctuant, transilluminates brilliantly, testis may be difficult to feel, new onset or rapidly recurrent hydrocele suggests an underlying testicular cause.
- Epididymal cyst: separate and behind the testis, transilluminates well, may be quite large.
- Varicocele: a collection of dilated and tortuous veins in the spermatic cord – 'bag of worms' on examination, more common on the left, associated with a dragging sensation, occasional haematospermia.

Key investigations

- FBC: infection.
- Ultrasound: painless, non-invasive imaging of testicle. Allows underlying pathology to be excluded in hydrocele. High sensitivity and specificity for tumours.
- Doppler ultrasound: may confirm presence of blood flow where torsion is thought unlikely.
- CT scan: staging for testicular tumours.
- Surgery: may be the only way to confirm or exclude torsion in a high-risk group. Should not be delayed for any other investigation if required.

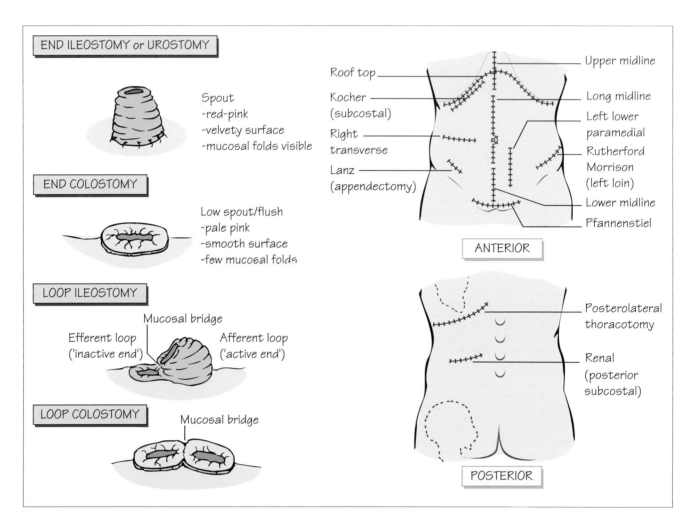

Definitions

Stomas

A *stoma* is an opening from a hollow viscus connecting it to the skin surface. A *gastrostomy* is an opening into the stomach which is maintained by inserting a tube. An *ileostomy* is an opening in the small intestine. A *colostomy* is an opening in the large intestine. A *urostomy* is an external opening in the urinary tract. The most common form is a short length of ileum formed into a stoma and connected to the urinary tract (ureters) to act as a conduit for urine (*ileal conduit*).

Incisions

A *laparotomy* is any incision in the abdominal wall but usually used to refer to anterior (para)midline approaches.

Key points

- Ileostomies and urostomies are usually spouted to reduce the risk of the output causing irritation of the surrounding skin.
- Colostomies are usually flush to the skin.
- Don't assume what type of stoma is present by its location.

Indications for common stomas

- Gastrostomy:
  temporary: inability to swallow (e.g. post CVA, during pharyngeal DXT)
  permanent: loss of swallowing (e.g. MS, MND)

- Ileostomy:

  permanent end: total proctocolectomy for ulcerative colitis

  temporary end: post-emergency right hemicolectomy/ileocaecal resection without anastomosis

  loop: relief of distal obstruction; protection of distal anastomosis, diversion of the faecal stream (may be temporary)

- Colostomy:

  permanent end: abdominoperineal resection of rectum and anal canal for very low rectal carcinoma

  temporary end: sigmoid colectomy for complications of carcinoma or diverticulitis (Hartmann's procedure)

  loop: relief of distal obstruction; protection of distal anastomosis, diversion of the faecal stream (may be temporary)

- Ileal conduit: urinary diversion after cystectomy.

Siting and care of a stoma

- Gastrostomy is created by placing a tube through the abdominal wall (LUQ) into the stomach usually by a percutaneous endoscopic technique (PEG).
- Electively formed stomas should be sited pre-operatively by the stoma specialist. Features to take into account are: abdominal size and shape, skin folds/creases (avoid), previous scars(avoid), level of the belt or dress line (place stomas above *or* below but not *on*), manual dexterity and visual impairment of patient.
- Stoma appliances are extremely varied: they may be one or two piece (separate bag and adherent flange), flat or convex, drainable or sealed, with or without odour filters.

Features to recognize a stoma

Spout

- Fully spouted stomas are almost always formed from ileum. They may be an ileostomy or a urostomy.
- Spouted stomas with two lumens are always loop ileostomies. Look carefully to identify a second lumen as it may not be obvious.
- Flush stomas are usually colostomies.

Position

- Although ileostomies are often placed in the right lower abdomen and colostomies are placed in the left lower abdomen, location is never a good indication of what type of stoma is present.

Contents

- Stoma appliance contents: ileostomies usually produce semi-liquid green-brown output, colostomies usually produce solid/semi-solid faecal output. Beware – this is often unreliable in disease processes or soon after formation where the outputs may be similar. Urostomies drain clear fluid, i.e. urine.

Complications of stomas

- Necrosis: acute early complication due to compromised blood supply – appears black or dark purple. Rx – re-operation to remake the stoma.
- Stenosis: narrowing of stoma or cutaneous orifice usually due to small skin defect or chronic ischaemia of stoma. Rx – dilatation by probe dilators or refashioning of stoma by surgery.
- Retraction: spout reduced/absent or stoma indrawn into abdominal wall, usually due to tension on the bowel used. Rx – convex stoma appliances, refashioning of stoma by surgery.
- Prolapse: excessive spout length, due to loose skin defect or chronic effect of bowel peristalsis. More common in loop stomas especially loop colostomies. Rx – stoma appliance change or refashioning of stoma.
- Herniation: presence of bowel in the subcutaneous tissues. Usually due to an oversized opening in the abdominal muscles wall. Most common long-term stoma complication. Often causes problems with stoma appliance adherence. Rx – repair hernia, resiting stoma.
- Peristomal dermatitis: due to contents spilling onto peristomal skin or trauma of appliance changes. Rx – better stoma care, change of appliance, topical anti-inflammatories.
- Fluid and electrolyte imbalances: usually only a problem in ileostomies (especially early after formation, if high in the small bowel or associated gastroenteritis). Caused by excessive wash-out of electrolyte rich fluid. Rx – control of high output (dietary modifications, use of anti-diarrhoeals, temporary use of isotonic oral fluids), intravenous fluid replacement if severe.

Abdominal and thoracic incisions

- Vertical incisions are usually non-muscle splitting but traverse several or many myotomes/dermatomes.
- Transverse incisions are usually muscle splitting but are placed to lie in one or two myotomes/dermatomes; Pfannansteil (transverse suprapubic) is the exception – no muscle division.
- Midline vertical incisions can easily be extended to improve access to all parts of the abdomen but are often larger than transverse incisions placed over the area to be operated on.
- Midline vertical incisions tend to be used where the extent or type of surgery is large or uncertain.
- Transverse incisions tend to have a lower risk of wound hernia formation.
- Thoracotomy incisions are placed between ribs and are muscle splitting.
- Thoracotomy incisions may involve division or disarticulation of the rib above or below the incision.

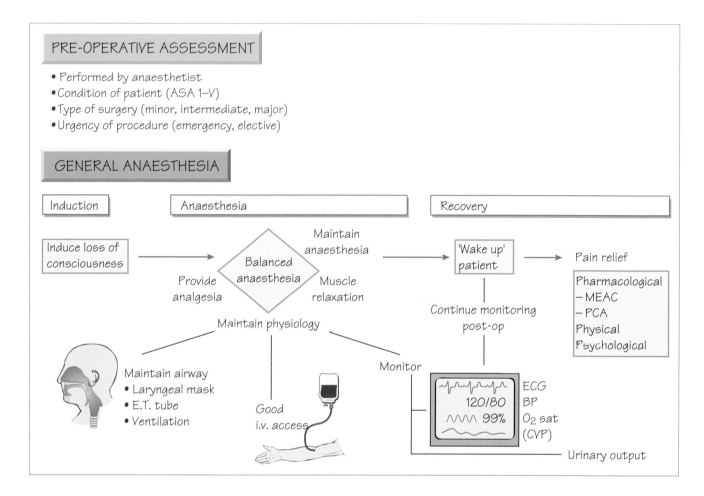

PRE-OPERATIVE ASSESSMENT

- Performed by anaesthetist
- Condition of patient (ASA 1–V)
- Type of surgery (minor, intermediate, major)
- Urgency of procedure (emergency, elective)

GENERAL ANAESTHESIA

Induction | Anaesthesia | Recovery

Induce loss of consciousness → Balanced anaesthesia (Maintain anaesthesia / Provide analgesia / Muscle relaxation) → 'Wake up' patient → Pain relief

Pharmacological
– MEAC
– PCA
Physical
Psychological

Continue monitoring post-op

Maintain physiology

Maintain airway
- Laryngeal mask
- E.T. tube
- Ventilation

Good i.v. access

Monitor

ECG
120/80 BP
99% O₂ sat (CVP)

Urinary output

Definitions

Anaesthesia (αναισθεσια = **without perception**): 1. a partial or complete loss of all forms of sensation caused by pathology in the nervous system; 2. a technique using drugs (inhalational, intravenous or local) that renders the whole or part of the organism insensible for variable periods of time. *Analgesia*: the loss of pain sensation. *Hypnotic agent*: a sleep-inducing drug. *Muscle relaxant*: a drug that reduces muscle tension by affecting the nerves that supply the muscles or the myoneuronal junction (e.g curare, succinylcholine). *Sedation*: the production of a calm and restful state by the administration of a drug.

General anaesthesia: relies upon generalized suppression of some functions of the cerebral cortex to induce a generalized state of insensibility.

Regional anaesthesia: relies upon blockage of nerve impulses or spinal transmission of impulses to induce analgesia and immobility.

Key points

- Fasting – while food should be avoided for several hours preoperatively, water may be given freely to most patients up to 2 hours before operation.
- Pre-operative assessment and risk is based on the ASA classification and the urgency and complexity of surgery.
- General anaesthesia comprises safe induction, active maintenance of anaesthesia and safe recovery.
- Regional anaesthesia is preferred for many procedures, e.g. obstetrics, eye surgery, orthopaedics.
- Spinal/epidural anaesthesia is contraindicated in the anticoagulated patients.

Pre-operative assessment

Prior to an operation the anaesthetist will assess the patient and devise a plan for anaesthesia based on the following:

- The condition of the patient (ASA classification) determined by:
  history
  physical examination
  selective investigations.
- The complexity of the surgery to be performed.
- The urgency of the procedure (emergency or elective).

Class	ASA pre-operative physical status classification
Class I	Fit and healthy
Class II	Mild systemic disease
Class III	Severe systemic disease that is not incapacitating
Class IV	Incapacitating systemic disease that is constantly life-threatening
Class V	Moribund – not expected to survive >24 hours without surgery

ASA = American Society of Anesthesiologists.

General anaesthesia
Pre-operative fasting
- Rationale:
  GA reduces reflexes that protect against aspiration of stomach contents into lungs
  fasting reduces volume and acidity of gastric contents.
- Adults:
  no *food* for 6 hours pre op
  may drink clear fluids up to 2 hours pre op – this may include carbohydrate supplements (as in ERAS programmes)
  caution in elderly, pregnant, obese and patients with stomach disorder.
- Children:
  no food for 6 hours pre op
  no breast milk for 4 hours
  may drink clear fluids (water, apple juice) for up to 2 hours pre op.
- Emergency surgery:
  cricoid pressure is applied as a part of 'rapid sequence' intubation – the cricoid cartilage is pushed against the body of the sixth cervical vertebra, compressing the oesophagus to prevent passive regurgitation.

Aims and technique
- To induce a loss of consciousness using hypnotic drugs which may be administered intravenously (e.g. propofol) or by inhalation (e.g. sevoflurane).

- To provide adequate operating conditions for the duration of the surgical procedure using *balanced anaesthesia*, i.e. a combination of hypnotic drugs to maintain anaesthesia (e.g. propofol, sevoflurane), analgesics for pain (e.g. opiates, NSAIDs) and, if indicated, muscle relaxants (e.g. suxamethonium, tubocurarine) or regional anaesthesia.
- To maintain essential physiological function by:
  providing a clear airway (laryngeal mask airway or tracheal tube ± IPPV)
  maintaining good oxygenation (inspired O_2 concentration should be 30%)
  maintaining good vascular access (large-bore IV cannula ± central venous catheter ± arterial cannula)
  monitoring vital functions:
    pulse oximetry (functional arterial O_2 saturation in %)
    capnography (expired respiratory gas CO_2 level)
    arterial blood pressure: non-invasive (sphigmomanometer) or invasive (arterial cannula) techniques
    temperature
    ECG
    ± hourly urinary output, CVP
    rarely: pulmonary arterial pressure, pulmonary capillary wedge pressure and cardiac output measured via a Swan–Ganz catheter or trans-oesophageal echocardiography.
- To awaken the patient safely at the end of the procedure. Immediately after the operation patients are admitted to a recovery room where airway, respiration, circulation, level of consciousness and analgesia requirements are monitored.

Enhanced recovery after surgery (ERAS)
A combined multidisciplinary approach to optimize return of normal bodily functions after general anaesthesia. An overall major tool is patient information and preparation for surgery and recovery. Key aspects of care are:
- Anaesthesia: short acting agents, avoidance of bolus intravenous opiates, use of regional anaesthesia (e.g. nerve blocks), goal-directed fluid replacement (to avoid over or under administration of crystalloids).
- Surgery: minimally invasive approaches (mini-laparotomy, laparoscopic), avoidance of bowel exposure/handling, avoidance of bowel preparation.
- Nutrition/fluids: pre-operative carbohydrate loading, early introduction of oral fluids and diet.
- Physiotherapy: goal-directed early mobilization.

Anaesthesia – regional

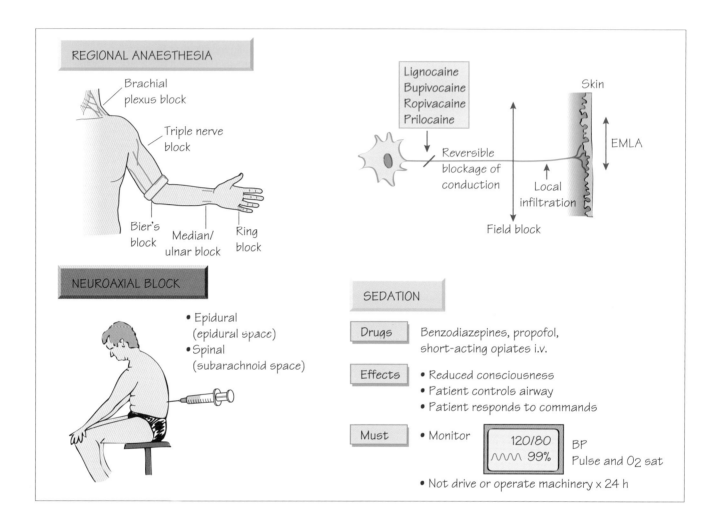

Regional anaesthesia
Aims and technique
• To render an area of the body completely insensitive to pain.
• Local anaesthetic agents (LA) prevent pain by causing a reversible block of conduction along nerve axons. Addition of a vasoconstrictor (e.g. epinephrine) reduces systemic absorption allowing more LA to be given and prolonging its duration of action.

	Dose, mg/kg (+ epinephrine)			Possible systemic toxicity of local anaesthetic agents
Lidocaine	3 (7)	}	{	CNS – drowsiness, confusion, visual disturbance, headache, nausea, vomiting, convulsions
Bupivacaine	2 (2)	}	{	
Ropivacaine	2 (2)	}	{	RS – respiratory arrest
Prilocaine	4 (7)	}	{	CVS – altered BP, arrhythmias, cardiac arrest

Regional anaesthetic techniques
• Topical administration of local anaesthetic (LA is placed on the skin – e.g. EMLA© (Eutectic Mixture of Local Anaesthetic) cream prior to venepuncture).
• Local infiltration of LA (subcutaneous infiltration around the immediate surrounding area – e.g. used for excision of skin lesions).
• Field block (subcutaneous infiltration of LA around an operative field to render the whole operative field anaesthetic – e.g. used for inguinal hernia repair).
• Local blocks of specific peripheral nerves (± ultrasound guidance) (e.g. sciatic nerve block, ring block of fingers/toes, intercostals nerve block).
• Local blocks of specific plexuses (± ultrasound guidance) (e.g. brachial plexus block for upper limb surgery, coeliac plexus block for cancer pain).
• Intravenous blocks (e.g. Bier's block of the upper limb – a short acting LA is injected via a cannula into an exsanguinated arm to which a tourniquet has been applied).

- Neuroaxial block:

  epidural anaesthesia – local anaesthetic is injected as a bolus or via a small catheter into the epidural space. It can be used as the sole anaesthetic for surgery below the waistline, especially useful in obstetrics, or as an adjunct to general anaesthesia.

  spinal anaesthesia – local anaesthetic is injected into the CSF in the subarachnoid space. The extent and duration of anaesthesia depend on the position of the patient, the specific gravity of the LA and the level of injection (usually lumbar spine level).

Sedation

Many minimally invasive procedures (e.g. colonoscopy) are performed under sedation only. Sedation is induced by administrating a drug or combination of drugs (e.g. benzodiazepines [*midazolam*], propofol ± short-acting opioids [*pethedine, fentanyl*]). During sedation the patient:

- has a reduced level of consciousness
- is free from anxiety
- is able to protect the airway
- is able to respond to verbal commands
- must be monitored (vital signs, pulse oximeter, ECG, level of consciousness)
- may be given an antagonist (*naloxone, flumazenil*) if oversedated (e.g. signs of respiratory depression).

After sedation the patient must be monitored until fully alert and must not drive or operate machinery for 24 hours.

Postoperative pain control

Pain is a complex symptom with physiological (*nociception* = neural detection of pain) and psychological (*anxiety, depression*) aspects. With modern analgesic techniques postoperative pain should not be considered an inevitable consequence of surgery. *Neuopathic* pain is caused by damage to the nerve pathways.

Analgesia in postoperative patients

- Opiates: powerful, highly effective if given by correct route (e.g. PCA) but antitussive, sedative only in overdose. Avoided where possible in ERAS.
- Epidural: excellent for upper abdominal/thoracic surgery, can cause hypotension by relative hypovolaemia.
- Patient controlled analgesia (PCA) is a system whereby the patient can self-administer parenteral opioids to achieve pain relief. The system requires careful patient selection and monitoring but is a very effective method of pain relief. Also patient controlled epidural anaesthesia (PCEA).
- Regional nerve blocks may augment systemic analgesia (opiate sparing), e.g. transversus abdominis percutaneous (TAP) block, LA infiltration.
- All hospitals should have an *acute pain team* to improve postoperative analgesia.

Methods of analgesia:

- Pharmacological – drugs must achieve **M**inimum **E**ffective **A**nalgesic **C**oncentration and may be administered:

oral	IV infusion
rectal	IV bolus
transdermal	IV patient controlled (PCA)
subcutaneous	epidural
intramuscular	nerve blocks
(inhalational	Entonox – 50:50 oxygen:nitrous oxide)

- Physical

  splinting, immobilization and traction

  physiotherapy

  transcutaneous electrical nerve stimulation (TENS).

- Psychological methods.

Type of analgesic	Effects and mode of action	Side-effects
Non-opioid		
Paracetemol	• Analgesic and antipyretic Inhibits prostaglandin production centrally	Hepatic necrosis in large doses
NSAID Salicylates Acetic acids Propionic acids	• Analgesic, anti-inflammatory, antipyretic, antiplatelet Inhibit COX enzyme in peripheral tissue thus reducing prostaglandin induced inflammation and nociceptor stimulation. COX 2 inhibitors do not impair beneficial COX 1 effects (e.g. cytoprotection)	Gastric irritation and ulceration, altered haemostasis, CNS toxicity, renal impairment, asthma
Opioid Morphine Diamorphine Pethidine Fentanyl Codeine Tramadol	• Act on opioid receptors μ, κ, δ Stimulation causes: μ-analgesia, RD, euphoria, dependence, N&V κ-spinal analgesia, sedation, miosiss δ-analgesia, RD euphoria, constipation	N&V, constipation, drowsiness, RD, tolerance, dependence
Adjuvant Antidepressants Anticonvulsants	• Analgesia (but not primary action of drug) Used mostly in chronic pain states	

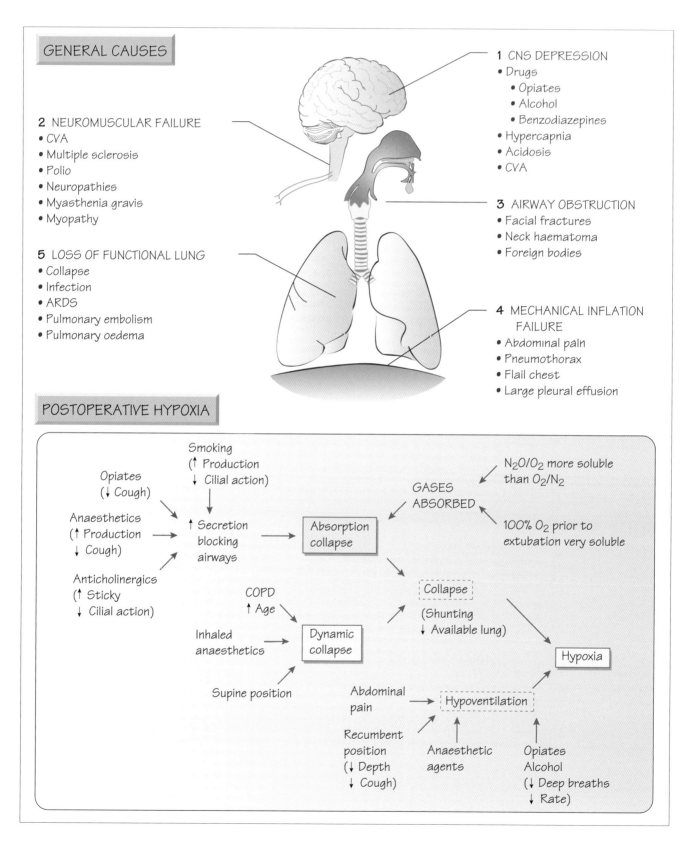

GENERAL CAUSES

2 NEUROMUSCULAR FAILURE
• CVA
• Multiple sclerosis
• Polio
• Neuropathies
• Myasthenia gravis
• Myopathy

5 LOSS OF FUNCTIONAL LUNG
• Collapse
• Infection
• ARDS
• Pulmonary embolism
• Pulmonary oedema

1 CNS DEPRESSION
• Drugs
  • Opiates
  • Alcohol
  • Benzodiazepines
• Hypercapnia
• Acidosis
• CVA

3 AIRWAY OBSTRUCTION
• Facial fractures
• Neck haematoma
• Foreign bodies

4 MECHANICAL INFLATION FAILURE
• Abdominal pain
• Pneumothorax
• Flail chest
• Large pleural effusion

POSTOPERATIVE HYPOXIA

Opiates
(↓ Cough)

Anaesthetics
(↑ Production
↓ Cough)

Anticholinergics
(↑ Sticky
↓ Cilial action)

Smoking
(↑ Production
↓ Cilial action)

↑ Secretion
blocking
airways

Absorption
collapse

GASES
ABSORBED

N₂O/O₂ more soluble
than O₂/N₂

100% O₂ prior to
extubation very soluble

COPD
↑ Age

Inhaled
anaesthetics

Dynamic
collapse

Supine position

Collapse

(Shunting
↓ Available lung)

Hypoxia

Abdominal
pain

Hypoventilation

Recumbent
position
(↓ Depth
↓ Cough)

Anaesthetic
agents

Opiates
Alcohol
(↓ Deep breaths
↓ Rate)

Definitions

Hypoxia is defined as a lack of O_2 (usually meaning lack of O_2 delivery to tissues or cells). *Hypoxaemia* is a lack of O_2 in arterial blood (low PaO_2). *Hypoventilation* is inadequate breathing leading to an increase of CO_2 (*hypercapnia*) and hypoxaemia. *Apnoea* means cessation of breathing in expiration.

Classification of hypoxia

- Hypoxic hypoxia: reduced O_2 entering the blood.
- Hypaemic/anaemic hypoxia: reduced capacity of blood to carry O_2.
- Stagnant hypoxia: poor oxygenation due to poor circulation.
- Histotoxic hypoxia: inability of cells to use O_2.

Common causes

Postoperative causes (usually hypoxic hypoxia)

- CNS depression, e.g. post-anaesthesia.
- Airway obstruction, e.g. aspiration of blood or vomit, laryngeal oedema.
- Poor ventilation, e.g. abdominal pain, mechanical disruption to ventilation.
- Loss of functioning lung, e.g. V/Q mismatch (pulmonary embolism, pneumothorax, collapse/consolidation).

General causes

- Central respiratory drive depression, e.g. opiates, benzodiazepines, CVA, head injury, encephalitis.
- Airway obstruction, e.g. facial fractures, aspiration of blood or vomit, thyroid disease or head and neck malignancy.
- Neuromuscular disorders (MS, myasthenia gravis).
- Sleep apnoea (obstructive, central or mixed).
- Chest wall deformities.
- COPD.
- Shock.
- Carboxyhaemoglobinaemia, methaemoglobinaemia.

Key points

- 80% of patients following upper abdominal surgery are hypoxic during the first 48 hours postoperatively. Have a high index of suspicion and treat prophylactically.
- Adequate analgesia is more important than the sedative effects of opiates – ensure good analgesia in all postoperative patients.
- Ensure the dynamics of respiration are adequate – upright position, abdominal support, humidified O_2.
- Acutely confused (elderly) patients on a surgical ward are hypoxic until proven otherwise.
- Pulse oximetry saturations <85% equate to an arterial PO_2 <8 kPa and are unreliable in patients with poor peripheral perfusion.

Clinical features

In the unconscious patient

- Central cyanosis.
- Abnormal respirations.
- Hypotension.

In the conscious patient

- Central cyanosis.
- Anxiety, restlessness and confusion.
- Tachypnoea.
- Tachycardia, dysrhythmias (AF) and hypotension.

Key investigations

- Pulse oximetry saturations: monitors the percentage of haemoglobin that is saturated with O_2 – gives a guide to arterial oxygenation. Very useful for patient monitoring.
- Arterial blood gases (PCO_2 PO_2 pH base excess): respiratory acidosis, metabolic acidosis later.
- Chest X-ray: ?collapse/pneumothorax/consolidation.
- ECG: AF.

Essential management

Airway control.
- Triple airway manoeuvre (mouth opening, head extension and jaw thrust), suction secretions, clear oropharynx.
- Consider endotracheal intubation in CNS depression/exhausted patients (rising PCO_2), neuromuscular failure.
- Consider surgical airway (cricothyroidotomy/minitracheostomy) in facial trauma, upper airway obstruction.

Breathing
- Position patient – upright.
- Adequate analgesia.
- Supplemental O_2 – mask/bag/ventilation.
- Support respiratory physiology – physiotherapy, humidified gases, encouraging coughing, bronchodilators.

Circulatory support.
- Maintain cardiac output.
- Ensure adequate fluid resuscitation.

Determine and treat the cause.

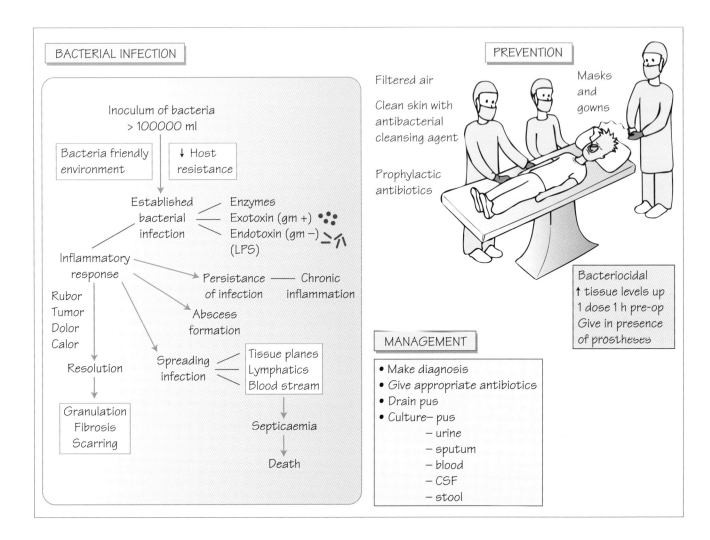

Definitions

Infection is the process whereby organisms (e.g. bacteria, viruses, fungi) capable of causing disease gain access and cause injury or damage to the body or its tissues. *Pus* is a yellow–green, foul-smelling, viscous fluid containing dead leucocytes, bacteria, tissue and protein. An *abscess* is a localized collection of pus, usually surrounded by an intense inflammatory reaction. Cellulitis is a spreading infection of subcutaneous tissue. *Necrotizing fasciitis* is progressive, infection located in the deep fascia, which spreads rapidly with secondary necrosis of the subcutaneous tissues.

Cleansing is the removal of gross surface contamination of an item, tissue or environment (e.g. simple hand washing). *Disinfection* is the reduction of infectious particles from an item or environment (e.g. surgical scrubbing). *Sterilization* is the removal/destruction of all infectious particles (spore and vegetative) from an item or environment (e.g. instrument autoclaving).

Key points

- An inoculum of >100000 bacteria/ml is required to establish an infection.
- Many features of gram-negative infection (fever, elevated WBC, hypotension and intravascular coagulation) are mediated by endotoxin.
- Narrow spectrum antibiotics are preferred where possible as they are less likely to induce resistance or *Clostridium difficile* infection.
- Abscesses should be drained either radiologically or surgically.

Pathophysiology of bacterial infection

Establishing a bacterial infection requires:
• An inoculum of bacteria.
• A bacteria-friendly environment (water, electrolytes, carbohydrate, protein digests, blood, warmth, oxygen rich (except anaerobic/microaerophilic organisms)).
• Diminished host resistance to infection (impaired physical barriers, reduced biochemical/humoral response, reduced cellular response).

Bacterial secretions

Bacteria cause some of their ill effects by releasing compounds:
• Enzymes (e.g. haemolysin, streptokinase, hyaluronidase).
• Exotoxin (released from intact bacteria, mostly gram-positive, e.g. tetanus, diphtheria).
• Endotoxin (LPS released from cell wall on death of bacterium).

Natural history of infection

• Inflammatory response is established (rubor/redness, tumor/swelling, dolor/pain, calor/heat).
• Resolution: inflammatory reaction settles and infection disappears.
• Spreading infection:
  direct to adjacent tissues
  along tissue planes
  via lymphatic system (lymphangitis)
  via blood stream (bacteraemia).
• Abscess formation: localized collection of pus.
• Organization: granulation tissue, fibrosis, scarring.
• Chronic infection: persistence of organism in the tissues elicits a chronic inflammatory response.

Koch's postulates for establishing a micro-organism as the cause of a disease.

The causative organism:
• is present in all patients with the disease
• must be isolated from lesions in pure culture
• must reproduce the disease in susceptible animals
• must be re-isolated from lesions in the experimentally infected animals.

Management of surgical infection
Preventive measures
• Short operations.
• Skin disinfection with antibacterial chemicals and detergents (patients', surgeons' and nurses' skin).
• Filtering of air in operating theatre.
• Occlusive surgical masks and gowns.
• Prophylactic antibiotics:
  should be bacteriocidal
  should have high tissue levels at time of contamination
  one pre-operative dose given 1 hour prior to surgery should suffice unless operation is heavily contaminated or dirty or the patient is immunocompromised
  specific antibiotics should be given to patients with implanted prosthetic materials, e.g. heart valves, vascular grafts, joint prostheses.

Management of established infection

Diagnosis: made by culture of appropriate specimens (pus, urine, sputum, blood, CSF, stool). Obtain appropriate specimens before giving antibiotics.

Antibiotics:
• Prescribe on basis of culture results and 'most likely organism' for initial empirical treatment while waiting for results.
• Certain antibiotics are reserved for serious infections – use the hospital policy wherever possible.
• Therapeutic monitoring of drug levels may be required, e.g. aminoglycosides.
• Synergistic combinations may be required in some infections, e.g. aminoglycoside, cephalosporin and metronidazole for faecal peritonitis.
• In serious, atypical or unresponsive infections seek advice from clinical microbiologist.
• Barrier nursing and isolation of patients with MRSA or VRE.

Drainage: surgical or radiological – is the most important treatment modality for an abscess or collections of infected fluid.

Wound classification	Definition	Example	Incidence of wound infection (%)
Clean	No contamination from GI, GU or RT	Thyroidectomy, elective hernia repair	1–5
Clean contaminated	Minimal contamination from GI, GU or RT	Cholecystectomy, TURP, pneumonectomy	7–10
Contaminated	Significantcontamination from GI, GU or RT	Elective colon surgery, inflamed appendicitis	15–20
Dirty	Infection present	Bowel perforation, perforated appendicitis, infected amputation	30–40

Surgical infection – specific

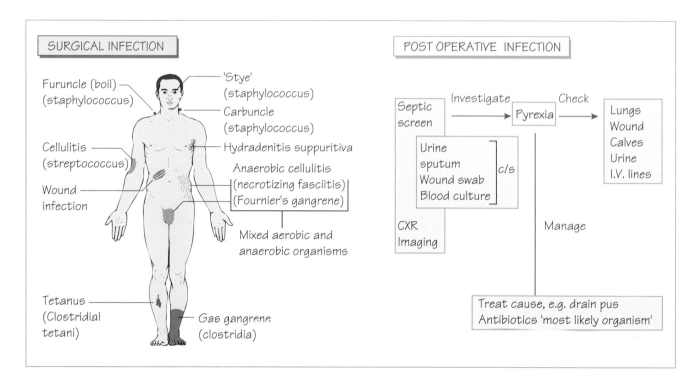

Specific surgical infections
Cellulitis
• Acute pyogenic cellulitis (*Streptococcus pyogenes*). Erysipelas (face) is most virulent form.
• Anaerobic cellulitis. Combination of aerobic (e.g. *β-hemolytic streptococci*) and anaerobic organisms (e.g *Bacteroides*). Two forms clinically:
   progressive bacterial syergistic gangrene (including Fournier's gangrene)
   necrotizing fasciitis.
   Rx: involves resuscitation, antibiotics (e.g. penicillin, metronidazole, gentamycin) and wide surgical debridement.
• Staphylococcal infections (*Staphlococcus aureus, Staphlococcus epidermis*).
   furuncle (a boil) – skin abscess involving hair follicle
   stye – infection of eyelash follicle
   carabuncle – subcutaneous necrosis with network of small abscesses
   sycosis barbae – infection of shaving area caused by infected razor.
• Hydradenitis suppuritiva – infection of apocrine glands in skin (axilla, groin).

Tetanus
• Clostridial infection caused by *C. tetani*.
• Penetrating dirty wounds.
• Most symptoms caused by exotoxin which is absorbed by motor nerve endings and migrates to anterior horn cells:
   spastic contractions and trismus (lockjaw)
   spasm of facial muscles (risus sardonicus)
   rigidity and extensor convulsions (opisthotonos).

Standard tetanus prophylaxis in the UK	Tetanus toxoid is given during 1st year of life as part of triple vaccine. Booster at 5 years and end of schooling
• Presentation with potentially contaminated wound + previous full immunization	Booster dose of tetanus toxoid given
• Presentation with potentially contaminated wound – previous immunization	Passive immunization with human antitetanus immunoglobin Full course of active immunization commenced

Gas gangrene
• Clostridial infection caused by *C. perfringes* (65%), *C. novyi* (30%), *C. septicum* (15%).
• Contamination of necrotic wounds with soil containing *Clostridia*.
• Spreading gangrene of muscles with crepitus from gas formation, toxaemia and shock.
• Rx: resuscitation, complete debridement and excision of ALL infected tissue (may require several operations).

Post-operative infections
Pyrexia is a common sign of infection. A mildly raised temperature is normal in the early post-operative period indicating response to major surgery.

Wound infections
• Incidence depends on wound classification (see above).
• Mild may settle with antibiotics but most need wound to be opened and drained.

Essential management of post-operative pyrexia

Note:
- Time of onset (1st 24 h usually atelectasis)
- Degree and type:
(Low persistent = low grade infectivity or inflammatory process, Intermittent = abscess ± rigors or haemodynamic change (bacteraemia/septicaemia)

Do:
- Septic screen
  – urine specimen
  – sputum sample
  – swabs of wounds or cannulae
  – blood cultures
- Chest X-ray (± other imaging as indicated, e.g. abdominal US or CT scan if peritonitis present)

Check:
- Lungs (atelectasis/pneumonia)
- Wound (infection)
- Calves (DVT)
- Urine (infection)
- IV or central lines

Give:
Antibiotics on basis of 'most likely organism'. (Refine treatment when septic screen results available)

Treat:
Cause as appropriate (e.g. remove infected cannula, drain abscess surgically or radiologically, give chest physiotherapy respiratory support, deal with anastomotic dehiscence, etc.)

Intra-abdominal infections
- Generalized peritonitis – pain, rigidity, absence of bowel sounds.
- Depends on cause – typically: *E coli*, *Klebsiella*, *Proteus*, *Strep. faecalis*, *Bacteroides*.
- Rx – resuscitation, broad-spectrum antibiotics, laparotomy and deal with cause if appropriate.

Intra-abdominal abscess
- Intermittent pyrexia, localized tenderness ± evidence of bacteraemia/septicaemia.
- Diagnosis by US or CT scanning.
- Rx – resuscitation, broad-spectrum antibiotics, drainage: either radiologically guided or open surgical.

Respiratory infections
- Predisposing factors:
  pre-existing pulmonary disease
  smoking
  starvation and fluid restriction
  anaesthesia
  post-operative pain.
- Prevention:
  pre-operative physiotherapy
  incentive spirometry
  stop smoking.
- Treatment:
  physiotherapy and appropriate antibiotics
  good post-operative analgesia
  keep well hydrated.

Urinary tract infections
- Often related to urinary catheter.
- Only catheterize when necessary.
- Use sterile technique and closed drainage.
- Treat with antibiotic on basis of urine culture.

Intravenous central line infection
- Prevention:
  use sterile technique when inserting line
  don't use line for giving IV drugs or taking blood samples especially if used for parenteral nutrition
  use single bag parenteral nutrition given over 24 hours
  never add anything to the parenteral nutrition bag.
- Diagnosis:
  suspect it with any fever in a patient with a central line.
- Treatment:
  remove the line if possible, send tip of catheter for culture, antibiotics (via the line if kept).

Pseudomembranous enterocolitis
- Caused by *Clostridium difficile*.
- Seen in patients who have been on antibiotics (esp. cephalosporins).
- Presents with diarrhoea, abdominal discomfort, leukocytosis.
- Dx: clinically – C. diff +ve with above clinical picture, pseudomembranous membrane in the colon at endoscopy.
- Rx: resuscitate, stop current antibiotics, oral vancomycin or metronidazole, rarely life-saving colectomy.

Multidrug-resistant organisms (MDRO)
- Microorganisms resistant to to one or more classes of antimicrobial drugs (e.g. Methicillin Resistant Staphylococcus aureus (MRSA), Vancomycin Resistant Enterococcus (VRE), extended spectrum beta-lactamase (ESBL) producing organisms esp. some gram-negative bacilli (GNB)).
- May arise in health facilities or *de novo* as community acquired (CA-MRSA).
- Cause same infections as other micro-organism but potentially more serious because of antimicrobial resistance
- Prevention and control:
  infection prevention
    improved hand hygiene
    contact precautions (isolate patient, use gloves/masks.
  accurate, prompt diagnosis and treatment – active MDRO surveillance cultures.
  judicious use of antimicrobials – MDROs are usually susceptible to certain antibiotics which should be reserved
  prevention of transmission
    enhanced environmental cleaning
    identify patients with MDROs
    decolonization of carriers (esp. MRSA).

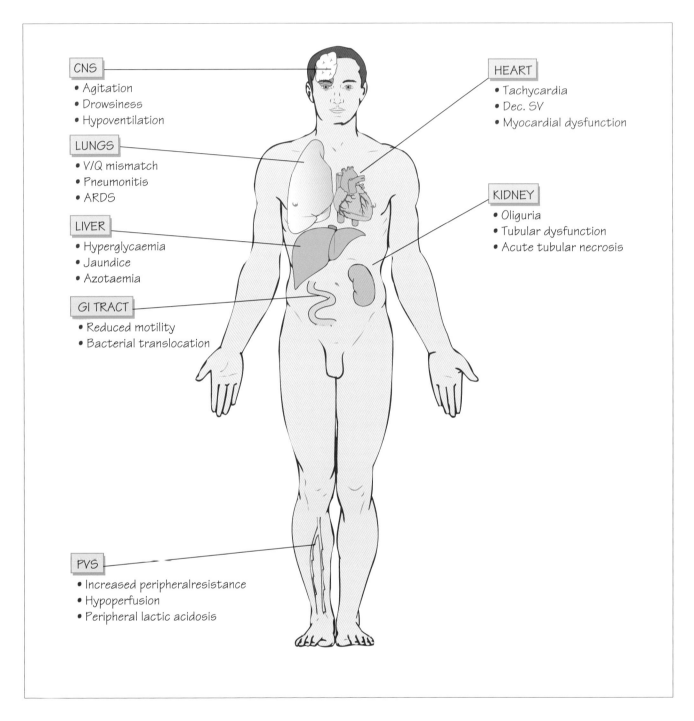

CNS
• Agitation
• Drowsiness
• Hypoventilation

LUNGS
• V/Q mismatch
• Pneumonitis
• ARDS

LIVER
• Hyperglycaemia
• Jaundice
• Azotaemia

GI TRACT
• Reduced motility
• Bacterial translocation

HEART
• Tachycardia
• Dec. SV
• Myocardial dysfunction

KIDNEY
• Oliguria
• Tubular dysfunction
• Acute tubular necrosis

PVS
• Increased peripheralresistance
• Hypoperfusion
• Peripheral lactic acidosis

Definitions

Sepsis is defined as the systemic response to the presence of various pathogenic organisms (bacteria – *bacteraemia*, viruses – *viraemia*, fungi – *fungaemia*) or their toxins (endotoxin – *lipopolysaccharide* or exotoxin – *tetanus/diphtheria toxin*) in the blood or tissues. Sepsis is a spectrum ranging from mild cellulitis to septic shock, with or without organ dysfunction.

Bacteraemia denotes the presence of bacteria in the blood stream. *Septicaemia* denotes the presence of large numbers of actively *dividing* bacteria in the blood stream, resulting in a systemic inflammatory response (SIRS, see Chapter 32) leading to organ dysfunction. *Pyaemia* is septicaemia caused by pus-forming bacteria (usually staphylococci) in the blood stream.

Severe sepsis denotes acute multiple organ dysfunction (MODS, see Chapter 32) secondary to infection.

Septic shock is severe sepsis plus hypotension not reversed with fluid resuscitation (Shock, see Chapter 33).

Epidemiology

The incidence of sepsis is 3/1000 worldwide and carries an overall mortality of 25%.

Risk factors

- Presence of an abscess or other source of infection (UTI, cholangitis, cellulitis, perforated viscus).
- Age: elderly and young most at risk.
- Immuno-compromised at risk:
  corticosteroids
  diabetes mellitus
  cancer chemotherapy
  burns.
- Surgery or instrumentation can precipitate sepsis:
  urinary catheterization
  cannulization of biliary tree
  prostatic biopsy.

Pathophysiology

The following may result from sepsis:
- Abnormal coagulation.
- Abnormal capillary permeability.
- Cell apoptosis.
- Endothelial cell injury.
- Elevated levels of TNF-α.
- Increased neutrophil activity.
- Poor glycaemic control.
- Reduced levels of steroid hormone.

Management		Supportive therapy	
Goal-directed early (first 6 hours) resuscitation	CVP 8–12 mmHg MAP ≥65 mmHg Urine output ≥0.5 mL/kg^{-1}/h^{-1} Mixed venous O_2 Sat ≥65%	Mechanical ventilation of ALI/ARDS	Tidal vol. 6 ml/kg Use PEEP Elevate head of bed 30°
Diagnosis	Cultures before antibiotics Imaging to identify source of infection	Sedation, analgesia and neuromuscular blockade	Achieve sedation for mechanical ventilation Do not use neuromuscular blockade
Antibiotic therapy	Early (within 1 hour) IV antibiotics Empirical Rx against all likely pathogens Review regime daily	Glucose control	Give IV insulin to achieve blood glucose of 8.3 mmol/L
Source control	Seek specific anatomical source of infection amenable to control Treat source with least physiological insult, e.g. percutaneous vs. surgical drainage of an abscess	Renal replacement	Use continuous renal replacement therapy
Fluid therapy	Give either crystalloids or colloids to achieve CVP ≥8 mmHg Give fluid challenges, e.g. 1000 ml crystalloid over 30 min	Bicarbonate therapy	Do not use
Vasopressors	Noradrenaline or dopamine to maintain MAP of ≥65 mmHg Patients on vasopressors should have BP measured by an arterial line	DVT prophylaxis	Use heparin (low molecular weight in preference to unfractionated) ± mechanical prophylaxis (compression stockings or devices)
Inotropes	Dobutamine infusion in the presence of myocardial dysfunction		
Steroids	IV hydrocortisone in adults only when BP not responsive to adequate fluid resuscitation and vasopressors		
Blood products	Maintain target Hb of 7.0–9.0 g/dl Do not use erythropoietin Only give FFP for coagulopathy in the presence of bleeding or prior to an invasive procedure Give platelets when ≤5000/mm^3 ≥50 000/mm^3 required for surgery	Consideration for limitation of support	Realistic outcomes should be discussed with patient and family Withdrawal of therapy may be in patient's best interest

Prognosis

Prognosis is related to the degree of sepsis but mortality is approximately 40% for established septic shock (see: www.survivingsepsis.org).

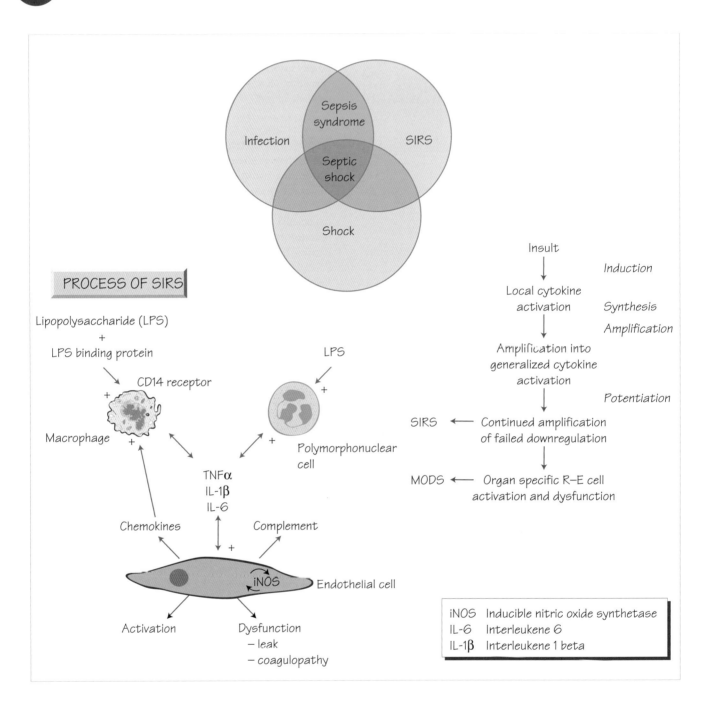

PROCESS OF SIRS

Lipopolysaccharide (LPS)
+
LPS binding protein

CD14 receptor

Macrophage

LPS

Polymorphonuclear cell

TNFα
IL-1β
IL-6

Chemokines

Complement

iNOS

Endothelial cell

Activation

Dysfunction
– leak
– coagulopathy

Insult

Induction

Local cytokine activation

Synthesis

Amplification

Amplification into generalized cytokine activation

Potentiation

SIRS ← Continued amplification of failed downregulation

MODS ← Organ specific R–E cell activation and dysfunction

iNOS	Inducible nitric oxide synthetase
IL-6	Interleukene 6
IL-1β	Interleukene 1 beta

Infection | Sepsis syndrome | SIRS

Septic shock

Shock

Definitions

Systemic inflammatory response syndrome (*SIRS*) is a systemic inflammatory response characterized by the presence of two or more of the following:

- Hyperthermia 38°C or hypothermia 36°C.
- Tachycardia > 90 beats/minute.
- Tachypnoea 20 beats/minute or PaCO$_2$ 4.3 kPa.
- Neutrophilia $\geq 12 \times 10^{-9}/L^{-1}$ or neutropenia $\leq 4 \times 10^{-9}/L^{-1}$.
  Severe SIRS is as above plus one of the following:
- Organ dysfunction (e.g. jaundice, hypoglycaemia, renal failure).
- Hypoperfusion (prolonged capillary refill time).
- Hypotension.

Sepsis syndrome is a state of SIRS with proven infection (SIRS + infection = sepsis). *Septic shock* is *sepsis* with systemic shock. *Multiple organ dysfunction syndrome* (*MODS*) is a state of progressive and potentially reversible physiological dysfunction such that organ function cannot maintain homeostasis. It usually involves two or more organ systems. The common terminal pathways for organ damage and dysfunction are vasodilatation, capillary leak, intravascular coagulation and endothelial cell activation. *CARS* is a *counter inflammatory response syndrome* that antagonizes SIRS.

Key points

- SIRS is more common in surgical patients than is diagnosed.
- Early treatment of SIRS may reduce the risk of MODS developing.
- The role of treatment is to eliminate any causative factor and support the cardiovascular, respiratory and renal physiology until the patient can recover.
- Overall mortality is 7% for a diagnosis of SIRS, 14% for sepsis syndrome and 40% for established septic shock.

Common surgical causes

- Perforated viscus with peritonitis.
- Fulminant colitis.
- Multiple trauma.
- Acute pancreatitis.
- Burns.
- Massive blood transfusion.
- Aspiration pneumonia, PE.
- Ischaemia reperfusion injury.
- Ruptured AAA.

Pathophysiology

Stage I: Insult (trauma, endotoxin or exotoxin) causes local cytokine (IL-1 and TNF-α) production.

Stage II: Cytokines released into circulation block nuclear factor-κB (NF-κB) inhibitor. NF-κB (via mRNA) induces the production of proinflammatory cytokines (IL-6, IL-8, IF-γ).

Stage III: Proinflammatory cytokines activate coagulation cascade (causing microvascular thrombosis), complement cascade (causing vasodilation and increased vascular permeability), release nitric oxide, platelet activating factor, prostaglandins and leucotrienes (cause endothelial damage). Unchecked the result is MODS.

CARS: The counter-inflammatory response syndrome counters the effects of SIRS through the action of IL-4 and IL-10, as well as antagonists to IL-1 and TNF-α.

The outcome depends on the balance between SIRS and CARS.

Treatment

- Treat the underlying cause, e.g. drain abscess, treat pneumonia, repair leaking AAA.
- Support patient in ICU with ventilation, circulatory support, control of hyperglycaemia and dialysis as indicated.
- Try to feed patients enterally whenever possible.
- No proven benefit for anticytokine therapy.

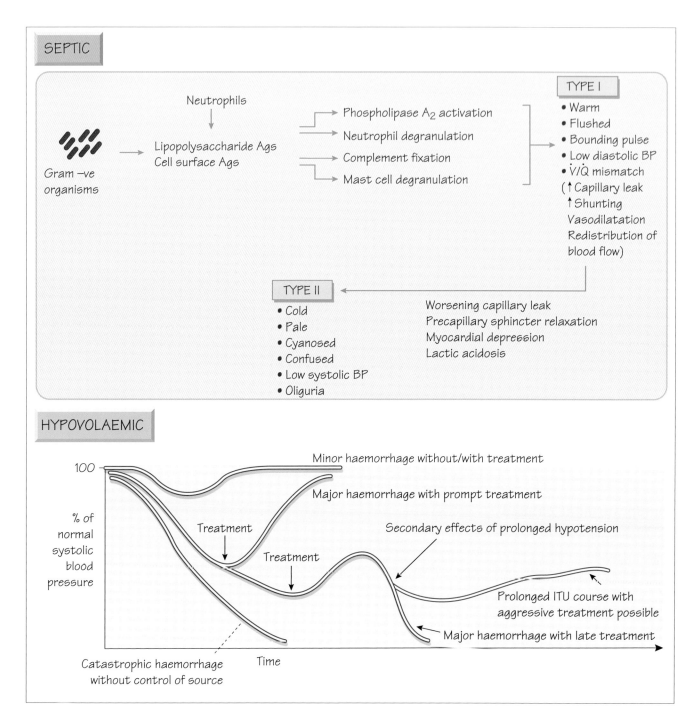

SEPTIC

Neutrophils

Gram −ve organisms → Lipopolysaccharide Ags
Cell surface Ags

- Phospholipase A$_2$ activation
- Neutrophil degranulation
- Complement fixation
- Mast cell degranulation

TYPE I
- Warm
- Flushed
- Bounding pulse
- Low diastolic BP
- V̇/Q̇ mismatch
  (↑ Capillary leak
   ↑ Shunting
   Vasodilatation
   Redistribution of
   blood flow)

Worsening capillary leak
Precapillary sphincter relaxation
Myocardial depression
Lactic acidosis

TYPE II
- Cold
- Pale
- Cyanosed
- Confused
- Low systolic BP
- Oliguria

HYPOVOLAEMIC

% of normal systolic blood pressure

100

Minor haemorrhage without/with treatment

Major haemorrhage with prompt treatment

Treatment

Treatment

Secondary effects of prolonged hypotension

Prolonged ITU course with aggressive treatment possible

Major haemorrhage with late treatment

Catastrophic haemorrhage without control of source

Time

Definition

Shock is defined as a state of acute inadequate or inappropriate tissue perfusion resulting in generalized cellular hypoxia and dysfunction.

Cellular shock is sometimes used to refer to the condition where adequate tissue distribution of nutrients is not accompanied by cellular utilization (can be caused by toxins, drugs and inflammatory mediators).

Key points

- Identify the cause early and begin treatment quickly.
- Shock in surgical patients is often overlooked – unwell, confused, restless patients may well be shocked.
- Unless a cardiogenic cause is obvious, treat shock with urgent fluid resuscitation.
- Worsening clinical status despite adequate volume replacement suggests the need for intensive care.

Common causes

Hypovolaemic

- Blood loss (trauma, ruptured abdominal aortic aneurysm, upper GI bleed, etc.).
- Plasma loss (burns, pancreatitis).
- Extracellular fluid losses (vomiting, diarrhoea, intestinal fistula).

Cardiogenic

- Myocardial infarction.
- Dysrhythmias (AF, ventricular tachycardia, atrial flutter).
- Pulmonary embolus.
- Cardiac tamponade.
- Valvular heart disease.

Septic

Gram-negative or, less often, gram-positive infections. Fungal – usually *Candida albicans*. Septic shock often caused by underlying GU or biliary problem.

Anaphylactic/distributive

Release of vasoactive substances when a sensitized individual is exposed to the appropriate antigen.

Clinical features

Hypovolaemic and cardiogenic

- Pallor, coldness, sweating, anxiety and restlessness.
- Tachycardia, tachypnoea, cyanosis, weak pulse, low BP, and oliguria.

Septic

- Initially warm, flushed skin, pyrexia and bounding pulse.
- Later confusion, low BP and low output picture.

Anaphylactic

- Dyspnoea, palpitation, itching, angioedema, stridor, palpitations, hypotension.

Investigations and assessment

Need to assess, resuscitate and treat the patient simultaneously (see Chapter 41):
- Monitor pulse, BP, temperature, respiratory rate and urinary output.
- Give O_2
- In anaphylaxis give injectable epinephrine (e.g. EpiPen®Auto-Injector).
- Establish good IV access and set up CVP line (± pulmonary artery catheterization with Swan–Ganz catheter – controversial). Intraosseous fluids can be used as a rescue technique when unable to establish IV access, especially in children. Give fluids based on monitoring.
- ECG, cardiac enzymes, echocardiography – transthoracic or transoesophageal – excellent in diagnosis and goal-directed management of shock.
- Hb, Hct, U+E, creatinine.
- Group and crossmatch blood: haemorrhage.
- Blood cultures: sepsis. Start broad spectrum antibiotic therapy after cultures taken.
- Arterial blood gases.
- Treat underlying cause of shock (e.g. trauma, myocardial infarction, choledocholithiasis, etc.).

Complications

- SIRS (see Chapter 32) may ensue if shock not corrected.
- Acute renal failure (acute tubular necrosis).
- Hepatic failure.
- Stress ulceration.
- Acalculous cholecystitis.

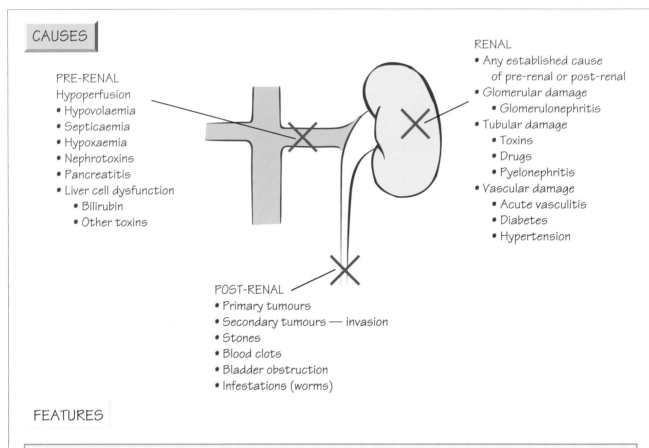

CAUSES

PRE-RENAL
Hypoperfusion
• Hypovolaemia
• Septicaemia
• Hypoxaemia
• Nephrotoxins
• Pancreatitis
• Liver cell dysfunction
  • Bilirubin
  • Other toxins

RENAL
• Any established cause
  of pre-renal or post-renal
• Glomerular damage
  • Glomerulonephritis
• Tubular damage
  • Toxins
  • Drugs
  • Pyelonephritis
• Vascular damage
  • Acute vasculitis
  • Diabetes
  • Hypertension

POST-RENAL
• Primary tumours
• Secondary tumours — invasion
• Stones
• Blood clots
• Bladder obstruction
• Infestations (worms)

FEATURES

	Normal	Prerenal	Renal	Postrenal
$U_{osmolality}$	Approx 400–500 mosm/kg	> 500	<400	Normal
U_{Na^+}	10–20 mmol/l	< 10	> 20	Normal
U_{urea}/P_{urea}	Approx 5/1	> 10/1	3/1 1/1	Normal
U_{osm}/P_{osm}	Approx 1.5/1	> 2/1	< 1.1/1	Normal
Findings	—	Concentrated urine ? Findings due to cause	Casts RBCs Protein	Normal urine ? Findings due to cause

Definitions

Acute kidney injury (AKI) is a sudden deterioration in renal filtration function. *Acute renal failure (ARF)* is AKI such that global renal function is no longer capable of excreting body waste products (e.g. urea, creatinine, potassium) that accumulate in the blood. It may be fatal unless treated. *Anuria* literally means no urine, but is considered to be present when <100 ml/day of urine is passed. *Oliguria* means that <0.5 ml/kg/hour (<400 ml/day) is passed. *Acute tubular necrosis (ATN)* is damage to the renal tubular cells caused by ischaemia, hypoxia or nephrotoxins which is usually reversible. *Acute cortical necrosis (ACN)* is advanced parenchymal destruction secondary to ischaemia, sepsis or toxins.

Key points

- Oliguria in a surgical patient is an emergency. The cause must be identified and treated promptly.
- Prompt correction of pre-renal causes may prevent the development of established renal failure.
- Ensure the oliguric patient is normovolaemic as far as possible before starting diuretics or other therapies.
- Don't use blind, large fluid challenges, especially in the elderly – if necessary use a CVP line or transfer to HDU.
- Established renal failure requires specialist support as electrolyte and fluid imbalances can be rapid in onset and difficult to manage.

Common causes

Pre-renal failure (volume depletion and hypotension, structurally intact nephrons)

- Shock from any cause causing reduced renal perfusion (hypovolaemia, haemorrhage, burns, pancreatitis, sepsis, anaphylaxis, heart failure).
- Arteriolar vasoconstriction leading to ARF can occur with hypercalcaemia, radio-contrast agents, NSAIDs, ACE inhibitors, angiotensin receptor blockers and the hepatorenal syndrome.

Intrinsic renal failure (structural and functional damage to kidney)

- Vascular: renal ischaemia (ATN).
- Glomerular: acute glomerulonephritis.
- Tubular (ATN):
  ischaemic
  cytotoxic (*aminoglycosides*, amphotericin B, radiocontrast agents, methotrexate, myoglobin).
- Interstitial:
  drugs (penicillins, NSAIDs, allopurinol)
  infection (severe pyelonephritis).
- Systemic: hypertension, diabetes mellitus, myeloma.

Post-renal failure (obstruction to the passage of urine)

- Urinary tract obstruction.
- Ureteric (fibrosis, stone disease).
- Bladder neck (common) (benign prostatic hypertrophy, cancer of the prostate, neurogenic bladder).
- Urethra (stricture, phimosis).

Clinical features

Oliguric phase

(May last hours/days/weeks.)
- Oliguria: passage of <0.5 ml/kg/hour urine.
- Uraemia: dyspnoea, confusion, drowsiness, coma.
- Nausea, vomiting, hiccoughs, diarrhoea.
- Anaemia, coagulopathy, GI haemorrhage.
- Fluid retention: hypervolaemia, hypertension.

- Hyperkalaemia: dysrhythmias.
- Metabolic acidosis.

Polyuric (recovery) phase

(May last days/weeks.)
- Polyuria: hypovolaemia, hypotension.
- Hyponatraemia.
- Hypokalaemia.

Investigations

- Urinalysis (see opposite page).
- U+E (especially K^+) and creatinine.
- Arterial blood gases: metabolic acidosis (normal PO_2, low PCO_2, low pH, high base deficit).
- ECG/chest X-ray/renal ultrasound/renal biopsy.

Prognosis

In hospital mortality 40–50%, ICU 70–80%.

Essential management

Prevention

- Keep at-risk patients (e.g. obstructive jaundice) well hydrated pre- and peri-operatively.
- Normal saline, sodium bicarbonate and *N*-acetyl cysteine have all been used to try to prevent radiocontrast nephropathy.
- Protect renal function in selected patients with drugs such as dopamine and mannitol.
- Monitor renal function regularly in patients on nephrotoxic drugs (e.g. aminoglycosides).

Identification

- Exclude urinary retention as a cause of anuria by catheterization.
- Correct hypovolaemia as far as possible. Use appropriate fluid boluses – if necessary guided by a CVP monitor on HDU.
- A trial of bolus high-dose loop diuretics may be appropriate in a normovolaemic patient.
- Dopamine infusions may be necessary but suggest the need for HDU or ICU care.

Treatment of established renal failure

- Maintain fluid and electrolyte balance.
- Water intake 400 mL/day + measured losses.
- Na^+ intake limited to replace loss only.
- K^+ intake nil (dextrose and insulin and/or ion-exchange resins are required to control hyperkalaemia).
- Diet: high calorie, low protein in a small volume of fluid.
- Acidosis: sodium bicarbonate.
- Treat any infection.
- Dialysis: peritoneal, haemofiltration, haemodialysis (usually indicated for hypervolaemia, hyperkalaemia or acidosis).

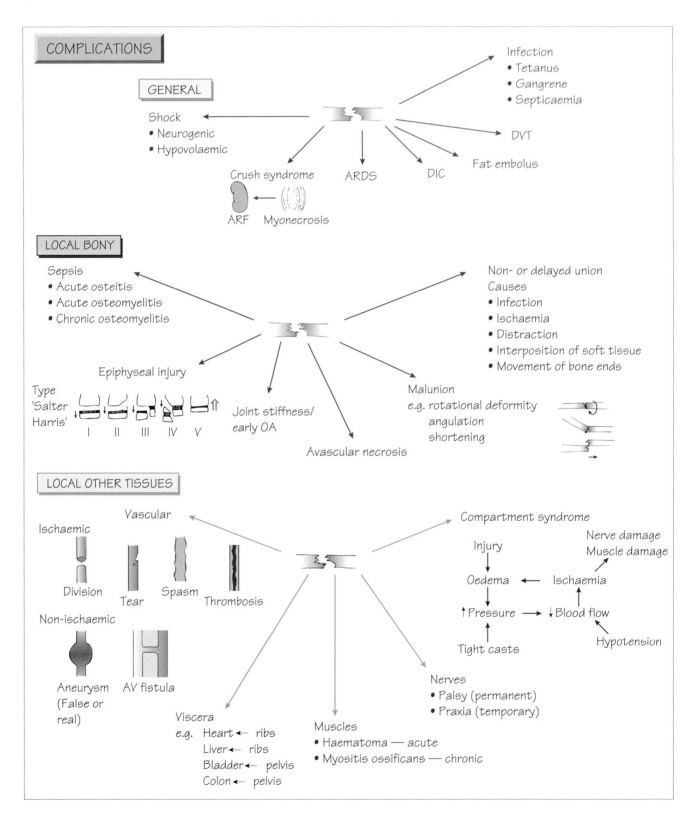

COMPLICATIONS

GENERAL

Infection
• Tetanus
• Gangrene
• Septicaemia

Shock
• Neurogenic
• Hypovolaemic

DVT

Crush syndrome   ARDS   DIC   Fat embolus

ARF   Myonecrosis

LOCAL BONY

Sepsis
• Acute osteitis
• Acute osteomyelitis
• Chronic osteomyelitis

Non- or delayed union
Causes
• Infection
• Ischaemia
• Distraction
• Interposition of soft tissue
• Movement of bone ends

Epiphyseal injury

Type
'Salter
Harris'
I   II   III   IV   V

Joint stiffness/
early OA

Malunion
e.g. rotational deformity
angulation
shortening

Avascular necrosis

LOCAL OTHER TISSUES

Vascular

Ischaemic

Division   Tear   Spasm   Thrombosis

Non-ischaemic

Aneurysm
(False or
real)   AV fistula

Compartment syndrome

Injury

Nerve damage
Muscle damage

Oedema ← Ischaemia

↑Pressure → ↓Blood flow

Tight casts   Hypotension

Viscera
e.g.   Heart ← ribs
        Liver ← ribs
        Bladder ← pelvis
        Colon ← pelvis

Muscles
• Haematoma — acute
• Myositis ossificans — chronic

Nerves
• Palsy (permanent)
• Praxia (temporary)

Definitions

A *fracture* is a break in the continuity of a bone. Fractures may be *transverse*, *oblique* or *spiral* in shape. In a *greenstick* fracture, only one side of the bone is fractured, the other simply bends (usually immature bones where cartilage is incompletely ossified). A *comminuted* fracture is one in which there are more than two fragments of bone. In a *complicated* fracture, some other structure is also damaged (e.g. a nerve or blood vessel). In a *compound* fracture, there is a break in the overlying skin (or nearby viscera) with potential contamination of the bone / fragments. A *pathological* fracture is one through a bone weakened by disease, e.g. a metastasis, osteopenia/osteoporosis.

Key points

- Always consider multiple injury in patients presenting with fractures.
- Remember there may significant blood loss in long bone fractures.
- Compound fractures are a surgical emergency and require appropriate measures to prevent infection, including tetanus prevention.
- Always image the joints above and below a long bone fracture.

Common causes

Fractures occur when excessive force is applied to a normal bone or moderate force to a diseased bone, e.g. osteoporosis.

Clinical features

- Pain.
- Loss of function.
- Deformity, tenderness and swelling.
- Discoloration or bruising.
- (Crepitus – not to be elicited!)

Investigations

- Radiographs in two planes (look for lucencies and discontinuity in the cortex of the bone).
- Tomography, CT scan, MRI scan.
- Ultrasonography and radioisotope bone scanning. (Bone scan is particularly useful when radiographs/CT scanning are negative in clinically suspect fracture.)

Complications

Early

- Blood loss.
- Infection
  soft tissue - cellulitis, myositis, fascitis
  bone – osteitis, osteomyelitis
  systemic – tetanus.
- Fat embolism.
- DVT and PE.
- Renal failure – esp. if associated with extensive muscle injury or rhabdomyolysis from compartment syndrome.
- Compartment syndrome.

Late

- Non-union (no sign of healing after 3–6 months, depending on fracture site).
- Delayed union (incomplete healing of a fracture at the expected time of healing).
- Malunion (bone fragments join in an unsatisfactory position).
- Growth arrest.
- Arthritis.
- Myositis ossificans (calcification within muscle especially in supracondylar humeral fracture).
- Post-traumatic sympathetic (reflex) dystrophy (Sudeck's atrophy).

Essential management

General

- Look for shock/haemorrhage and check ABC (see Chapter 41).
- Look for injury in other areas at risk (head and spine, ribs and pneumothorax, femoral and pelvic injury).

The fracture
Immediate
- Relieve pain (opiates IV, nerve blocks, splints, traction).
- Establish good IV access and send blood for group and crossmatch.
- Open (compound) fractures require débridement, antibiotics and tetanus prophylaxis.

Definitive
- Reduction (closed or open).
- Immobilization (casting, functional bracing, internal fixation, external fixation, traction).
- Rehabilitation (aim to restore the patient to pre-injury level of function with physiotherapy and occupational therapy).

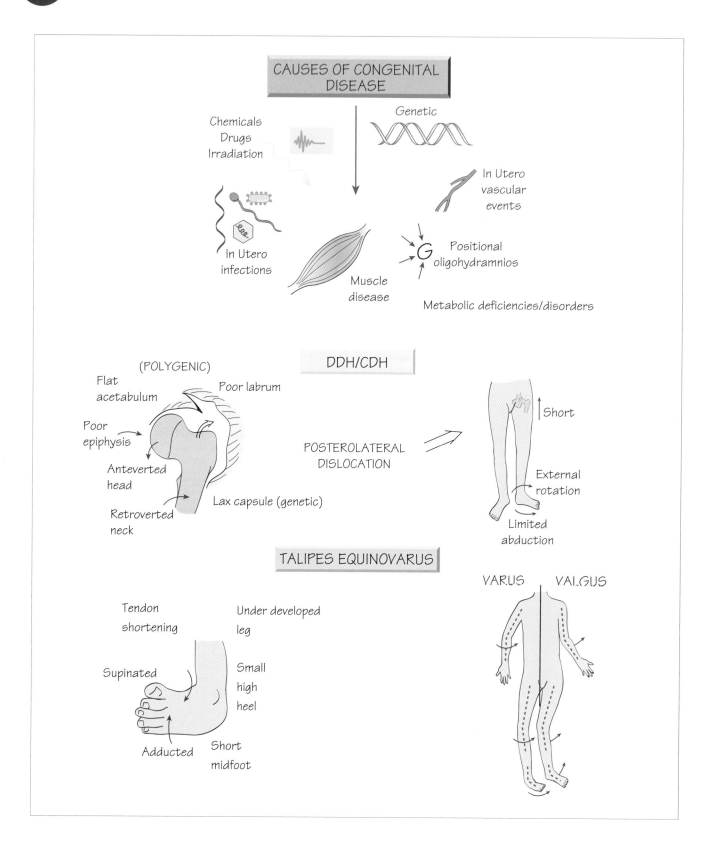

CAUSES OF CONGENITAL DISEASE

Chemicals
Drugs
Irradiation

Genetic

In Utero vascular events

In Utero infections

Muscle disease

Positional oligohydramnios

Metabolic deficiencies/disorders

DDH/CDH

(POLYGENIC)

Flat acetabulum

Poor labrum

Poor epiphysis

Anteverted head

Retroverted neck

Lax capsule (genetic)

POSTEROLATERAL DISLOCATION

Short

External rotation

Limited abduction

TALIPES EQUINOVARUS

Tendon shortening

Under developed leg

Supinated

Small high heel

Adducted

Short midfoot

VARUS   VALGUS

Definitions

Orthopaedics: Branch of surgery concerned with the skeletal system (*ortho-* [straight] + *paes* [child] = straightening the child. *Varus deformity*: the inward angulation of the distal segment of a bone or joint. *Valgum deformity*: the outward angulation of the distal segment of a bone or joint.

Orthotics: specialty concerned with the design, manufacture and application of *orthoses* which are devices that support or correct the function of a limb or the torso e.g. spinal brace. *Prosthesis*: an artificial device that replaces a missing part e.g. artificial limb.

Key points

- Multidisciplinary approach is essential in the management of childhood orthopaedics.
- Cerebral palsy is the leading cause of childhood disability affecting function and development and a major social, medical and educational problem.
- DDH (CDH) a very serious condition if not diagnosed and treated early.
- Slipped capital femoral epiphysis is uncommon but requires emergency surgery to stabilize hip joint.

Classification

General abnormalities

- Cerebral palsy: damage to the brain at birth leading to muscle weakness, spacticity, loss of voluntary control, deformity, seizures and intellectual impairment (40%). Rx:multidisciplinary approach: speech therapy, muscle training, splinting ± botulinum toxin, surgery to tendons, bone, nerves.
- Achondroplasia: dwarfing because of poor epiphyseal growth. Normal trunk and head.
- Osteochondroma: bony exostoses on shaft of long bone. No treatment required.
- Dyschondroplasia: cartilaginous cysts in bone (enchondroma) – thickening and shortening.
- Rare abnormalities:
  osteogenesis imperfecta: collagen deficiency causing fragile bones – fractures, blue sclera
  arthrogryposis multiplex congenita – multiple joint contractures producing severe deformity
  craniocleidal dysostosis – failure of development of membranous bone, clavicles and skull.

Specific abnormalities

Hip joint

- Developmental dysplasia of the hip (DDH) (congenital dislocation of the hip (CDH)): 1.5/1000 births. F:M = 8:1. Screening by Barlow test ('clunk' heard on abduction). U/S in infants <6 months, radiographs >6 months. Rx: Early: Maintain hips in abduction (double nappies or splint); Late: Surgery. May develop adult osteoarthritis.
- Legg–Calvé–Perthes disease: Osteochondritis of the femoral head caused by avascular necrosis. Boys 4–10 years. Pain and limping. Radiographs show collapse of femoral head. Rx: Minimize weight bearing and protect joint. Surgery to contain head of femur in acetabulum. May develop adult osteoarthritis.
- Slipped capital femoral epiphysis (SCFE): a serious condition of adolescence with displacement of the femoral neck off the femoral head through a weakened epiphyseal plate. Cause unknown. M:F = 2.5:1 Age 10–16 years. Obesity and metabolic endocrine disorders predispose. Hip or knee pain, intermittent limp. Limited range of movement. Rx: Immediate surgical internal fixation of the femoral head to prevent further slippage. Avascular necrosis of the head of the femur is a very serious complication needing total hip replacement eventually. May develop adult osteoarthritis.

Knee joint

- *Genu varus* (bow legs) and *genu valgum* (knock knees). Usually not serious.
- Osgood–Schlatter's disease: Bony outgrowth caused by traction on the tibial tubercle.

Foot disorders

- Congenital *talipes equino varus* (CTEV) (club foot) and *talipes calcaneo valgus* (CTCV – reverse of CTEV). Rx: by strapping or plaster of Paris. Surgery sometimes.
- *Metatarsus adductus (varus)* (hooked foot). 90% correct spontaneously.
- *Pes cavus* (high arched foot) always neurological cause, e.g. muscular dystrophy.
- Flat foot. Usually due to ligament laxity. No Rx required.

Neck

- Torticollis: Damage to sternocleidomastoid during delivery. Rx: Surgical release.

Spine

- Spina bifida and meningomyelocele: vertebral arch fails to close leaving the spinal cord exposed. Motor, sensory and viceral paralysis ± hydrocephalus (Arnold–Chiari malformation).
- Scoliosis: Idiopathic lateral curvature of the spine. Rx: casts/braces/ surgery.

Miscellaneous

- Osteomyelitis: see Chapter 37.
- Bone tumours in children: see Chapter 39.

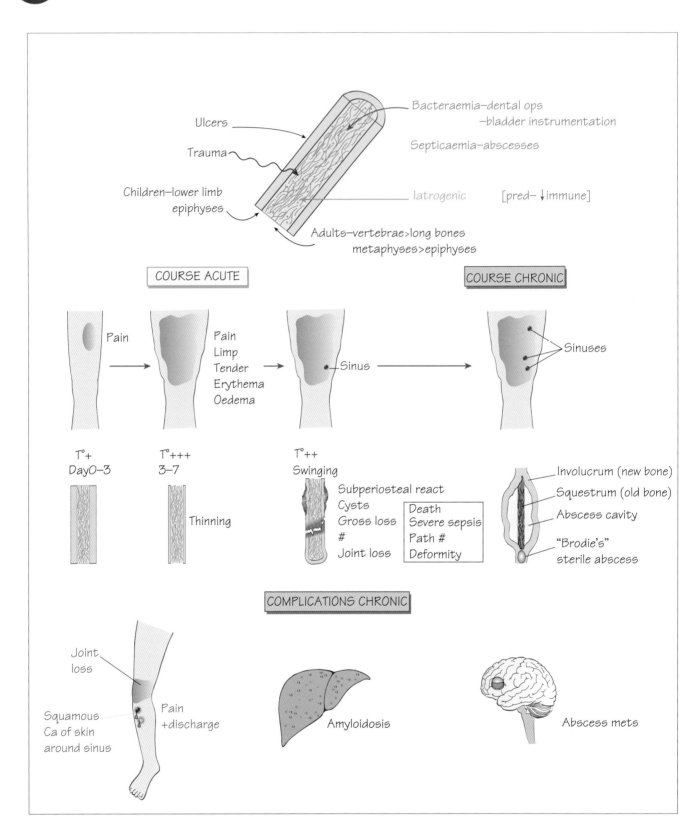

Definitions

Metabolic bone diseases: disorders of bone which may be attributed to cellular changes or to dietary deficiencies, genetic defects or lack of exposure to sunlight. They are characterised by bone loss or dysplasia. They include osteoporosis, rickets and osteomalacia, Paget's disease of bone and hyperparathyroidism.

Osteoblasts: bone cells responsible for bone formation. *Osteoclasts:* bone cells responsible for bone resorption.

Key points

- 98% of calcium is stored in bones with equal flux into and out of skeleton maintained by parathormone, vitamin D and calcitonin.
- 30% of women in developed countries will sustain an osteoporotic fracture during their lifetime.
- Acute osteomyelitis should be diagnosed early and treated aggressively with IV antibiotics.

Bone loss

Osteoporosis

Primary

- Systematic skeletal disorder common in postmenopausal women.
- Characterized by low bone mass, micro-architectural deterioration of bone tissue, and susceptibility to fracture.
- Oestrogen reduction causes reduced collagen in bone with decreased bone mineral density (BMD) leading to fracture – especially hips and vertebrae.
- Presents with progressive kyphosis, hip or wrist fracture.
- Diagnosis by bone densitometry (DXA scan).
- Rx: lifestyle changes – stop smoking, exercise, calcium and vitamin D supplements.
- Medications: bisphosphonates reduce risk of fracture; HRT, selective oestrogen receptor modulators (SERM) and anabolic agents (e.g. hPTH promotes new bone growth) are all used.
- Hip protectors.

Secondary

Cushing's disease, steroids, rheumatoid arthritis, malabsorption, chronic renal failure, immobilization, weightlessness (astronauts).

Osteopenia

(DXA scan diagnosis) BMD less than normal but not osteoporosis.

Rickets/osteomalacia

- Skeletal deformity due to impaired matrix mineralization.
- Reduced vitamin D (diet or sunlight) leads to disordered calcium/phosphate metabolism and defective mineralization of bone.
- Rickets: deformity and growth disturbance in children.
- Osteomalacia: bone pain and tenderness, fractures and proximal myopathy.
- Radiographs: widened irregular epiphyses in rickets, pseudofractures in osteomalacia.
- Rx: vitamin D and calcium supplements.

Osteolysis

Osteoclastic absorption of bone from malignant deposits or post joint replacement.

Hyperparathyroidism

Resorption of calcium leading to bone cysts (see Chapter 63).

Dysplasia

- Paget's disease of bone: localized disorder of bone remodelling resulting in disorganized woven and lamellar bone with increased blood supply. Older males. Local bone pain, commonly pelvis, lumbar spine and femur. Complications: 'sabre tibia', increasing head size, deafness, vertebral fracture, osteosarcoma, high output cardiac failure, hypercalcaemia. Radiology: expansion and deformity of long bones, widening of skull vault. Rx: bisphosphonates – suppress osteoclastic activity. With treatment disease is controlled, but risk of osteosarcoma remains.
- Marble bone disease (osteopetrosis): rare congenital disease characterized by hard dense bone liable to fracture, anaemia, neurological problems due to defective osteoclast function.
- Fibrous dysplasia: rare genetic disorder that causes bone to be replaced by fibrous tissue.

Infections

- Acute osteomyelitis: blood-borne infection of long bone metaphysis with *Staphylococcus aureus/Haemophilus influenzae*. Tibia/femur/humerus. Children/pain/fever/tenderness. Rx: IV antibiotics ± surgery to release pus and relieve pain.
- Chronic osteomyelitis: sequel to acute osteomyelitis. Chronic discharging sinus between skin and dead bone (*sequestrum*) surrounded by new bone (*involucrum*). *Brodie's abscess* is a chronic abscess in the metaphysis. Successful Rx depends on eradication of the dead bone.
- Septic arthritis: infection of joint by direct or haematogenous spread. Swollen, red, painful, hot, tender joint. Effusion. Rx: antibiotics/joint lavage.
- Tuberculous: haematogenous spread. Frequently affects hip and spine (Pott's disease) causing kyphosis. Rx: antituberculous drugs (rifampisin + isoniasid + pirasinamide + etambutol) for up to 18 months. Occasionally spinal surgery for instability.
- Poliomyelitis: viral infection of anterior horn cells. Muscle weakness and paralysis ± altered bone growth and deformity. Rx: orthoses (appliances) to support joints. Surgery: arthrodeses, tendon transfer.

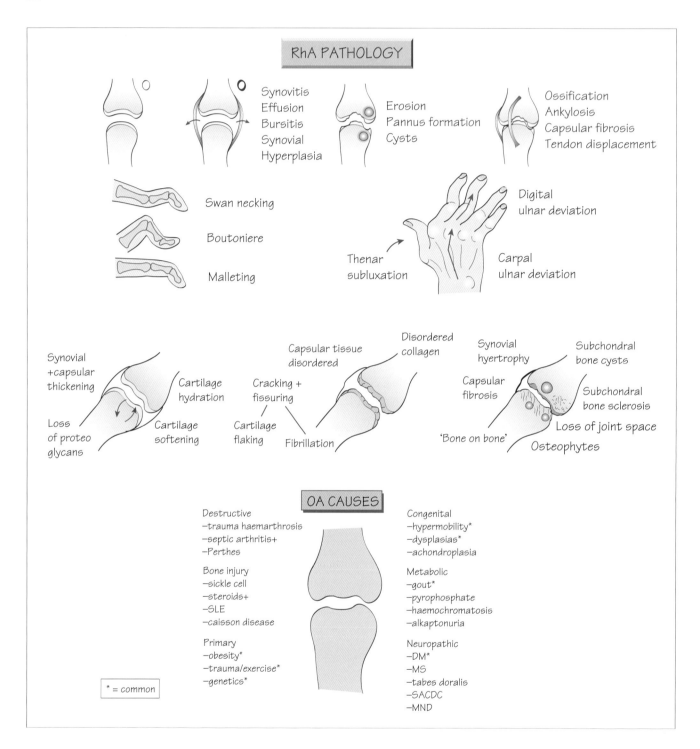

Definitions

Arthritis: (*arthro-* [joint] + *itis* [inflammation] = joint inflammation). Inflammation of a joint characterised by pain, swelling, and stiffness, resulting from degenerative changes, metabolic disturbances or infection.

Osteoarthritis (OA)

Definition

Degenerative condition with mechanical damage to articular cartilage.

Aetiology

'Wear and tear'. Excessive joint wear from joint instability, loose body in joint, obesity, previous fracture or other pathology.

Pathology

Usually lower limb joints. Breakdown of articular cartilage exposing underlying bone. Bone surface becomes dense (sclerotic) with cysts underneath and growth of new bone at the peripheries (osteophytes). Fibrosis in capsule restricts movement.

Clinical features

Pain and stiffness developing insidiously in middle-aged or elderly. If hip or knee affected, gait will be abnormal. Movement is restricted and eventually a fixed deformity may develop. Ankylosis of a joint may relieve the pain. Muscle wasting, crepitus and decreased range of movement are clinical signs.

Investigations

Blood investigations: all normal. Radiograph: joint space narrowing, bone sclerosis with cysts in subchondral bone and osteophyte formation at the joint margin.

Essential management

Depends on joint involved, symptoms and disability.

Non-surgical management
Non-weight bearing exercise (swimming/cycling), local heat, simple analgesics, weight loss, walking stick. Intra-articular steroids and arthroscopic washout may relieve pain (especially in the knee).

Surgical Rx
Arthrodesis = fusion of joint, e.g. 'triple arthrodesis' for osteoarthritis of ankle, *Arthroplasty* = making a new artificial joint, e.g. total hip or knee replacement. *Osteotomy* = cutting a bone to realign the stress across the joint, e.g. tibial wedge osteotomy to correct varus or valgus knee deformity.

Prognosis
Symptoms of osteoarthritis fluctuate but overall there is a steady deterioration over time. Knee and hip arthroplasty have >80% success rate.

Rheumatoid arthritis (RA)

Definition

A chronic systemic autoimmune disease of unknown cause that results in inflammation and deformity of the joints ± subcutaneous nodules, anaemia, kerato-conjunctivitis, pleural and cardiac disease and vasculitis.

Aetiology

Unknown but genetic, immunological, infectious, environmental and hormonal factors all implicated.

Pathology

A trigger induces an auto-immune reaction causing an inflammatory response resulting in synovial hypertrophy (pannus), cartilage and bone destruction, laxity of ligaments and joint deformity as well as extra-articular manifestations.

Clinical features

F>M. Age: 15–35 years. Insidious onset, fever, malaise, symmetrical polyarthritis mostly affecting small joints of hands and feet especially MCP, wrist, PIP. Any joint may be affected. Morning stiffness. Joint swelling, tenderness, warmth and decreased range of motion. Ulnar deviation of wrist, boutonniere and swan-neck deformity of fingers, subcutaneous nodules on extensor surface of ulna. Synovial thickening and knee effusion. Neck stiffness and occipital headache.

Investigations

Diagnosis is made on clinical, laboratory (markers of inflammation: ESR, CRP; haematological parameters: FBC (anaemia, thrombocytosis); immunological markers: rheumatoid factor (RF), antinuclear antibody (ANA), anti-citrullinated peptide antibody (anti-CCP) and anti RA33 antibody) and imaging (X-ray, MRI, U/S) features.

Essential management

An integrated approach should be adopted.

Non-pharmacological Rx
Exercise, diet, massage, stress reduction, physical therapy (active + passive exercise, application of heat/cold/ultrasound, hydrotherapy) occupational therapy, orthotics and splints.

Pharmacological Rx
Early treatment with disease-modifying antirheumatic drugs (DMARDs) retards the disease and induces remissions. (Xenobiotic DMARDs: methotrexate, hydroxychloroquine, sulfasalazine, minocycline, leflunomide. Biological DMARDs: etanercept, infliximab, and adalimumab are all TNF antagonists). Glucocorticoids and NSAIDs have been mostly displaced by DMARDs.

Surgical Rx
Aim is to achieve pain relief, correct deformity and improve function. Procedures include synovectomy, tenosynovectomy, tendon realignment, reconstructive surgery, arthroplasty and arthrodesis.

Prognosis

RA is progressive and cannot be cured. However in some patients the disease gradually becomes less aggressive.

Other types of arthritis
Gout

Deposition of uric acid crystals (from breakdown of purines) causes intense pain, swelling, tenderness, heat and discolouration of the affected joint, usually the MTP joint of the big toe. Middle aged/elderly. Patients usually have elevated serum uric acid but diagnosis is made by seeing uric acid crystals on microscopy of joint fluid. Gouty tophi and renal calculi may occur. Rx of acute attack: NSAIDs, colchicine, corticosteroids. Rx to prevent further attacks: colchicine, probenecid, allopurinol, febuxostat. In 'pseudogout' calcium pyrophosphate crystals are deposited instead of uric acid.

Psoriatic arthritis

An autoimmune disease that causes an aggressive inflammatory arthritis usually associated with skin psoriasis. Fingers and toes, wrists and ankles, spine. Rx: NSAIDs for arthropathy and topical, photo or systemic therapy for skin. Ultimately leads to joint damage and disability.

Ankylosing spondylitis

Arthritis involving the axial skeleton (spine, sacroiliac joints, hips and shoulders). Young adults, M:F = 3:1, back stiffness and pain. HLA-B27 positive in 90% of patients. Many have uveitis. Rx: exercise to maintain mobility, NSAIDs, corticosteroids, DMARDs, TNF antagonists.

Reactive arthritis or Reiter's syndrome

Aseptic inflammatory polyarthritis usually triggered by non-gonococcal urethritis (*Chlamydia trachomatis*) or infectious dysentery (*Salmonella* or *Shigella*). Leads to chronic disease in over 50% of cases. Classic triad of arthritis, conjunctivitis and urethritis. HLA-B27 positive in 65% of patients. Rx: initially NSAIDs and doxycycline for chlamydia. Persistent arthritis may need DMARDs.

Haemophillic arthritis

Repeated haemarthrosis leads to chronic synovitis and destruction of cartilage. Usually weight bearing joints involved. May eventually need athroplasty.

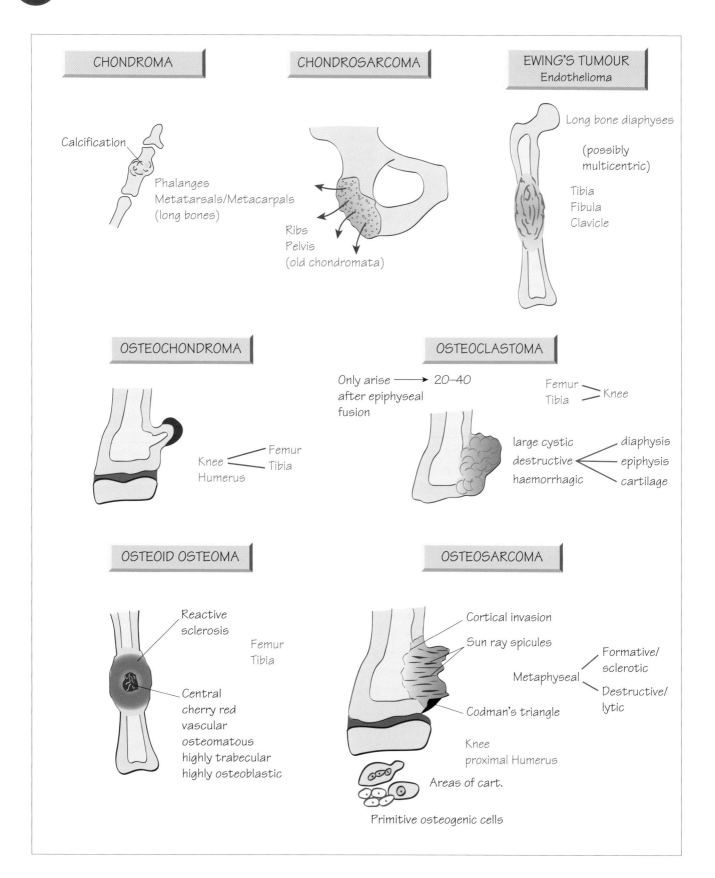

CHONDROMA

Calcification

Phalanges
Metatarsals/Metacarpals
(long bones)

CHONDROSARCOMA

Ribs
Pelvis
(old chondromata)

EWING'S TUMOUR
Endothelioma

Long bone diaphyses

(possibly
multicentric)

Tibia
Fibula
Clavicle

OSTEOCHONDROMA

Knee — Femur
Tibia
Humerus

OSTEOCLASTOMA

Only arise → 20–40
after epiphyseal
fusion

Femur
Tibia ⟩ Knee

large cystic
destructive — diaphysis
haemorrhagic — epiphysis
cartilage

OSTEOID OSTEOMA

Reactive
sclerosis

Femur
Tibia

Central
cherry red
vascular
osteomatous
highly trabecular
highly osteoblastic

OSTEOSARCOMA

Cortical invasion

Sun ray spicules

Metaphyseal — Formative/
sclerotic
Destructive/
lytic

Codman's triangle

Knee
proximal Humerus

Areas of cart.

Primitive osteogenic cells

Definitions

Sarcoma: a malignant tumour arising from connective (*mesodermal*) tissue. (Carcinoma arises from *epithelial* tissue.)

Epidemiology

Musculoskeletal tumours are uncommon – 1% of adult and 12% of paediatric malignancies – may occur at any age from youth (e.g. Ewing's sarcoma) to old age (e.g. multiple myeloma) and may be benign (e.g osteoid osteoma) or malignant (e.g. chondrosarcoma).

Key points

- May affect extremities (50%), trunk and retroperitoneum (40%), or head and neck (10%).
- Benign soft tissue lesions are 100 times more common than malignant soft tissue lesions.
- Surgery and systemic chemotherapy are the mainstays of treatment for patients with osteosarcomas, malignant fibrous histiocytoma and fibrosarcoma.
- Surgery alone is the mainstay of treatment for chondrosarcoma and chordoma.
- Radiation therapy has role in the management of Ewing's sarcoma.
- Some benign tumours (e.g. lipoma) can safely be observed.

Classification of musculoskeletal tumours

Cell of origin	Benign	Malignant
Primary bone tumours		
Fibroblast	Bone cysts	Malignant fibrous hystiocytoma (MFH) Fibrosarcoma
Chondrocyte	Chondroma (exostosis)	Chondrosarcoma
Bone cells	Osteoma Osteoid osteoma Osteoblastoma	Osteosarcoma
Marrow		Myeloma, lymphoma
Unknown		Giant cell tumour Ewing's sarcoma
Secondary bone tumours		
Bronchus, breast, renal		Osteoclastic lesions
Prostate		Osteosclerotic lesions
Soft tissue tumours		
Fatty tissue	Lipoma	Liposarcoma
Neural tissue	Neurofibroma	Neurofibrosarcoma Neurilemmoma
Interstitial cells of Cajal		Gastrointestinal stromal tumour (GIST)
Muscle	Leiomyoma	Leiomyosarcoma Rhabdomyosarcoma
Vascular	Haemangioma	Angiosarcoma
Synovium	Giant cell synovioma	Synovial sarcoma

Clinical features

- Pain. Bone tumours cause dull aching pain that is worse at night and aggravated by exercise.
- Minor trauma may initiate symptoms.
- Enlarging painless mass in extremity or trunk is characteristic of soft tissue sarcoma.

Investigations

- Establish tissue diagnosis, evaluate the extent of disease and feasability of resection.
- Imaging: radiographs, CT, MRI, nuclear medicine and PET scanning are all used.
- Biopsy: needle, trephine or incisional. (The biopsy track must be excised with the tumour if positive.)
- Staging: Stage I: low grade, no spread. Stage II: high grade, no spread. Stage III: high grade, spread to lymph nodes. Stage IV: high grade, metastatic spread.

Essential management

- Surgery: limb sparing surgery with clear margins is the aim. Amputation may be indicated.
- Neoadjuvant chemotherapy is effective in shrinking osteosarcomas and increasing numbers suitable for limb-sparing surgery.
- Radiotherapy: most bone tumours are radioresistant with the exception of Ewing's sarcoma.
- Rehabilitation: very important in restoring patients to the best quality of life achievable.

Specific bone tumours

Multiple myeloma

- Malignancy characterized by the proliferation of immunoglobulin-producing *plasma cells* in bone marrow.
- Elderly patients.
- Anemia, fatigue, bone pain, elevated creatinine or serum protein, and hypercalcemia.
- Diagnostic criteria: (1) serum or urinary monoclonal protein; (2) clonal plasma cells in the bone marrow or a plasmacytoma; (3) end organ damage, e.g. lytic bone lesions, renal failure.
- Rx: chemotherapy alone or chemotherapy plus haematopoietic cell transplantation (HCT).
- Prognosis: almost all patients eventually relapse. Overall 5-year survival is 35%.

Osteosarcoma

- Most common primary malignant *bone* tumour.
- Any age, but most frequent at 10–20 years.
- Pain, limp or pathological fracture ± palpable mass.
- Diagnosis: radiographs show periosteal elevation (Codman's Δ) and bony destruction. CT lesion and chest (pulmonary metastases). MRI for staging. Biopsy (open, trephine or needle).
- Rx: neoadjuvant chemotherapy (80% have micro-metastases) and surgery with clear margins (limb sparing or amputation). Pulmonary metastases can be cured by resection.
- Prognosis: 5-year survival is 70% in patients without detectable metastases and 30% with resectable pulmonary metastases.

Chondrosarcoma

- Second commonest primary malignant tumour of bone. *Cartilage* is tissue of origin. Usually large >5 cm. Variable aggressiveness.
- Pain (often at night).
- Age 50–70 years.
- Diagnosis: radiography, MRI, needle or open biopsy.
- Rx: surgery with clear margins. Limited role for chemo or radiotherapy.
- Prognosis: 50–60% 5-year survival.

Ewing's sarcoma family of tumours

- A group of tumours derived from *neural crest cells*.
- Age 5–30 years.
- Pain, palpable mass ± fever and weight loss.
- Diagnosis: radiographs and MRI, CT and radionucleotide scans for metastases. Biopsy. Neoadjuvant chemotherapy and surgery for resectable tumours. If not resectable radiotherapy is indicated.
- Prognosis: overall 5-year survival 65%.

40 Burns

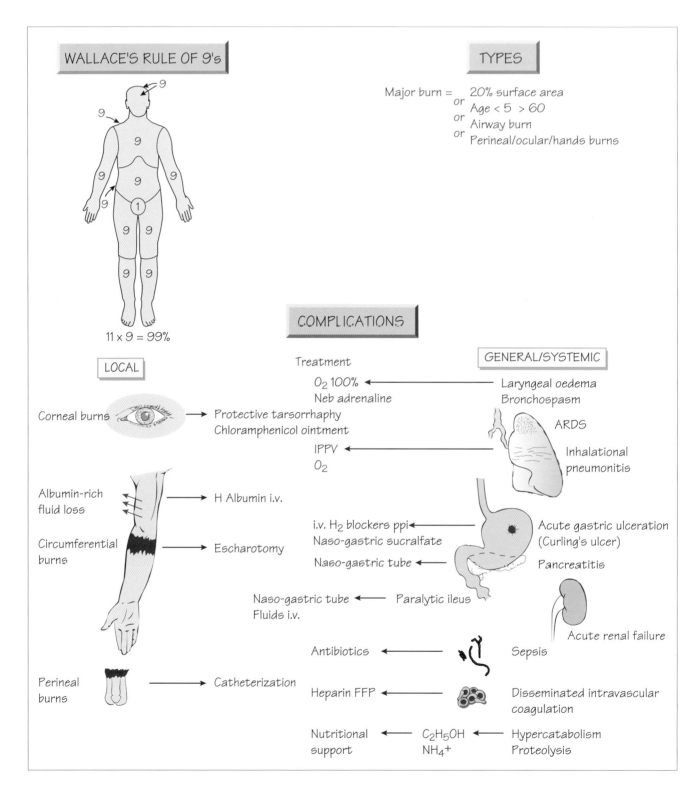

WALLACE'S RULE OF 9's

$11 \times 9 = 99\%$

TYPES

Major burn = 20% surface area
or Age < 5 > 60
or Airway burn
or Perineal/ocular/hands burns

COMPLICATIONS

LOCAL

Corneal burns → Protective tarsorrhaphy
Chloramphenicol ointment

Albumin-rich fluid loss → H Albumin i.v.

Circumferential burns → Escharotomy

Perineal burns → Catheterization

Treatment

O_2 100%
Neb adrenaline

IPPV
O_2

i.v. H_2 blockers ppi
Naso-gastric sucralfate

Naso-gastric tube

Naso-gastric tube
Fluids i.v.

Antibiotics

Heparin FFP

Nutritional support ← C_2H_5OH
NH_4^+

GENERAL/SYSTEMIC

Laryngeal oedema
Bronchospasm

ARDS

Inhalational pneumonitis

Acute gastric ulceration (Curling's ulcer)

Pancreatitis

Paralytic ileus

Acute renal failure

Sepsis

Disseminated intravascular coagulation

Hypercatabolism
Proteolysis

Definitions

A *burn* is the response of the skin, mucous membranes and subcutaneous tissues to thermal injury. A *partial thickness* burn does not destroy the skin epithelium or destroys only part of it, sub-classified into *superficial* and *deep partial thickness*. A *full thickness* burn destroys all sources of skin epithelial regrowth.

Common causes

- Thermal injury: dry – flame, hot metal, sunburn; moist – hot liquids or gases.
- Electricity (deep burns at entry and exit sites, may cause cardiac arrest).
- Chemicals (usually industrial accidents with acid or alkali).
- Radiation (partial thickness initially, chronic deeper injury later).

Clinical features
General

Classification	Appearance	Sensation	Healing	Scarring
Superficial	Dry, red, blanches on pressure	Painful	3–6 days Rx: medical	None
Superficial partial	Blisters, moist, blanches on pressure	Painful	7–20 days Rx: medical	Unusual
Deep partial	Blisters, wet or waxy, no blanching	None	>21 days Rx: surgical	Severe
Full thickness	Waxy white to black, dry no blanching on pressure	None	Never Rx: surgical	Very severe

Specific

- Evidence of smoke inhalation (soot in nose or sputum, burns in the mouth, hoarseness).
- Eye or eyelid burns (early ophthalmological opinion).
- Circumferential burns (will need escharotomy).
- Hands, feet, genitalia, joints (will need specialist care).

Investigations

- FBC, U+E.
- If inhalation suspected: chest X-ray, arterial blood gases, CO estimation.
- Blood group and crossmatch.
- ECG/cardiac enzymes with electrical burns.

Complications
Immediate

- Smoke inhalation: commonest cause of death from burns.
- Circumferential burns → compartment syndrome (limbs → limb ischaemia; thorax → restrictive respiratory failure). Rx: escharotomy.

Early

- Hyperkalaemia (from cytolysis in large burns). Rx: insulin and dextrose.
- Acute renal failure (combination of hypovolaemia, sepsis, tissue toxins). Rx: aggressive early resuscitation, ensuring high GFR with fluid loading and diuretics, treat sepsis.
- Infection (*Staphlococcus* and MRSA, *Streptococcus*, *E. coli*, *Klebsiella*, *Pseudomonas*, yeasts). Treat established infection (10^6 organisms present in wound biopsy) with systemic antibiotics. Early surgical excision.
- Stress ulceration (Curling's ulcer). Prevent with PPI prophylaxis.

Late

Contractures.

41 Major trauma – basic principles

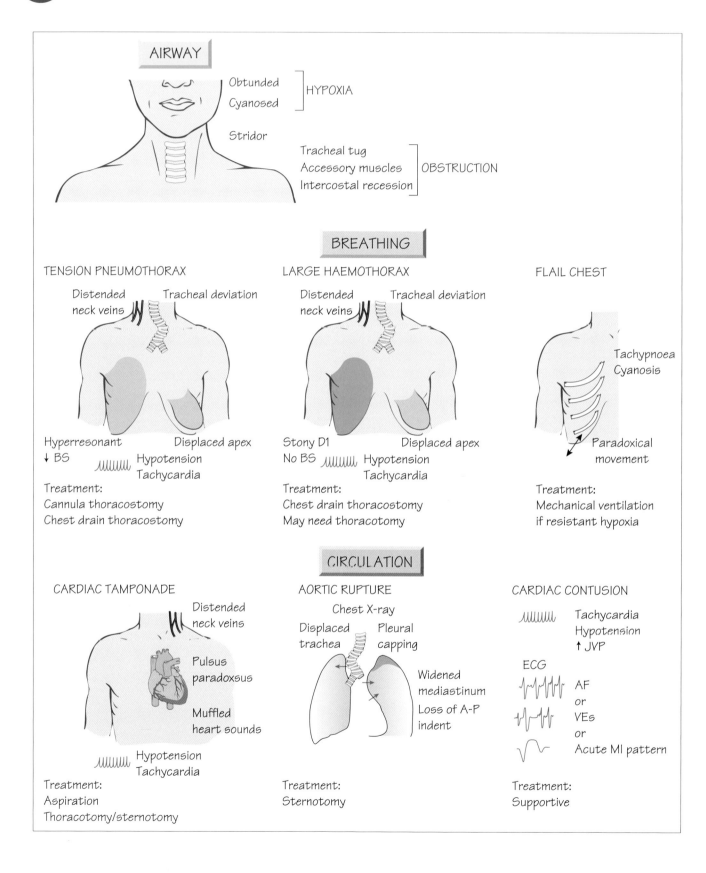

AIRWAY

Obtunded ⎤ HYPOXIA
Cyanosed ⎦

Stridor

Tracheal tug ⎤
Accessory muscles ⎬ OBSTRUCTION
Intercostal recession ⎦

BREATHING

TENSION PNEUMOTHORAX

Distended neck veins   Tracheal deviation

Hyperresonant   Displaced apex
↓ BS   Hypotension
    Tachycardia
Treatment:
Cannula thoracostomy
Chest drain thoracostomy

LARGE HAEMOTHORAX

Distended neck veins   Tracheal deviation

Stony D1   Displaced apex
No BS   Hypotension
    Tachycardia
Treatment:
Chest drain thoracostomy
May need thoracotomy

FLAIL CHEST

Tachypnoea
Cyanosis

Paradoxical movement

Treatment:
Mechanical ventilation
if resistant hypoxia

CIRCULATION

CARDIAC TAMPONADE

Distended neck veins

Pulsus paradoxsus

Muffled heart sounds

Hypotension
Tachycardia
Treatment:
Aspiration
Thoracotomy/sternotomy

AORTIC RUPTURE

Chest X-ray
Displaced   Pleural
trachea   capping

Widened mediastinum
Loss of A-P indent

Treatment:
Sternotomy

CARDIAC CONTUSION

Tachycardia
Hypotension
↑ JVP

ECG

AF
or
VEs
or
Acute MI pattern

Treatment:
Supportive

Definition

Major trauma (MT) can be defined as injury (or injuries) of organs of severity sufficient to present an immediate threat to life. MT often involves multiple injuries. The majority of patients who reach hospital alive following MT have potentially survivable injuries if detected and treated early.

Key points

- Treat all MT patients as having a potentially unstable cervical spine.
- Treat life-threatening injuries identified in the primary survey immediately upon discovery.
- Undiagnosed hypotension is due to occult haemorrhage unless proven otherwise.
- Commence rapid IV infusion immediately (warmed if possible).
- Emergency surgery may be part of the resuscitation of patients suffering from internal haemorrhage.

Principles of management

Management for MT is divided into two categories.

- **'First aid'** – 'roadside' given by paramedics or on-site medical teams. Aims to maintain life during extraction and evacuation of patient.
- **Primary survey** – in hospital performed by accident and emergency or trauma teams. Aims to identify and treat immediately life-threatening injuries to airways, respiratory and cardiovascular systems using **ABCDE** (see below). Important to: reassess repeatedly, treat life-threatening conditions as soon as diagnosed, leave penetrating wounds and implements for formal surgical exploration, stop external bleeding by direct pressure.
- **Secondary survey** – aim to document any other injuries, take history, examine patient from head to toe, document GCS, assess neck (clinical and radiology to include C7–T1) and perform major skeletal radiology.
- **Definitive treatment** – follows primary and secondary surveys and will depend on what injuries are present.

Patterns of injury

Some of the major injuries that may be encountered in the primary survey are shown opposite. Mechanisms of injury and patterns of injury may be associated, e.g.

Restrained RTA	Pedestrian collision
Cervical spine injury	Long bone fractures
Sternal fracture	Knee ligamentous injury
Cardiac contusion	Rib fractures
Liver laceration	Pneumothorax
	Facial fractures
	Head injury

Timing of death following trauma

- 1st peak: immediately at time of injury due to primary injury.
- 2nd peak: up to several hours post injury due to secondary injury, e.g. hypoxia, haemorrhage. Secondary injuries are frequently avoidable or treatable (e.g. chest drain for pneumothorax).
- 3rd peak: days or weeks post injury due to sepsis or multiple organ failure.

Essential management of trauma

Cervical spine
- Stabilize with in-line manual traction.
- Lateral C spine/X-ray (must include C7–T1).
- Secure with hard collar, head supports and tape.
- Can only be 'cleared' by normal examination in a fully conscious patient or normal X-rays.

A Airway management (see opposite for major abnormalities)
- Clear obstructions by hand and suction and lift chin (jaw thrust) in obtunded patients.
- Secure airway with oropharyngeal or nasopharyngeal airway (obtunded patients).
- Definitive airway (endotracheal intubation) for: *apnoea/(risk of) upper airway obstruction/(risk of) aspiration/need for mechanical ventilation.*
- Surgical airway (cricothyroidotomy) indicated by: *maxillofacial injuries/laryngeal disruption/failure to intubate.*

B Breathing (see opposite for some major abnormalities)
- Administer supplemental O_2.
- Assess respiratory rate/air entry CXR (symmetry)/chest wall motion (symmetry)/tracheal position.
- Monitor with pulse oximetry and observations.

C Circulation (see opposite for some major abnormalities)
- Assess capillary refill, pulse /blood pressure/apex beat/JVP/heart sounds/evidence of blood loss.
- Insert two large bore IV lines. (Intraosseus fluids if IV access not readily available, e.g. children.)
- Draw blood for crossmatch, FBC & U+E.
- Insert urinary catheter and monitor urinary output.

D Dysfunction of the CNS
- Assess GCS (see Chapter 42)/pupil reactivity/limb gross motor and sensory function where possible.

E Exposure of extremities
- Assess limbs for major long bone injuries and sites of major blood loss/pelvic X-ray.

42 Traumatic brain injury (head injury)/1

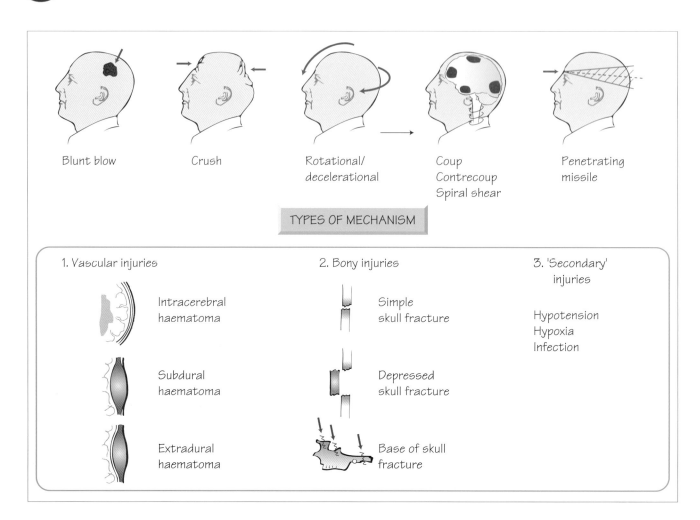

Blunt blow Crush Rotational/decelerational Coup Contrecoup Spiral shear Penetrating missile

TYPES OF MECHANISM

1. Vascular injuries

Intracerebral haematoma

Subdural haematoma

Extradural haematoma

2. Bony injuries

Simple skull fracture

Depressed skull fracture

Base of skull fracture

3. 'Secondary' injuries

Hypotension
Hypoxia
Infection

Surgery at a Glance, Fifth Edition. Pierce A. Grace and Neil R. Borley. © 2013 John Wiley & Sons, Ltd. Published 2013 by John Wiley & Sons, Ltd.

Definitions

A *traumatic brain injury (TBI)* or *head injury* is the process whereby trauma to the head results in skull and/or brain inury. *Primary brain injury* is the damage that occurs to the brain immediately as the result of the trauma. The degree of primary brain injury is directly related to the location of injury, the amount of energy transfered to the head and the rate of energy transfer. Prevention (e.g. helmets, airbags) is the only way to reduce primary injury (deflecting penetration/energy and slowing energy transfer).

Secondary brain injury is the damage that develops later as a result of complications. Secondary damage results from *hypoxia* and/or *hypercarbia* (respiratory complications, e.g. *airway obstruction*), hypovolaemic shock, intracranial bleeding, cerebral oedema, epilepsy, infection and hydrocephalus. *Brain death* is defined as the absence of brain function.

Key points

- Prevention of secondary brain injury caused by hypoxia and hypotension is the most important objective of head injury care.
- A full trauma survey (see Chapter 41) must be carried out on all patients with head injuries.
- Head injury does not cause hypovolaemic shock – look for another cause.
- The GCS provides a simple method of monitoring global CNS function over a period rather than a precise index of brain injury at any one time.
- CT scanning is the investigation of choice to assess the head/brain but transfer to CT scan is complex and requires optimum stabilization of the patient to perform.
- 100% of those with severe head injury and 60% of those with moderate head injury will be permanently disabled.

Epidemiology

Head injury is very common. RTAs, falls, assaults and sports injuries are common causes. A million patients each year present to emergency departments in the UK with head injury and about 5000 patients die each year following head injuries.

Pathophysiology

Closed head injury

Direct blow

May cause damage to the brain at the site of the blow (*coup injury*) or to the side opposite the blow when the brain moves within the skull and hits the opposite wall (*contrecoup injury*).

Rotation/deceleration

Neck flexion, extension or rotation results in the brain striking bony points within the skull (e.g. the wing of the sphenoid bone). Severe rotation also causes shear injuries within the white matter of the brain and brainstem, causing axonal injury and intracerebral petechial haemorrhages.

Crush

The brain is often remarkably spared direct injury unless severe (especially in children with elastic skulls).

Penetrating head injury

Missiles tend to cause loss of tissue with injury proportionate. Brain swelling – less of a problem due to the skull disruption automatically decompressing the brain. High velocity injuries (bullets) worse than low velocity due to shock wave disruption of brain tissue.

Clinical features

- History of direct trauma to head or deceleration.
- Patient must be assessed fully for other injuries.
- Level of consciousness determined by GCS.
- Headache, nausea, vomiting, a falling pulse rate and rising BP indicate cerebral oedema.
- Neurological assessment: motor exam, sensory exam, reflex exam, cranial nerves.
- Brainstem tests: pupillary exam, ocular movements, corneal reflex, gag reflex;

Investigations

- CT/MRI scan: show contusions, haematomas, hydrocephalus, cerebral oedema. CT is the diagnostic study of choice.
- Skull X-ray: no benefit if CT is being performed. If CT unavailable two views should be obtained. Plain radiographs are used to exclude cervical spine injury.

Glasgow Coma Scale						
Eye opening		Voice response		Best motor response	
Spontaneous	4	Alert and orientated	5	Obeys commands	6
To voice	3	Confused	4	Localizes pain	5
To pain	2	Inappropriate	3	Flexes to pain	4
No eye opening	1	Incomprehensible	2	Abnormal flexion to pain	3
		No voice response	1	Extends to pain	2
				No response to pain	1

Fully conscious: GCS = 15; deep coma: GCS = 3.

Traumatic brain injury (head injury)/2

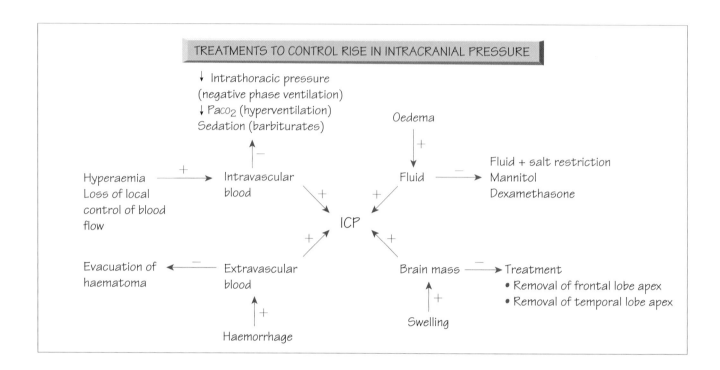

TREATMENTS TO CONTROL RISE IN INTRACRANIAL PRESSURE

↓ Intrathoracic pressure
(negative phase ventilation)
↓ Pa_{CO_2} (hyperventilation)
Sedation (barbiturates)

Surgery at a Glance, Fifth Edition. Pierce A. Grace and Neil R. Borley. © 2013 John Wiley & Sons, Ltd. Published 2013 by John Wiley & Sons, Ltd.

Essential management

Trivial head injury

The patient is conscious, may be history of period of LOC. Retrograde amnesia for events prior to head injury is significant.

Indications for CT scan

- LOC or amnesia/GCS ≤14.
- Neurological signs.
- CSF leakage.
- Suspected penetrating injury.
- Alcohol intoxication.
- Difficulty in assessing patient.

Indications for admission

- Confusion or reduced GCS.
- Abnormalities on imaging.
- Neurological signs or headache or vomiting.
- Difficulty in assessing patient.
- Coexisting medical problem.
- Inadequate social conditions or lack of responsible adult to observe patient.

Indications for neurosurgical referral

- Skull fracture + confusion/decreasing GCS.
- Focal neurological signs or fits.
- Persistence of neurological signs or confusion for >12 hours.
- Persisting coma (GCS ≤8) after resuscitation.
- Definite or suspected penetrating injury.
- Depressed skull fracture or CSF leak.
- Deterioration.

Severe head injury

- Patient will arrive unconscious to emergency department. May be multiple trauma.
- ABC (see Chapter 41). Intubate and ventilate unconscious patients to protect airway and prevent secondary brain injury from hypoxia.
- Resuscitate patient and look for other injuries, especially if the patient is in shock. Head injury may be accompanied by cervical spine injury and the neck must be protected by a cervical collar in these patients.
- Treat life-threatening problems (e.g. ruptured spleen) and stabilize patient before transfer to neurosurgical unit. Ensure adequate medical supervision (anaesthetist + nurse) during transfer.

Complications

Skull fractures

Indicate severity of injury. No specific treatment required unless compound, depressed or associated with chronic CSF loss (e.g. anterior cranial fossa basal skull fracture).

Intracranial haemorrhage

- Extradural haemorrhage: tear in middle meningeal artery. Haematoma between skull and dura. Often a 'lucid interval' before signs of raised ICP ensue (falling pulse, rising BP, ipsilateral pupillary dilatation, contralateral paresis or paralysis). Treatment is by evacuation of haematoma via burr holes.
- Acute subdural haemorrhage: tearing of veins between arachnoid and dura mater. Usually seen in elderly. Progressive neurological deterioration. Treatment is by evacuation but even then recovery may be incomplete.
- Chronic subdural haematoma: tear in vein leads to subdural haematoma which enlarges slowly by absorption of CSF. Often the precipitating injury is trivial. Drowsiness and confusion, headache, hemiplegia. Treatment is by evacuation of the clot.
- Intracerebral haemorrhage: haemorrhage into brain substance causes irreversible damage. Efforts are made to avoid secondary injury by ensuring adequate perfusion oxygenation and nutrition.

Raised intracranial pressure

Cerebral oedema is an increase in brain volume caused by an absolute increase in cerebral water content and results in raised ICP. Frequently, raised ICP complicates closed head injury. Management may involve some of the following: ICP monitoring, head elevation, maintenance of cerebral perfusion (BP >90 mmHg) and oxygenation (PaO_2 – 8 kPa), CSF drainage by ventriculostomy, hyperventilation, hypothermia, diuretics (mannitol), barbiturates and decompressive craniectomy.

Prognosis

Prognosis is related to level of consciousness on arrival in hospital.

GCS on admission	Mortality
13–15 (mild TBI)	1%
9–12 (moderate TBI)	5%
<8 (severe TBI)	40%

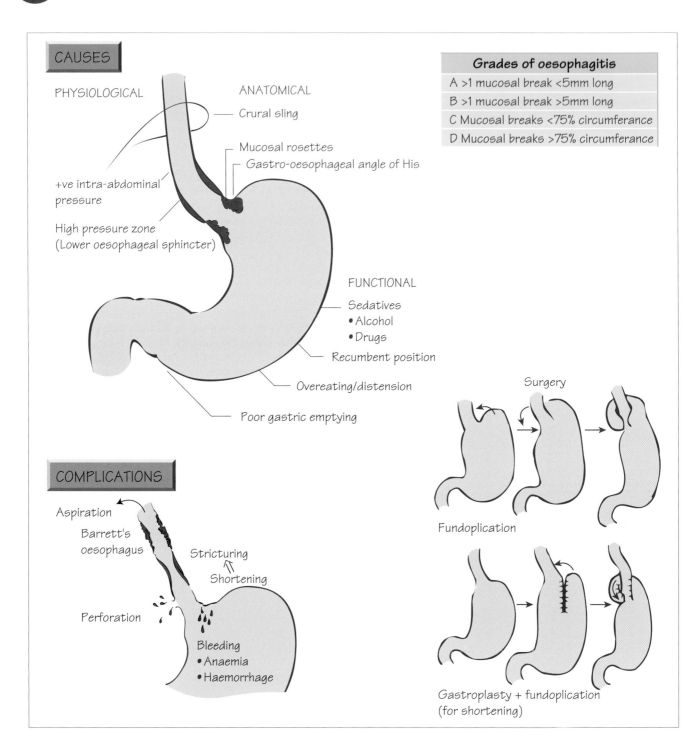

CAUSES

PHYSIOLOGICAL

ANATOMICAL
- Crural sling
- Mucosal rosettes
- Gastro-oesophageal angle of His

+ve intra-abdominal pressure

High pressure zone (Lower oesophageal sphincter)

FUNCTIONAL
- Sedatives
  - Alcohol
  - Drugs
- Recumbent position
- Overeating/distension
- Poor gastric emptying

Grades of oesophagitis

A	>1 mucosal break <5mm long
B	>1 mucosal break >5mm long
C	Mucosal breaks <75% circumferance
D	Mucosal breaks >75% circumferance

COMPLICATIONS

- Aspiration
- Barrett's oesophagus
- Stricturing
- Shortening
- Perforation
- Bleeding
  - Anaemia
  - Haemorrhage

Surgery

Fundoplication

Gastroplasty + fundoplication (for shortening)

Definitions

Gastro-oesophageal reflux disease (GORD) is a condition caused by the retrograde passage of gastric contents into the oesophagus resulting in inflammation (*oesophagitis*), which manifests as dyspepsia. A *hiatus hernia* is an abnormal protrusion of the proximal stomach through the oesophageal opening in the diaphragm resulting in a more proximal positioning of the oesophagogastric junction and predisposition to GORD. *Sliding* (common) and *rolling* or *para-oesophageal* (rare) hiatus hernias are recognized.

Key points

- The majority of GORD is benign and uncomplicated.
- Barrett's oesophagus is a recognized association predisposing to adenocarcinoma of the oesophagus.
- Consider malignancy in patients >55 years or with GORD symptoms.
- Surgery for GORD indicated for complications or patients resistant to medical therapy.

Common causes

- tLOSRs: transient lower esophageal sphincter relaxation (normal continence mechanisms: LOS pressure, length of intra-abdominal LOS, angle of His, sling fibres around the cardia, the crural fibres of the diaphragm, the mucosal rosette).
- LOS pressure reduced by smoking, alcohol and coffee and some drugs (calcium-channel blockers, nitrates, beta-blockers, progesterone).
- Anatomical disruption of sphincter by hiatus hernia.

Clinical features

- Retrosternal burning pain, radiating to epigastrium, jaw and arms. (Oesophageal pain is often confused with cardiac pain.)
- Regurgitation of acid contents into the mouth (waterbrash).
- Back pain (a penetrating ulcer in Barrett's oesophagus).
- Dysphagia from a benign stricture.
- Coughing or wheezing, hoarseness (due to aspiration of gastric contents).

Investigations

- Oesophagoscopy: assess oesophagitis, biopsy for histology, dilate stricture if present.
- Barium swallow and meal: sliding hiatus hernia, oesophageal ulcer, stricture.
- Ambulatory 24-hour pH monitoring: assess the degree of reflux.
- Oesophageal manometry.

Essential management

General

- Lose weight, avoid smoking, coffee, alcohol, chocolate, tomatoes and citrus juices.
- Avoid tight garments, stooping and large meals. Elevate head of bed.

Medical

- Exclude carcinoma by OGD in patients > 55 years and symptoms suspicious of malignancy.
- Control acid secretion (H_2 receptor antagonists (e.g. ranitidine) or PPIs (e.g. omeprazole)). Antacids may be effective in controlling symptoms in mild disease.
- Minimize effects of reflux (give alginates to protect oesophagus).
- Prokinetic agents (e.g. bethanechol, metoclopramide, domperidone) improve LOS tone and promote gastric emptying.

Surgical

- Antireflux surgery (e.g. laparoscopic Nissen fundoplication) gives excellent results. Indicated in approximately 20% of patients with GORD:
  failed optimum medical treatment
  complications of reflux (benign stricture, Barrrett's oesophagus)
  severe oesophagitis on endoscopy
  'large volume' reflux.

Complications

- Benign stricture of the oesophagus.
- Barrett's oesophagus (see below).
- Bleeding.

Barrett's oesophagus

Definition and aetiology

Segment of columnar metaplasia of any length visible endoscopically above the gastro-oesophageal junction. Related to increasing incidence of GORD.

Diagnosis (two criteria)

- Columnar epithelium lines the distal oesophagus on endoscopy.
- Biopsy of the columnar epithelium shows intestinal metaplasia.

Complications

Risk of adenocarcinoma:

- 2% – no dysplasia present.
- 20% – low-grade dysplasia present.
- 50% – high-grade dysplasia present.
  Screening of patients with GORD symptoms for Barrett's oesophagus is advocated.

Management

- Follow-up OGD (surveillance endoscopy 6–12 monthly with four quadrant biopsy).
- Treat GORD with PPIs (possibly laparoscopic fundoplication).
- Low-grade dysplasia: radiofrequency ablation may be used.
- High-grade dysplasia: endoscopic eradication therapy (endoscopic mucosal resection + radiofrequency ablation or photodynamic therapy) or surgery (oesophagectomy).

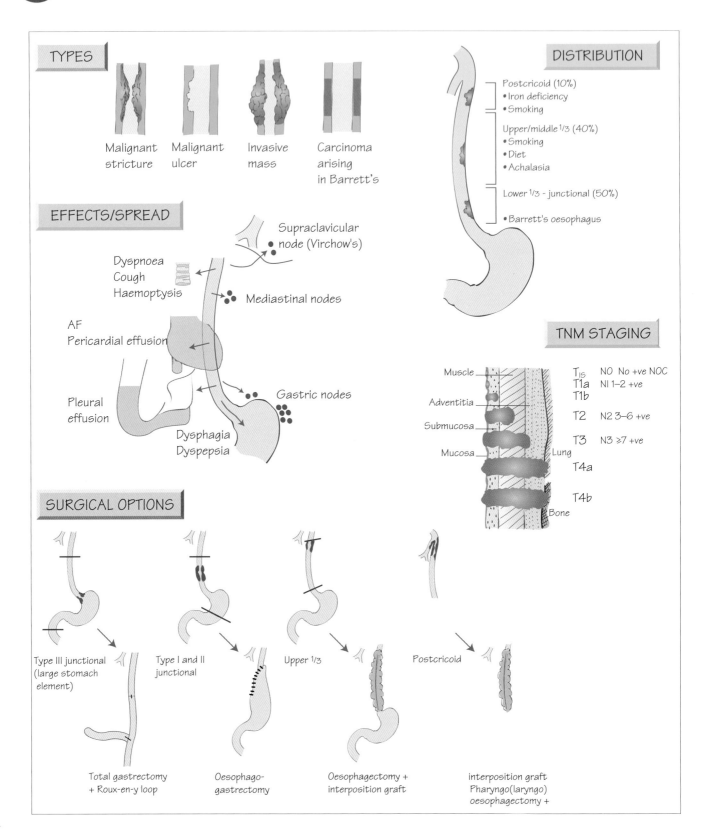

TYPES

Malignant stricture

Malignant ulcer

Invasive mass

Carcinoma arising in Barrett's

DISTRIBUTION

Postcricoid (10%)
• Iron deficiency
• Smoking

Upper/middle 1/3 (40%)
• Smoking
• Diet
• Achalasia

Lower 1/3 - junctional (50%)

• Barrett's oesophagus

EFFECTS/SPREAD

Supraclavicular node (Virchow's)

Dyspnoea
Cough
Haemoptysis

Mediastinal nodes

AF
Pericardial effusion

Pleural effusion

Gastric nodes

Dysphagia
Dyspepsia

TNM STAGING

Muscle

Adventitia

Submucosa

Mucosa

T_{IS} N0 No +ve NOC
T1a   N1 1–2 +ve
T1b

T2   N2 3–6 +ve

T3   N3 ⩾7 +ve

Lung
T4a

T4b
Bone

SURGICAL OPTIONS

Type III junctional (large stomach element)

Total gastrectomy + Roux-en-y loop

Type I and II junctional

Oesophago-gastrectomy

Upper 1/3

Oesophagectomy + interposition graft

Postcricoid

interposition graft Pharyngo(laryngo) oesophagectomy +

Definition

Malignant lesion of the epithelial lining of the oesophagus.

Key points

- All new symptoms of dysphagia should raise the possibility of oesophageal carcinoma.
- Adenocarcinoma of the oesophagus is increasingly common.
- Only a minority of tumours are successfully cured by surgery.

Epidemiology

- Male:female 3:1, peak incidence 50–70 years. High incidence in areas of China, Russia, Scandinavia, among the Bantu in South Africa and black males in the USA.
- Adenocarcinoma has the fastest increasing incidence of any carcinoma in the UK.

Aetiology

Predisposing factors:

- Alcohol consumption and cigarette smoking.
- Chronic oesophagitis and Barrett's oesophagus – possibly related to biliary reflux.
- Stricture from corrosive (lye) oesophagitis.
- Achalasia.
- Plummer–Vinson syndrome (oesophageal web, mucosal lesions of mouth and pharynx, iron deficiency anaemia).
- Nitrosamines.
- Elevated BMI – increased risk for adenocarcinoma.

Pathology

- Histological type: squamous carcinoma (upper two-thirds of oesophagus); adenocarcinoma (middle third, lower third and junctional). Worldwide squamous carcinoma is commonest (80%) but adenocarcinoma accounts for >50% in USA and UK.
- Spread: lymphatics, direct extension, vascular invasion.

Clinical features

- Dysphagia progressing from solids to liquids.
- Weight loss and weakness.
- Aspiration pneumonia.
- Supraclavicular/cervical adenopathy (advanced disease).

Investigations

Aim is to confirm diagnosis, stage the tumour and assess suitablity for resection.

- Oesophagoscopy and biopsy (minimum of eight biopsies): malignant stricture.
- Barium swallow (if high lesion suspected or OGD contraindicated): narrowed lumen with 'shouldering'.
- Contrast-enhanced abdominal and chest CT scanning/MRI: assess degree of spread if surgery is being contemplated – especially metastases (M staging).
- EUS: useful in staging disease (depth of penetration [T staging] and perioesophageal nodes [N staging]).
- CT PET scanning: increasingly used.
- Laparoscopy to assess liver and peritoneal involvement prior to proceeding to surgery.
- Bronchoscopy: assess if bronchial invasion suspected with upper third lesions.

Essential management

Curative treatment

- Stage I (T1a/N0/M0) – Endoscopic Mucosal Resection.
- Stage I and IIA disease (T1/N0/M0 – T2/N0/M0) – Surgical resection is potentially curative only if lymph nodes are not involved and clear tumours margins can be achieved.
- Stage IIB and III (T1/N1/M0 – T4/anyN/M0) – Surgery or neoadjuvant (pre-operative) chemotherapy (cisplatin and fluorouracil) or chemoradiation followed by surgery or definitive chemoradiation.
- The role of neoadjuvant or adjuvant (postoperative) chemotherapy or chemoradiotherapy continues to be explored in clinical trials.
- Chemoradiotherapy and radiotherapy are occasionally used with curative intent in patients deemed not suitable for surgery.
- Reconstruction is by jejunal or gastric 'pull-up' or rarely colon interposition.

Palliation (Stage IV disease – anyT/anyN/M1)

- Partially covered self-expanding metal stents are the intubation of choice for obstructive symptoms – especially useful when tracheo-oesophageal fistula present ± laser therapy.
- Radiotherapy – external beam DXT or endoluminal brachytherapy.
- Laser resection (Nd:YAG laser) of the tumour to create lumen.
- Photodynamic therapy: photosensitizing agents (given IV) are taken up by dysplastic malignant tissue which is damaged when photons (light) is applied.

Prognosis

Following resection, 5-year survival rates are about 20%, but up to 45% in some patients with neoadjuvant chemoradiation. 5-year survival for disease confined to oesophagus – 37%, involving nodes – 18%, disseminated – 3%, all stages combined – 20%.

2-week wait referral criteria for suspected upper GI cancer

- New-onset dysphagia (any age).
- Dyspepsia + 'alarm symptoms': weight loss/anaemia/vomiting.
- Dyspepsia + FHx/Barrett's oesophagus/previous peptic ulcer surgery/atrophic gastritis/pernicious anaemia.
- New dyspepsia >55 years.
- Jaundice.
- Upper abdominal mass.

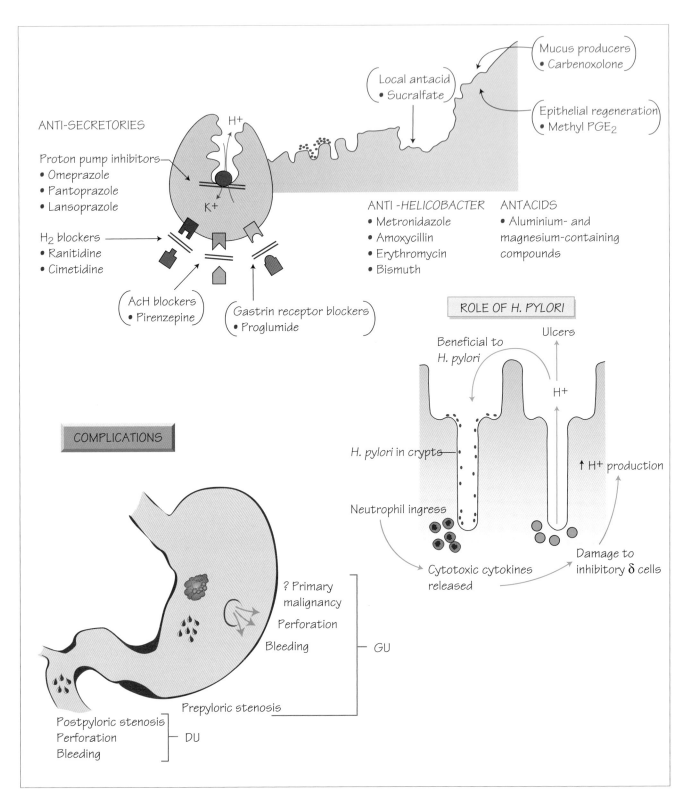

Definition

A *peptic ulcer* is a break in the epithelial surface of the stomach or duodenum (or Meckel's diverticulum) caused by the action of gastric secretions (acid and pepsin) and infection with *Helicobacter pylori*.

Key points

- Not all dyspepsia is due to peptic ulcer disease (PUD).
- The majority of chronic duodenal ulcers are related to *H. pylori* infection and respond to eradication and antisecretory therapy.
- Patients ≥45 years or with suspicious symptoms require endoscopy to exclude malignancy.
- Surgery is limited to complications of ulcer disease.

Common causes

- Infection with *H. pylori* (gram-negative spirochete).
- NSAIDs.
- Imbalance between acid/pepsin secretion and mucosal defence.
- Alcohol, cigarettes and 'stress'.
- Hypersecretory states e.g. gastrin hypersecretion in the ZE-syndrome or antral G cell hyperplasia).

Clinical features

Duodenal ulcer and type II gastric ulcer (i.e. prepyloric and antral)

- Male : female 1:1, peak incidence 25–50 years.
- Epigastric pain during fasting (hunger pain), relieved by food/antacids, often nocturnal, typically exhibits periodicity (i.e. recurs at regular intervals).
- Boring back pain if ulcer is penetrating posteriorly.
- Haematemesis from ulcer penetrating gastroduodenal artery posteriorly.
- Peritonitis if perforation occurs with anterior DU.
- Vomiting if gastric outlet obstruction (pyloric stenosis) occurs (note succussion splash and watch for hypokalaemic, hypochloraemic alkalosis).

Type I gastric ulcer (i.e. body of stomach)

- Male : female 3:1, peak incidence 50+ years.
- Epigastric pain induced by eating.
- Weight loss.
- Nausea and vomiting.
- Anaemia from chronic blood loss.

Investigations

- FBC: to check for anaemia.
- U+E.
- Faecal occult blood.
- OGD:
  necessary to exclude malignant gastric ulcer in:
    patients over 45 years at first presentation
    concomitant anaemia
    short history of symptoms
    other 'alarm' symptoms suggestive of malignancy
  useful to obtain biopsy for CLO and rapid urease test.
- Barium meal: best for patients unable to tolerate OGD or evaluation of the duodenum in cases of pyloric stenosis.
- Carbon 13-urease breath test/*H. pylori* serology: non-invasive method of assessing the presence of *H. pylori* infection. Used to direct therapy or confirm eradication.

Essential management

Medical

- Triple therapy: *H. pylori* eradication (Rx: 1 g amoxicillin 500 mg, and clarithromycin 500 mg) and PPI (20 mg omeprazole or 30 mg lansoprazole b.d.) for 7–14 days. Metronidazole may replace amoxicillin in penicillin-allergic patients).
- Quadruple therapy: bismuth, metronidazole, tetracycline and PPI for 7–14 days.
- NSAID-induced ulcers: PPIs – 4 weeks for DU, 8 weeks for GU.
- Re-endoscope patients with GU after 6 weeks because of risk of malignancy.
- Patient with complication (bleeding perforation) should undergo *H. pylori* eradication.

Other therapy:
- Avoid smoking and foods that cause pain.
- Avoid NSAIDs.
- Antacids for symptomatic relief.
- H_2 blockers (ranitidine, cimetidine).

Surgical

- Only indicated for failure of medical treatment and complications.
- Elective for intractable DU: highly selective vagotomy (may be laparoscopic).
- Elective for intractable GU: Billroth I gastrectomy.
- Perforated DU/GU: simple closure of perforation and biopsy (may be laparoscopic).
- Haemorrhage: high dose intravenous PPI infusion ± endoscopic control by:
  adrenaline injection, thermal coagulation, argon plasma coagulation
  haemoclips, application of fibrin sealant or sclerosants (e..g. polidocanol)
  surgery: undersewing bleeding vessel ± vagotomy.
- Pyloric stenosis: gastroenterostomy ± truncal vagotomy.

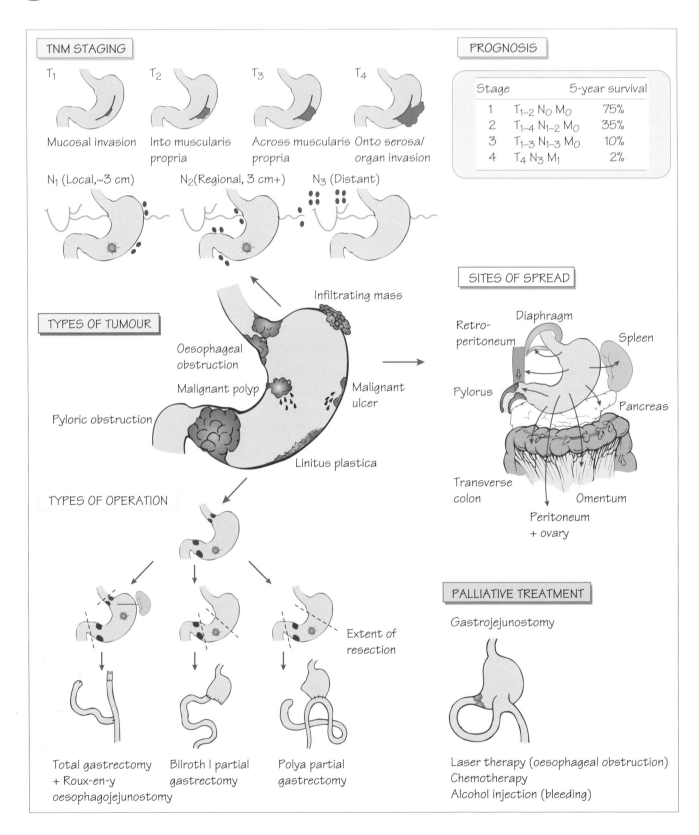

TNM STAGING

T_1 — Mucosal invasion
T_2 — Into muscularis propria
T_3 — Across muscularis propria
T_4 — Onto serosal/organ invasion

N_1 (Local,~3 cm) N_2 (Regional, 3 cm+) N_3 (Distant)

PROGNOSIS

Stage		5-year survival
1	T_{1-2} N_0 M_0	75%
2	T_{1-4} N_{1-2} M_0	35%
3	T_{1-3} N_{1-3} M_0	10%
4	T_4 N_3 M_1	2%

TYPES OF TUMOUR

Infiltrating mass
Oesophageal obstruction
Malignant polyp
Pyloric obstruction
Malignant ulcer
Linitus plastica

SITES OF SPREAD

Retro-peritoneum
Diaphragm
Spleen
Pylorus
Pancreas
Transverse colon
Omentum
Peritoneum + ovary

TYPES OF OPERATION

Extent of resection

Total gastrectomy + Roux-en-y oesophagojejunostomy

Bilroth I partial gastrectomy

Polya partial gastrectomy

PALLIATIVE TREATMENT

Gastrojejunostomy

Laser therapy (oesophageal obstruction)
Chemotherapy
Alcohol injection (bleeding)

Definition

Malignant lesion of the stomach epithelium.

Key points

- Second most common cause of cancer-related death worldwide.
- Most tumours are unresectable at presentation. Only 10% have early-stage disease.
- Tumours considered candidates for resection should be staged with CT and laparoscopy to reduce the risk of an 'open and shut' laparotomy.
- Locally advanced tumours may respond to chemo(radio)therapy.

Epidemiology

Male : female 2:1. Age: 50+ years. Associated with poor socioeconomic status. Dramatic difference in incidence according to geography/genetics (population). Incidence has decreased in Western world over last 75 years. Still common in Japan, Chile and Scandinavia.

Aetiology

Predisposing factors:
- *H. pylori*: ×2 – ×3 increase of gastric cancer in infected individuals.
- Diet (smoked fish, pickled vegetables, benzpyrene, nitrosamines), smoking, alcohol.
- Atrophic gastritis, pernicious anaemia, previous partial gastrectomy.
- Familial hypogammaglobulinaemia.
- Positive family history (possibly related to E-cadherin gene mutation).
- Blood group A.

Pathology

- Histology: adenocarcinoma (intestinal and diffuse).
- Advanced gastric cancer (penetrated muscularis propria) may be polypoid, ulcerating or infiltrating (i.e. linitus plastica).
- Early gastric cancer (confined to mucosa or submucosa).
- Spread: lymphatic (e.g. Troisier's sign in Virchow's node); haematogenous to liver, lung, brain; transcoelomic to ovary (Krukenberg tumour).
- *GastroIntestinal Stromal Tumours* (GIST) arise in the muscle wall of the GI tract, most commonly the stomach, and have an overall better survival after surgery than adenocarcinomas. Neoadjuvant and adjuvant treatment with the tyrosine kinase inhibitor (TKI) imatinib is indicated for GIST with good results. Resistant to standard chemo- and radiotherapy.

Clinical features

- Dyspepsia (epigastric discomfort, postprandial fullness, loss of appetite).
- Anaemia.
- Dysphagia.
- Vomiting.
- Anorexia and weight loss.
- The presence of physical signs usually indicates advanced (incurable) disease.

Investigations

- FBC, U+E., LFTs.
- OGD (see the lesion and obtain biopsy to distinguish from benign gastric ulcer).
- Barium meal (space-occupying lesion/ulcer with rolled edge). Best for patients unable to tolerate OGD. Less sensitive than OGD for detecting early malignancy.
- CT scan (helical)/MRI: stages disease locally and systemically.
- PET scanning: no advantage over standard imaging in locating occult metastatic disease.
- Endoscopic ultrasound: more accurate than CT for T and N staging.
- Laparoscopy: used to exclude undiagnosed peritoneal or liver secondaries prior to consideration of resection.

Essential management

Curative treatment

- Stage I (T1a/b/N0/M0 – T1/N1/M0). Surgical resection + regional lymphadenectomy ± adjuvant chemoradiation. Endoscopic mucosal resection for mucosal disease (T1a/b/N0/M0).
- Stage II (T1/N2/M0 – T2/N2/M0). Surgical resection + regional lymphadenectomy + neoadjuvant chemotherapy + adjuvant chemoradiation.
- Stage III (T3/N0/M0 – T4/N3/M0). Surgical resection (if possible) + regional lymphadenectomy + neoadjuvant chemotherapy + adjuvant chemoradiation.

Palliation (Stage IV disease – anyT/anyN/M1)
- Palliative chemotherapy (e.g. ECF regimen: epirubicin, cisplatin, and 5-FU).
- Endoluminal laser therapy or stent placement if obstructed.
- Palliative radiotherapy for bleeding pain or obstruction.
- Palliative surgery (for continued bleeding or obstruction).

Prognosis

Following 'curative' resection, 5-year survival rates are 50% for distal and 10% for proximal gastric cancer. Overall 5-year survival (palliation and resection) is only about 5%.

2-week wait referral criteria for suspected upper GI cancer

- New-onset dysphagia (any age).
- Dyspepsia + weight loss/anaemia/vomiting.
- Dyspepsia + FHx/Barrett's oesophagus/previous peptic ulcer surgery/atrophic gastritis/pernicious anaemia.
- New dyspepsia >55 years.
- Jaundice.
- Upper abdominal mass.

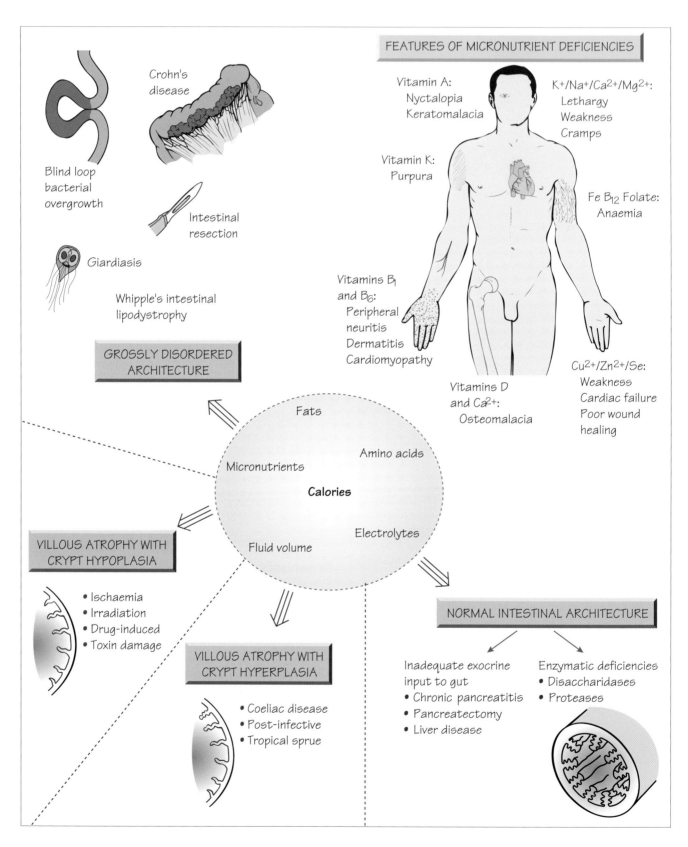

FEATURES OF MICRONUTRIENT DEFICIENCIES

Crohn's disease

Blind loop bacterial overgrowth

Intestinal resection

Giardiasis

Whipple's intestinal lipodystrophy

GROSSLY DISORDERED ARCHITECTURE

Vitamin A: Nyctalopia Keratomalacia

Vitamin K: Purpura

$K^+/Na^+/Ca^{2+}/Mg^{2+}$: Lethargy Weakness Cramps

Fe B_{12} Folate: Anaemia

Vitamins B_1 and B_6: Peripheral neuritis Dermatitis Cardiomyopathy

Vitamins D and Ca^{2+}: Osteomalacia

$Cu^{2+}/Zn^{2+}/Se$: Weakness Cardiac failure Poor wound healing

Fats

Micronutrients

Amino acids

Calories

Fluid volume

Electrolytes

VILLOUS ATROPHY WITH CRYPT HYPOPLASIA
- Ischaemia
- Irradiation
- Drug-induced
- Toxin damage

VILLOUS ATROPHY WITH CRYPT HYPERPLASIA
- Coeliac disease
- Post-infective
- Tropical sprue

NORMAL INTESTINAL ARCHITECTURE

Inadequate exocrine input to gut
- Chronic pancreatitis
- Pancreatectomy
- Liver disease

Enzymatic deficiencies
- Disaccharidases
- Proteases

Definition

Malabsorption is the failure of the body to acquire and conserve adequate amounts of one or more essential dietary elements. Encompasses a series of defects occurring during the digestion and absorption of nutrients from the GI tract. The cause may be localized or generalized.

Key points

- Malabsorption usually affects several nutrient groups.
- Coeliac disease is a common cause and may present with obscure, vague abdominal symptoms.
- Always consider micronutrients and trace elements in malabsorption.

Clinical features

- Diarrhoea (often watery from increased osmotic load).
- Steatorrhoea (from fat malabsorption).
- Weight loss and fatigue.
- Flatulence and abdominal distension (bacterial action on undigested food products).
- Oedema (hypoalbuminaemia).
- Anaemia (Fe^{2+}, vitamin B_{12}), bleeding disorders (vitamin K, vitamin C), bone pain, pathological fracture (vitamin D, Ca^{2+}).
- Neurological (Ca^{2+}, Mg^{2+}, folic acid, vitamin A, vitamin B_{12}).

Differential diagnosis

Coeliac disease

- Classically presents as sensitivity to gluten-containing foods with diarrhoea, steatorrhoea and weight loss in early adulthood.
- Mild forms may present later in life with non-specific symptoms of malaise, anaemia (including iron deficiency picture), abdominal cramps and weight loss.

Crohn's disease

- Most common presenting symptoms are colicky abdominal pains with diarrhoea and weight loss.
- Malabsorption is an uncommon presenting symptom but may accompany stenosing disease (secondary overgrowth from obstruction), inflammatory disease (widespread loss of functioning ileum) or after extensive or repeated resection.

Cystic fibrosis

- Most patients with CF have insufficiency of the exocrine pancreas from birth.
- Insufficient secretion of digestive enzymes (lipase) leads to malabsorption of fat (with steatorrhea) and protein.

Intestinal resection

- Global malabsorption may develop after small bowel resections leaving <50 cm of functional ileum. Water and electrolyte balance is most disordered but fat, vitamin and other nutrient absorption is also affected with lengths progressively <50 cm.
- Specific malabsorption may result from relatively small resection (e.g. fat and vitamin B_{12} malabsorption after terminal ileal resection, vitamin B_{12} and iron malabsorption after gastrectomy).

Whipple's disease (intestinal lipodystrophy)

- Intestinal infection *with Tropheryma whipplei* resulting in thickened club like villi and bacteria.
- Presents with steatorrhoea associated with arthralgia and malaise.

Bacterial overgrowth

- Malabsorption caused by bacterial metabolism of nutrients and production of breakdown products such as CO_2 and H_2.
- Usually a result of exclusion of a loop of ileum (e.g. in Crohn's disease, postsurgery, intestinal fistulation) with consequent bacterial overgrowth, although can occur in chronically damaged or dilated bowel.

Radiation enteropathy

- Slow onset, progressive global malabsorption. Usually only if large areas of ileum affected.
- May occur many years after original radiotherapy exposure.

Chronic ischaemic enteropathy

Rare cause of malabsorption. Usually accompanied by chronic intestinal ischaemia causing 'mesenteric angina/claudication' upon eating.

Parasitic infection

Common in tropics but rare in the UK.

Investigations

- FBC, U+E, LFTs, Ca: general nutritional status.
- Trace elements (Zn, Se, Mg, Mn, Cu).
- 72-hour faecal fat collection (detects fat malabsorption).
- Faecal calprotectin (detects chronic mucosal inflammation).
- D-xylose test (integrity of intestinal mucosa) (carbohydrate malabsorption).
- Hydrogen (lactose non-absorption) and bile salt (bile salt metabolism) breath tests.
- Schilling test (vitamin B_{12} deficiency) – intrinsic factor, pancreatic insufficiency, ileal resection/disease.
- Anti-tissue trans-glutaminase (ATA) and antigliadin antibodies (ATA) (serum assays); D2 biopsies (for coeliac disease).
- CT scan/MR enterography: best for Crohn's disease, radiation or ischaemic enteropathy and blind loop formation.
- Wireless capsule endoscopy.

Essential management

- Major deficiencies should be corrected by supplementation (oral or parenteral) (e.g. Pancrease or Creon for pancreatic exocine deficiency).
- Infectious causes should be excluded or (consider probiotics) treated promptly.
- Coeliac disease: gluten-free diet.
- Crohn's disease: usually requires resection of affected segment. Course of systemic steroids or immunosuppressive agents may help.
- Radiation or ischaemic malabsorption rarely responds to any medical therapy – often requires parenteral nutrition.

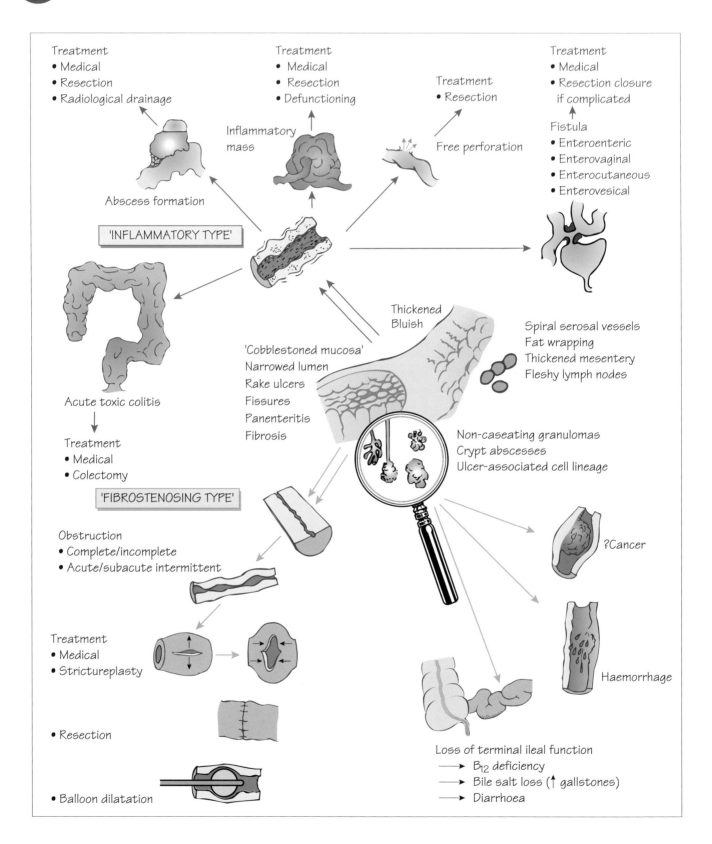

Treatment
- Medical
- Resection
- Radiological drainage

Abscess formation

Inflammatory mass

Treatment
- Medical
- Resection
- Defunctioning

Treatment
- Resection

Free perforation

Treatment
- Medical
- Resection closure if complicated

Fistula
- Enteroenteric
- Enterovaginal
- Enterocutaneous
- Enterovesical

'INFLAMMATORY TYPE'

Acute toxic colitis

Treatment
- Medical
- Colectomy

'FIBROSTENOSING TYPE'

Thickened
Bluish

'Cobblestoned mucosa'
Narrowed lumen
Rake ulcers
Fissures
Panenteritis
Fibrosis

Spiral serosal vessels
Fat wrapping
Thickened mesentery
Fleshy lymph nodes

Non-caseating granulomas
Crypt abscesses
Ulcer-associated cell lineage

?Cancer

Haemorrhage

Obstruction
- Complete/incomplete
- Acute/subacute intermittent

Treatment
- Medical
- Strictureplasty

- Resection

- Balloon dilatation

Loss of terminal ileal function
→ B_{12} deficiency
→ Bile salt loss (↑ gallstones)
→ Diarrhoea

Definition

Crohn's disease is a chronic transmural inflammatory disorder of unknown cause affecting the alimentary tract (any part from mouth to anus). Crohn's disease and ulcerative colitis together are referred to as *idiopathic inflammatory bowel disease.*

Key points

- May present with acute, subacute or chronic manifestations.
- Perianal disease is common and may be the presenting feature.
- Increasingly seen in children of all ages.
- Immunomodulation and biological agents are the mainstay of Rx.
- Surgery is common but not curative and should be used sparingly.
- Chronic disabling disease with recurrent relapses. 10% of sufferers disabled by the disease.

Epidemiology

Male:female 1:1.6. Young adults. High incidence among Europeans and Jewish people. Family tendency to the disease.

Aetiology

- Unknown.
- Genetic link probable. Following genes may be involved: *NOD2/CARD-15, IBD-3, IBD-5, IL23R, ATg16L1.*
- Impaired cell-mediated immunity. Chronic inflammation from Th-1 cell activation producing IL-12, TNF-α, IFN-γ.
- Smoking doubles the risk of relapse of Crohn's disease.
- No proven link to mycobacterial infection or measles virus hypersensitivity.

Pathology

Macroscopic

- May affect any part of the alimentary tract.
- Skip lesions in bowel (affected bowel wall and mesentery are thickened and oedematous, frequent fistulae).
- Affected bowel characteristically 'fat wrapped' by mesenteric fat.
- Perianal disease characterized by perianal induration (blue skin discoloration) and sepsis with fissure, sinus and fistula formation.

Histology

- Transmural inflammation in the form of lymphoid aggregates.
- Non-caseating epithelioid cell granulomas with Langhans giant cells. Regional nodes may also be involved.

Clinical features

Acute presentations (uncommon)

- RIF peritonitis (like appendicitis picture).
- Generalized peritonitis (due to free perforation).
- Acute colitis: uncommon as primary presentation.

Subacute presentations (common)

- RIF inflammatory mass (often ± fistulae or abscesses).
- Widespread ileal inflammation: general ill health, malnutrition, anaemia, abdominal pain.
- Colitis: abdominal pain and bloody diarrhoea.

Chronic presentations

- Strictures: intermittent colicky abdominal pains associated with eating – 'food fear'.
- Malabsorption (due to widespread disease often with previous resections).
- Growth retardation in children (due to chronic malnutrition and chronic inflammatory response suppressing growth).

Perianal disease

- Up to one-third of patients may have perianal disease.
- Large, oedematous, 'blueish' skin tags typical.
- Fissure-*in-ano*, fistula-*in-ano*, perianal sepsis.

Extraintestinal features

- Eye: episcleritis, uveitis.
- Acute phase proteins, e.g. CRP.
- Joints: arthritis (sacroiliac joint arthritis, ankylosing spondylitis).
- Skin: erythema nodosum, pyoderma gangrenosum.
- Liver: sclerosing cholangitis, cirrhosis.

Investigations

- FBC: macrocytic anaemia, WBC raised, ESR raised.
- Acute phase proteins, e.g. CRP.
- Small bowel enema: narrowed terminal ileum, 'string sign' of Kantor, stricture formation, fistulae.
- Abdominal ultrasound: RIF mass, abscess formation.
- CT scan: RIF mass, abscess formation.
- Colonoscopy and intubation of terminal ileum and biopsy.
- Indium-labelled white-cell scan: areas of inflammation.
- Video capsule endoscopy.

Essential management

Aims of treatment

There is no cure for Crohn's disease. Rx aims to induce and maintain remission, minimize side effects of therapy and improve QoL.

Medical – 'Step up' approach
- Step 1. Nutritional support (enteral and parenteral feeding, (semi)elemental diet):
  anti-inflammatory drugs: 5-ASA (mesalazine)
  antibiotics (metronidazole, ciprofloxin) (complicating bacterial infection).
- Step 2. Immunodulation:
  corticosteroids – systemic (prednisone) or topical (budesonide) inhibitors of DNA synthesis (6-mercaptopurine, azathioprine, methotrexate).
- Step 3. Biological therapy (anti-TNF-α agents: infiximab, adalimumab and certolizumab-pegol) or surgery.

Surgical

For:
- Complications (peritonitis, obstruction, abscess, fistula).
- Failure of medical treatment and persisting symptoms.
- Growth retardation in children.
- Principles – resect minimum necessary, conserve length (e.g. strictureplasty). Stomas (often temporary) may be treatment (to defunction-involved distal bowel) or necessary (anastomosis unsafe). Laparoscopic surgery increasing used.

Prognosis

- Crohn's disease is a chronic problem, and recurrent episodes of active disease are common.
- 75% of patients will require surgery at some time.
- 60% of patients will require more than one operation.
- Crohn's disease patients have normal life expectancy.

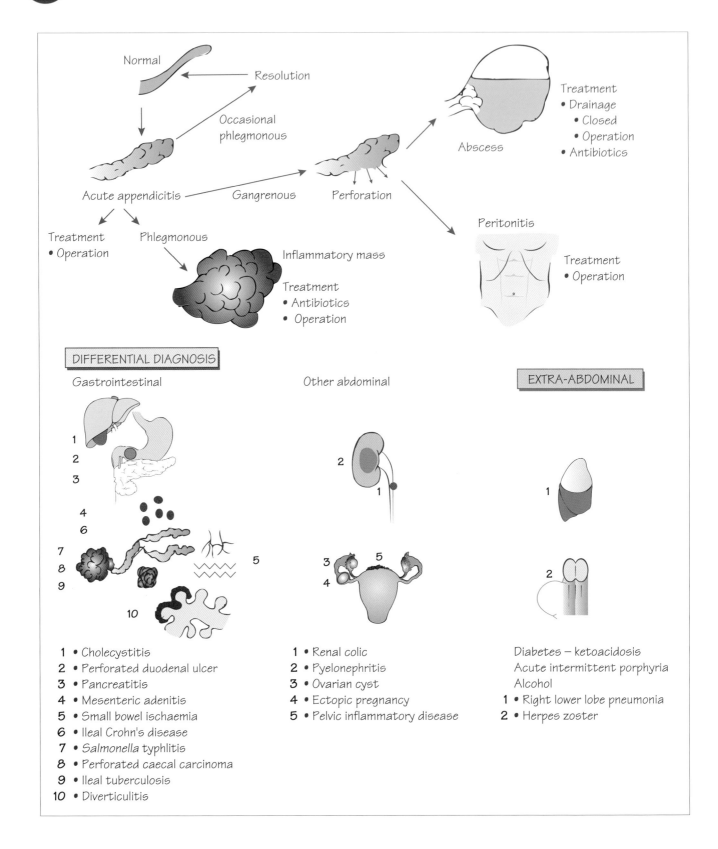

Normal

Resolution

Occasional
phlegmonous

Acute appendicitis

Gangrenous

Perforation

Abscess

Treatment
• Drainage
  • Closed
  • Operation
• Antibiotics

Treatment
• Operation

Phlegmonous

Inflammatory mass

Treatment
• Antibiotics
• Operation

Peritonitis

Treatment
• Operation

DIFFERENTIAL DIAGNOSIS

Gastrointestinal

Other abdominal

EXTRA-ABDOMINAL

1 • Cholecystitis
2 • Perforated duodenal ulcer
3 • Pancreatitis
4 • Mesenteric adenitis
5 • Small bowel ischaemia
6 • Ileal Crohn's disease
7 • Salmonella typhlitis
8 • Perforated caecal carcinoma
9 • Ileal tuberculosis
10 • Diverticulitis

1 • Renal colic
2 • Pyelonephritis
3 • Ovarian cyst
4 • Ectopic pregnancy
5 • Pelvic inflammatory disease

Diabetes – ketoacidosis
Acute intermittent porphyria
Alcohol
1 • Right lower lobe pneumonia
2 • Herpes zoster

Definition

Acute appendicitis is an inflammation of the vermiform appendix.

Key points

- 70% of cases of RIF pain in children <10 years are non-specific and self-limiting.
- The most common differential diagnosis in young women is ovarian pathology.
- RIF peritonism >55 years should raise the suspicion of other causes.
- CT imaging should be obtained whenever there is real concern about the diagnosis to prevent inappropriate surgical exploration.
- Laparoscopy is the diagnostic and therapeutic option of choice when the diagnosis is strongly suspected.

Epidemiology

Most common surgical emergency in the Western world. Rare <2 years, common in second and third decades, can occur at any age.

Pathology

- 'Obstructive': infection superimposed on luminal obstruction from any cause.
- 'Phlegmonous': viral infection, lymphoid hyperplasia, ulceration, bacterial invasion without obvious cause.
- 'Necrotic': usually secondary to obstructive causes with secondary infarction.

Clinical features

- Periumbilical abdominal pain, nausea, vomiting.
- Localization of pain to RIF.
- Mild pyrexia.
- Patient is flushed, tachycardia, furred tongue, halitosis.
- Tender (usually with rebound) over McBurney's point.
- Right-sided pelvic tenderness on PR examination (not indicated in children or most adults).
- Peritonitis if appendix perforated.
- Appendix mass if patient presents late (>5 days).

Investigations

- Diagnosis is a clinical diagnosis, but WCC (almost always leucocytosis) and CRP (usually raised) are helpful.
- Laparoscopy commonly used to exclude ovarian pathology in young women.
- Ultrasound: may show appendix mass or other pelvic pathology (e.g. ovarian cyst). May confirm appendicitis but *cannot* rule it out.
- CT scan: most accurate non-invasive test for appendicitis. Use when diagnosis unclear but care in young adults (radiation exposure).
- Colonoscopy – to exclude underlying caecal pathology in adults with an appendix mass.

Differential diagnosis

- Mesenteric lymphadenitis and acute non-specific abdominal pain (ANSAP) in children.
- Pelvic disease in women (e.g. PID, UTIs, ectopic pregnancy, ruptured corpus luteum cyst).
- Occasionally: perforated caecal carcinoma, sigmoid diverticulitis, caecal diverticulitis in elderly patients.
- More rarely: Crohn's disease, cholecystitis, perforated duodenal ulcer, right basal pneumonia, torsion of the right testis, diabetes mellitus, appendiceal carcinoma/mucinous adenoma.

Essential management

- Acute appendicitis: appendicectomy, laparoscopic (open if large phlegmon or complicated) after IV fluids and peri-operative antibiotics for gram-negative and anaerobic pathogens
- Appendix mass: IV fluids, antibiotics, close observation. Then: if symptoms resolve observe ± interval appendicectomy after 2–3 months (after colonoscopy in adults) (trend is towards *not performing* interval appendicectomy routinely) if symptoms progress, urgent appendicectomy ± drainage.

Complications

- Wound infection.
- Intra-abdominal abscess (pelvic, RIF, subphrenic).
- Adhesions.
- Abdominal actinomycosis (rare).
- Portal pyaemia.

50 Diverticular disease

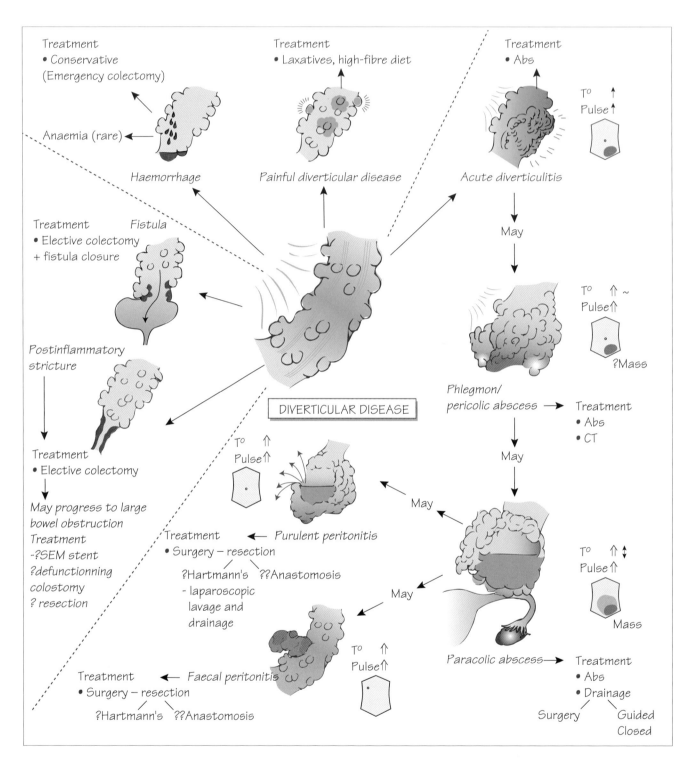

Treatment
• Conservative
(Emergency colectomy)

Anaemia (rare)

Haemorrhage

Treatment
• Laxatives, high-fibre diet

Painful diverticular disease

Treatment
• Abs

T° ↑
Pulse ↑

Acute diverticulitis

May

T° ↑ ~
Pulse ↑

?Mass

Phlegmon/
pericolic abscess → Treatment
• Abs
• CT

Treatment   Fistula
• Elective colectomy
+ fistula closure

Postinflammatory
stricture

Treatment
• Elective colectomy

May progress to large
bowel obstruction
Treatment
-?SEM stent
?defunctionning
colostomy
? resection

DIVERTICULAR DISEASE

May

T° ↑
Pulse ↑

Treatment   ← Purulent peritonitis
• Surgery – resection
   ?Hartmann's   ??Anastomosis
   - laparoscopic
   lavage and
   drainage

May

T° ↑ ↕
Pulse ↑

Mass

Paracolic abscess → Treatment
• Abs
• Drainage
Surgery   Guided
                Closed

T° ↑
Pulse ↑

Treatment   ← Faecal peritonitis
• Surgery – resection
   ?Hartmann's   ??Anastomosis

 Surgery at a Glance, Fifth Edition. Pierce A. Grace and Neil R. Borley. © 2013 John Wiley & Sons, Ltd. Published 2013 by John Wiley & Sons, Ltd.

Definition

Diverticular disease (or diverticulosis) is a condition in which many sac-like mucosal projections (diverticula) develop in the large bowel, especially the sigmoid colon. Acute inflammation of a diverticulum causes *diverticulitis*.

Key points

- Most diverticular disease is asymptomatic.
- The majority of acute attacks resolve with non-surgical Rx.
- Emergency surgery for complications has a high morbidity and mortality and often involves an intestinal stoma.
- Elective surgery should be reserved for recurrent proven symptoms and complications (e.g. stricture).
- 'Diverticular' strictures should be biopsied in case of underlying colon carcinoma.

Epidemiology

Male:female 1:1.5, peak incidence 40s and 50s onwards. High incidence in the Western world where it is found in 50% of people over 60 years.

Aetiology

- Low fibre in the diet causes an increase in intraluminal colonic pressure, resulting in herniation of the mucosa through the muscle coats of the wall of the colon.
- Weak areas in wall of colon where nutrient arteries penetrate to submucosa and mucosa.
- Occasional family history especially in pan-colonic disease.

Pathology

Macroscopic

- Diverticula can be anywhere in the colon but mostly in the sigmoid colon.
- Emerge between the taenia coli and may contain faecoliths.

Histological

Projections are *acquired diverticula* as they contain only mucosa, submucosa and serosa and not all layers of intestinal wall.

Clinical features

- Mostly asymptomatic.
- Painful diverticulosis: LIF pain, constipation, diarrhoea.
- Acute diverticulitis: malaise, fever, LIF pain and tenderness ± palpable mass and abdominal distension.
- Perforation: peritonitis + features of diverticulitis.
- Large bowel obstruction: absolute constipation, distension, colicky abdominal pain and vomiting.
- Fistula: to bladder (cystitis/pneumaturia/recurrent UTIs); to vagina (faecal discharge PV); to small intestine (diarrhoea).
- Lower GI bleed: painless spontaneous – distinguish from angiodysplasia.
- Diverticular colitis (segmental colitis) – rare.

Investigations

- Diverticulosis: colonoscopy or barium enema + flexible sigmoidoscopy.
- Diverticulitis: FBC, WCC, U+E, chest X-ray, CT scan.
- ? Diverticular mass/paracolic abscess: CT scan.
- ? Perforation: plain film of abdomen, CT scan.
- ? Obstruction: water soluble contrast enema, CT scan, colonoscopy to exclude underlying malignancy if no LBO.
- ? Fistula:
  colovesical: MSU, cystoscopy, barium enema, CT scan.
  colovaginal: colposcopy, flexible sigmoidoscopy, CT scan.
- Haemorrhage: colonoscopy, selective angiography.

Essential management

Medical
Painful or asymptomatic
High-fibre diet (fruit, vegetables, wholemeal breads, bran). Increase fluid intake.

Acute diverticulitis

- Antibiotics (e.g. amoxicillin-clavulanate + metronidazole × 7–10 days).
- Radiologically guided drainage for localized abscess. Usually for complications/recurrent, proven acute attacks or failed medical treatment.
- Elective surgery: resect diseased colon and primary anastomosis, may be laparoscopic.
- Emergency left colon surgery with *diffuse* peritonitis: resect diseased segment, oversew distal bowel (i.e. upper rectum) and bring out proximal bowel as end-colostomy (Hartmann's procedure).
- Emergency left colon surgery with *limited or no* peritonitis: laparoscopic peritoneal lavage and drainage or resect diseased segment and primary anastomosis with defunctioning proximal stoma.
- Complicated left colon surgery (e.g. colovesical fistula): resection, primary anastomosis (may have defunctioning proximal stoma) may be laparoscopic.

Prognosis

Diverticular disease is a 'benign' condition, but there is significant mortality and morbidity from the complications.

Hinchey classification of acute diverticulitis

- Ia – localized colic sepsis (e.g. phlegmon).
- Ib – localized paracolic sepsis (e.g. peri-colic or intramesenteric abscess).
- II – localized intrapelvic sepsis (e.g. pelvic abscess).
- III – purulent peritonitis (free gas and purulent fluid).
- IV – faeculent peritonitis (free faeces or faeculent fluid).

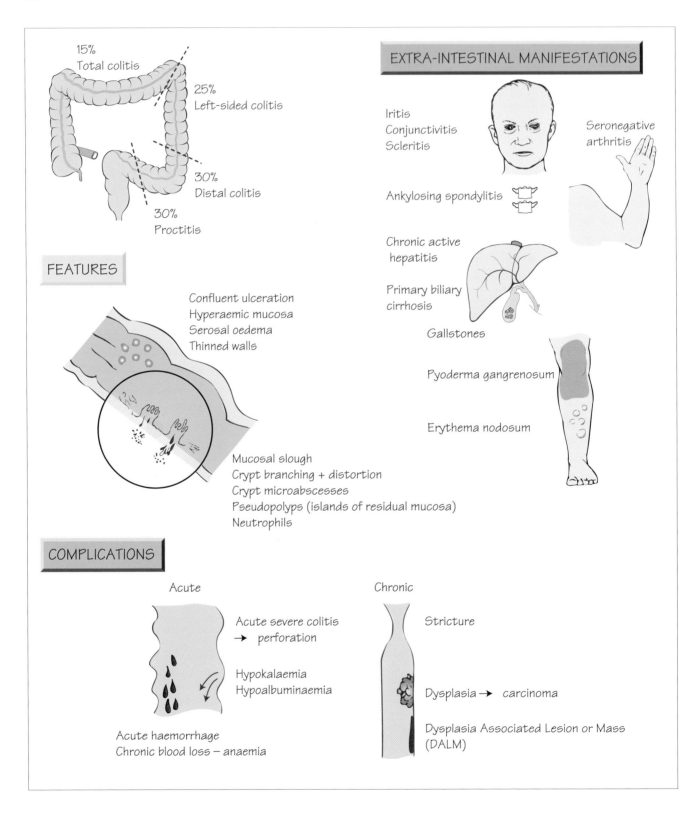

15%
Total colitis

25%
Left-sided colitis

30%
Distal colitis

30%
Proctitis

EXTRA-INTESTINAL MANIFESTATIONS

Iritis
Conjunctivitis
Scleritis

Seronegative arthritis

Ankylosing spondylitis

Chronic active hepatitis

Primary biliary cirrhosis

Gallstones

Pyoderma gangrenosum

Erythema nodosum

FEATURES

Confluent ulceration
Hyperaemic mucosa
Serosal oedema
Thinned walls

Mucosal slough
Crypt branching + distortion
Crypt microabscesses
Pseudopolyps (islands of residual mucosa)
Neutrophils

COMPLICATIONS

Acute

Acute severe colitis
→ perforation

Hypokalaemia
Hypoalbuminaemia

Acute haemorrhage
Chronic blood loss – anaemia

Chronic

Stricture

Dysplasia → carcinoma

Dysplasia Associated Lesion or Mass (DALM)

Definition

A chronic inflammatory disorder of unknown cause of the colonic mucosa, usually beginning in the rectum and extending proximally to a variable extent. Ulcerative colitis and Crohn's disease together are referred to as *idiopathic inflammatory bowel disease.*

Epidemiology

Male:female 1:1.6, peak incidence 30–50 years. High incidence among relatives of patients (up to 40%) and among Europeans and people of Jewish descent.

Aetiology

- Uncertain but definite genetic linkage: increased prevalence (10%) in relatives, associated with HLA-B27 phenotype. Similar genes implicated in UC and Crohn's disease.
- Autoimmune basis – autoantibodies against intestinal epithelial cells, ANCA, ASCA.
- Association with increased sulphide in GI tract, decreased vitamins A and E, NSAID use, milk consumption.
- Smoking 'protects' against relapse.

Pathology

Disease confined to colon, rectum always involved, may be 'backwash' ileitis.

Macroscopic

In simple disease, only the mucosa is involved with superficial ulceration, exudation and pseudopolyposis. In severe disease, the full thickness of the colon wall may become involved in inflammation.

Histological

Mucin depletion, crypt abscess formation, acute neutrophilic infiltrate in severe disease, inflammatory pseudopolyps and highly vascular granulation tissue. Epithelial dysplasia with long-standing disease. (Sub)mucosal atrophy and fibrosis in chronic, 'burnt out' disease.

Clinical features

Disease distribution is 'distal to proximal'; rectum almost always involved with (sequentially) sigmoid, left side, pan colon involvement. Rectum rarely spared. Caecum may have isolated 'patch' of inflammation.

Proctitis

- Mucus, pus and blood PR.
- Urgency and frequency (diarrhoea less prominent).

Left-sided colitis → total colitis

Symptoms of proctitis + increasing features of systemic upset, abdominal pain, anorexia, weight loss and anaemia with more extensive disease.

Extraintestinal features

Percentage involved:
- Joints: arthritis (25%).
- Eye: uveitis (10%).
- Skin: erythema nodosum, pyoderma gangrenosum (10%).

- Liver: pericholangitis, fatty liver (3%), primary sclerosing cholangitis.
- Blood: thromboembolic disease (rare).

Severe/fulminant disease

- 6–20 bloody bowel motions per day/dehydration.
- Fever, anaemia, dehydration, electrolyte imbalance.
- Colonic dilatation/perforation – 'toxic megacolon'/shock.

Investigations

- FBC: iron deficiency anaemia. WBC raised, ESR raised.
- Serological markers: ANCA and pANCA as with UC, ASCA more with Crohn's disease.
- Stool culture + C. difficile toxin: exclude infective colitis before treatment.
- Plain abdominal radiograph: colonic dilatation or air under diaphragm indicating perforation in fulminant colitis.
- Double-contrast barium enema: loss of haustrations, shortened 'lead pipe' colon.
- Radionuclide studies useful in acute fulminant colitis.
- Sigmoidoscopy: inflamed friable mucosa, bleeds to touch.
- Colonoscopy: extent of disease at presentation, evaluation of response to treatment after exacerbations, screening of long-standing disease for dysplasia.
- Biopsy: typical histological features.

Prognosis

Ulcerative colitis is a chronic problem that requires constant surveillance unless surgery, which is drastic but curative, is performed.

52 Colorectal carcinoma

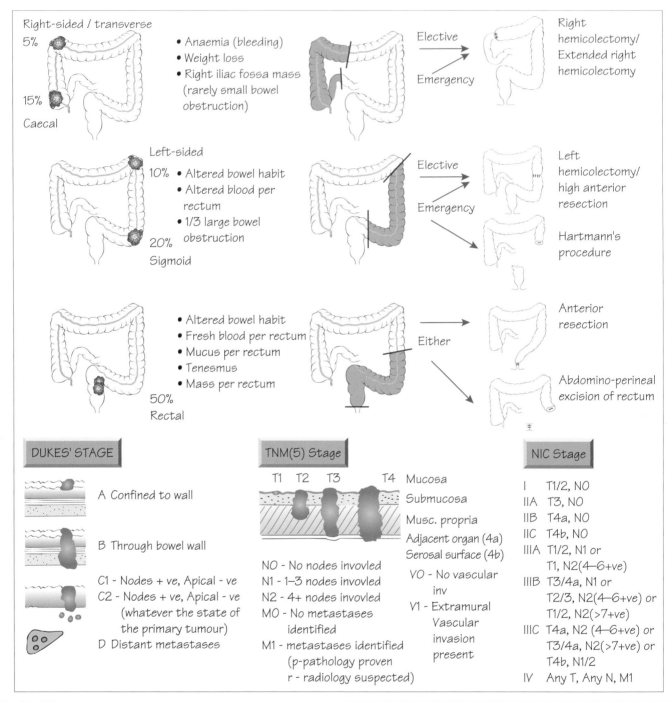

Right-sided / transverse
5%
15%
Caecal

- Anaemia (bleeding)
- Weight loss
- Right iliac fossa mass (rarely small bowel obstruction)

Elective
Emergency

Right hemicolectomy/ Extended right hemicolectomy

Left-sided
10%
20%
Sigmoid

- Altered bowel habit
- Altered blood per rectum
- 1/3 large bowel obstruction

Elective
Emergency

Left hemicolectomy/ high anterior resection

Hartmann's procedure

- Altered bowel habit
- Fresh blood per rectum
- Mucus per rectum
- Tenesmus
- Mass per rectum

50%
Rectal

Either

Anterior resection

Abdomino-perineal excision of rectum

DUKES' STAGE

A Confined to wall

B Through bowel wall

C1 - Nodes + ve, Apical - ve
C2 - Nodes + ve, Apical - ve (whatever the state of the primary tumour)
D Distant metastases

TNM(5) Stage

T1   T2   T3   T4   Mucosa
Submucosa
Musc. propria
Adjacent organ (4a)
Serosal surface (4b)

NO - No nodes invovled
N1 - 1–3 nodes invovled
N2 - 4+ nodes invovled
MO - No metastases identified
M1 - metastases identified (p-pathology proven r - radiology suspected)

VO - No vascular inv
V1 - Extramural Vascular invasion present

NIC Stage

I   T1/2, NO
IIA   T3, NO
IIB   T4a, NO
IIC   T4b, NO
IIIA T1/2, N1 or T1, N2(4–6+ve)
IIIB T3/4a, N1 or T2/3, N2(4–6+ve) or T1/2, N2(>7+ve)
IIIC T4a, N2 (4–6+ve) or T3/4a, N2(>7+ve) or T4b, N1/2
IV   Any T, Any N, M1

Definition

Colorectal carcinoma (CRC) describes malignant lesions in the mucosa of the colon (65%) or rectum (35%).

Key points

- Genetic factors have an important role in the pathogenesis of CRC.
- Sequence of progression from normal mucosa to adenoma-carcinoma

- Most colorectal cancers are left-sided with symptoms of, pain, bleeding or altered bowel habit.
- Prognosis depends mainly on stage at diagnosis.
- Surgery is the only curative treatment. Chemotherapy and radiotherapy are (neo)adjuvant therapies.
- Screening with guaiac faecal occult blood testing (gFOBT) reduces mortality from CRC.
- 20% of patients with CRC present as emergencies.

 Surgery at a Glance, Fifth Edition. Pierce A. Grace and Neil R. Borley. © 2013 John Wiley & Sons, Ltd. Published 2013 by John Wiley & Sons, Ltd.

Epidemiology

Male:female 1.3:1, peak incidence 50+ years increasing in the West.

Aetiology

Predisposing factors in decreasing importance:
- Personal history of CRC or adenomatous polyps.
- Hereditary syndromes (e.g. familial adenomatous polyposis (FAP), Lynch syndrome (HNPCC), juvenile polyposis syndrome,).
- Family history of CRC: having single first degree relative with CRC increases risk × 2
- Inflammatory bowel disease, especially UC.
- Acromegaly – increased colonic adenomas and CRC.
- Obesity, alcohol, smoking, diabetes mellitus, coronary heart disease, renal transplantation, cholecystectomy all associated with increased risk of CRC.
- NSAIDs protect against CRC, as may physical activity, calcium, statins and diet high in vegetables and low in processed/charred red meat.

Pathology

Macroscopic

- Polypoid, ulcerating, annular, infiltrative.
- 75% of lesions are within rectum, sigmoid or left colon.
- 3% are synchronous (i.e. 2nd lesion found at the same time) and 3% are metachronous (i.e. 2nd lesion found later).

Histological

- Adenocarcinoma (10–15% are mucinous adenocarcinoma).
- Staging by TNM classification (Dukes [A–D] not used anymore).
- Spread: lymphatic, haematogenous, peritoneal.

Clinical features

- Colicky abdominal pain (44%) – tumours which are causing partial obstruction, e.g. transverse or descending colonic lesions
- Alteration in bowel habit (43%) – either constipation or diarrhoea.
- Bleeding (40%), passage of mucus PR, *tenesmus* (frequent or continuous desire to defaecate) – rectal tumour.
- Weakness (20%).
- Anaemia (11%) – caecal cancers often present with anaemia.
- Weight loss (6%).

Investigations

- Digital rectal examination and faecal occult blood.
- FBC: anaemia.
- U+E: hypokalaemia, LFTs: liver metastases.
- Endoscopy: sigmoidoscopy (rigid to 30 cm/flexible to 60 cm) and colonoscopy (whole colon) – see the lesion, obtain biopsy.
- Double-contrast barium enema – 'apple core lesion', polyp.
- CT colonography ('virtual colonoscopy') with air or CO_2 pneumocolon.
- Preoperative CEA measured for prognostic significance and measure of surgical clearance.
- Trans rectal ultrasound (TRUS) ± MRI to assess primary tumour invasion in rectal cancer.

Essential management

Surgery (potentially curative)

Resection of the tumour with adequate margins to include regional lymph nodes is definitive treatment. Sentinel node biopsy not accurate in CRC.

Procedures

- Resections may be open or laparoscopic ± mechanical bowel preparation.
- Right hemicolectomy: lesions from caecum to hepatic flexure.
- Extended right hemicolectomy: lesions of the transverse colon.
- Left hemicolectomy (rare): lesions of the descending colon.
- Anterior resection excision for sigmoid colon and rectal tumours (total mesorectal excision for rectal tumours) ± proximal defunctioning stoma.
- Abdomino-perineal resection and colostomy for very low rectal lesions.
- Hartmann's procedure or resection with primary anastomosis for emergency surgery to left-sided colon tumours.
- Resection should be considered for liver or lung metastases if anatomically resectable with no evidence of other disseminated disease.
- Some rectal tumours are amenable to local excision (e.g. early T1, polyp cancer).

Surgery/interventions (palliative)

- Resection of the tumour (with anastomosis or stoma) for obstructing or symptomatic cancers despite metastases.
- Surgical bypass or defunctioning stoma for obstructing inoperable cancers.
- Transanal resection for symptomatic inoperable rectal cancer.
- Intraluminal stents for obstructing cancers.

Other treatment

- Neoadjuvant chemoradiotherapy indicated for T3–T4/N0/M0 or T1–T2/N1/M0 *rectal* cancers.
- Adjuvant radiotherapy should be offered to T4 *colon* cancers or positive resection margin.
- Adjuvant chemotherapy for Stage III (node positive) *colon* cancer – reduces recurrence and mortality. Benefit in Stage II disease controversial – *Oncotype DX®* colon cancer 12 gene assay may help.
- Palliative chemotherapy used to prolong survival in patients with unresectable CRC.

Prognosis

- 5-year survival depends on staging – Stage I (75%), Stage II (55%), Stage III (45%), Stage IV (6%). Stages II and III have subgroups with slightly better (A) or worse (B, C) outcomes.
- 25% 5-year survival after successful resections of liver metastases.

2-week wait referral criteria for suspected colorectal cancer

- Rectal bleeding + increased frequency or loose stools >6 weeks.
- Rectal bleeding without anal symptoms.
- Increased frequency or looser stools ?6 weeks.
- Rectal mass.
- Right-sided abdominal mass.
- Iron deficiency anaemia without obvious cause.

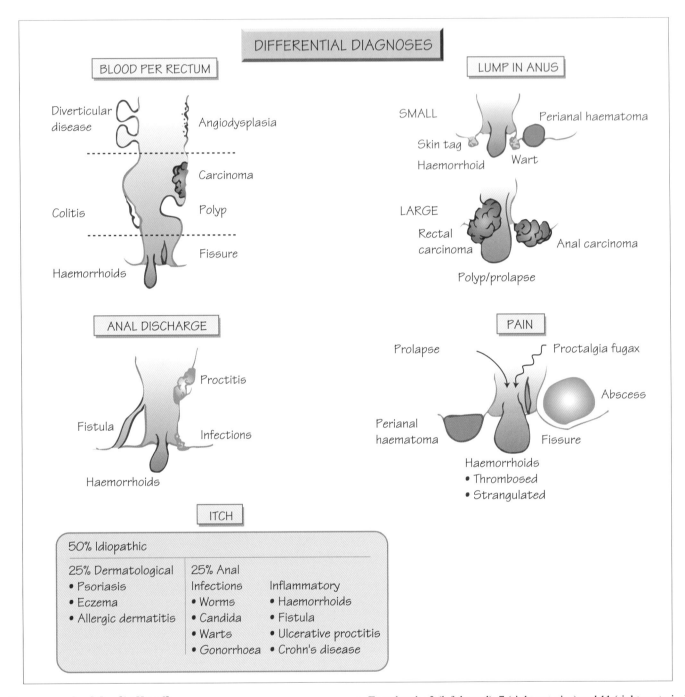

Haemorrhoids ('piles')

Definition

A submucosal swelling in the anal canal consisting of a dilated venous plexus, a small artery and areolar tissue. *Internal*: only involves tissue of upper anal canal above dentate line. *External*: involves tissue of lower anal canal below dentate line.

Aetiology

• Increased venous pressure from straining (low-fibre diet) or altered haemodynamics (e.g. during pregnancy) causes chronic dilation of submucosal venous plexus.

• Found at the 3 (left lateral), 7 (right anterior) and 11 (right posterior) o'clock positions in the anal canal.

Classification

• First degree: bulge into lumen but do not prolapse.

• Second degree: prolapse during defaecation with spontaneous reduction.

• Third degree: prolapse during defaecation and require manual reduction.

• Fourth degree: irreducible and may strangulate.

Clinical features
- Bright red bleeding – on toilet tissue or staining toilet.
- Pruritus – may be leakage of rectal contents.
- Pain – associated with thrombosis.
- Prolapse – the haemorrhoid prolapses out of the anal canal.
- Thrombosis – very painful when in external haemorrhoid

Treatment
- 1st degree: bulk laxatives, high fluid and fibre diet.
- 2nd degree (some 3rd degree): rubber band (Barron's) ligation, injection sclerotherapy, cryosurgery.
- 4th degree: haemorrhoidectomy (closed/open/stapled) (complications: bleeding, anal stenosis, pain). Haemorrhoidal artery ligation operation (HALO) – uses Doppler to identify haemorrhoidal artery which is then ligated – no need for general anaesthetic.

Rectal prolapse
Definition
The protrusion from the anus to a variable degree of the rectal mucosa (partial) or rectal wall (full thickness).

Aetiology
Rectal intussusception, poor sphincter tone, chronic straining, pelvic floor injury.

Clinical features
Faecal incontinence, constipation, mucous discharge, bleeding, tenesmus, obvious prolapse. 10% of children with prolapse have cystic fibrosis.

Treatment
Manual reduction. Treat underlying cause. Prolapse in young children is normally self-resolving and associated with straining. Surgery: Delorme's perianal mucosal resection, laparoscopic or open surgical rectopexy ± sigmoid resection (rectum is 'hitched' up on to sacrum).

Perianal haematoma
Very painful subcutaneous haematoma caused by rupture of small blood vessel in the perianal area. Evacuation of the clot provides instant relief.

Anal fissure
Definition
Longitudinal tear in the mucosa of the anal canal, in the midline posteriorly (90%) or anteriorly (10%).

Aetiology
- 90% caused by local trauma during passage of hard stool and potentiated by spasm of the exposed internal anal sphincter.
- Other causes: pregnancy/delivery, Crohn's disease, sexually transmitted infections (often lateral position), carcinoma of the anus.

Clinical features
Exquisitely painful on passing bowel motion, small amount of bright red blood on toilet tissue, severe sphincter spasm, skin tag at distal end of tear ('sentinel pile').

Treatment
- First-line: stool softeners/bulking agents, LA gels, 0.2/0.4 % nitroglycerine ointment.

- Second-line: botulinum toxin injection (especially in women), topical calcium-channel blockers, lateral internal sphincterotomy (cures 95% but may result in minor incontinence in 10% of patients).
- EUA and biopsy for atypical/suspicious abnormal fissures (e.g. Crohn's disease).

Perianal abscess
Aetiology
Focus of infection starts in anal glands ('cryptoglandular sepsis') and spreads into perianal tissues to cause:
- Perianal abscess: adjacent to anal margin.
- Ischioanal abscess: in ischioanal fossa.
- Para-rectal abscess: above levator ani.
  Recurrent abscesses are likely to be due to underlying fistula *in ano*.

Clinical features
Painful, red, tender, swollen mass ± fever, rigors, sweating, tachycardia.

Treatment
Incision and drainage, antibiotics.

Fistula-in-ano
Definition and aetiology
Abnormal communication between the perianal skin and the anal canal. Commonest cryptoglandular, also associated with Crohn's and TB.
- Low: below 50% of the EAS.
- High: crossing 50% or more of the EAS.

Clinical features
Chronic perianal discharge, external orifice of track with granulation tissue seen perianally.

Treatment
- Low: probing and laying open the track (fistulotomy).
- High: seton insertion, core removal of the fistula track, fibrin glue, collagen plug.
- Complex fistulas may need endoanal or endorectal advancement flap to close internal opening of fistula, cutting seton/staged surgery.

Pilonidal sinus
Definition
A blind-ending track containing hairs in the skin of the natal cleft. *Pilus* = hair, *nidus* = nest.

Aetiology
May be trauma (promotes hair migration into the skin) or congenital (natal cleft sinus).

Clinical features
May present as: natal cleft abscess, discharging sinus in midline posterior to anal margin with hair protruding from orifice, natal cleft itch/pain. May occur on dorsum of hands between fingers in barbers or shepherds.

Treatment
Good personal hygiene and removal of hair. Incision and drainage of abscesses, excision of sinus network with primary or delayed closure or tissue flap (asymmetric cleft closure).

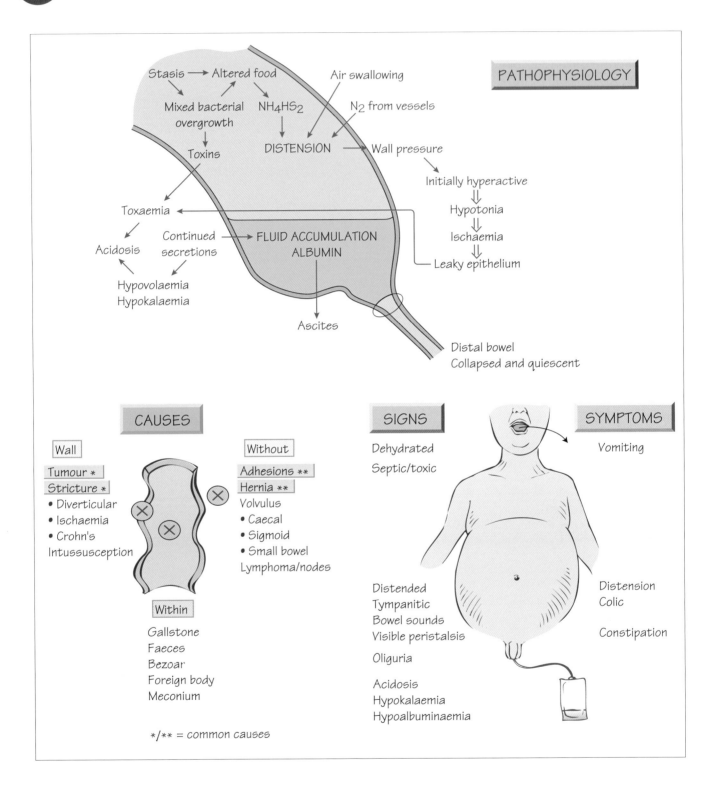

PATHOPHYSIOLOGY

Stasis → Altered food   Air swallowing

Mixed bacterial overgrowth NH_4HS_2 N_2 from vessels

Toxins   DISTENSION → Wall pressure

Initially hyperactive

⇓

Hypotonia

⇓

Ischaemia

⇓

Leaky epithelium

Toxaemia ←

Acidosis   Continued secretions → FLUID ACCUMULATION ALBUMIN

Hypovolaemia
Hypokalaemia

Ascites

Distal bowel
Collapsed and quiescent

CAUSES

Wall

Tumour *
Stricture *
• Diverticular
• Ischaemia
• Crohn's
Intussusception

Within

Gallstone
Faeces
Bezoar
Foreign body
Meconium

Without

Adhesions **
Hernia **
Volvulus
• Caecal
• Sigmoid
• Small bowel
Lymphoma/nodes

*/** = common causes

SIGNS

Dehydrated
Septic/toxic

Distended
Tympanitic
Bowel sounds
Visible peristalsis

Oliguria

Acidosis
Hypokalaemia
Hypoalbuminaemia

SYMPTOMS

Vomiting

Distension
Colic

Constipation

Definitions

Complete intestinal obstruction indicates total blockage of the intestinal lumen, whereas *incomplete* denotes only a partial blockage. Obstruction may be *acute* (hours) or *chronic* (weeks), *simple (mechanical)*, i.e. blood supply is not compromised, or *strangulated*, i.e. blood supply is compromised. A *closed loop obstruction* indicates that both the inlet and outlet of a bowel loop is closed off. A *volvulus* is an abnormal twisting of a segment of the bowel causing intestinal obstruction and possible ischaemia and gangrene of the twisted segment.

> ### Key points
> - Small bowel obstruction is often rapid in onset and commonly due to adhesions or hernia.
> - Large bowel obstruction may be gradual or intermittent in onset, is often due to carcinoma or strictures and never due to adhesions alone.
> - All obstructed patients need fluid and electrolyte replacement.
> - Many patients with adhesion small bowel obstruction will settle on conservative Rx.
> - The cause should be sought and confirmed wherever possible prior to operation.
> - Tachycardia, pyrexia and abdominal tenderness indicate the need to operate whatever the cause.

Common causes

- Extramural: adhesions, bands, volvulus, hernias (internal and external), compression by tumour (e.g. frozen pelvis).
- Intramural: inflammatory bowel disease (Crohn's disease), tumours, carcinomas, lymphomas, strictures, paralytic: (adynamic) ileus, intussusception.
- Intraluminal: faecal impaction, foreign bodies, bezoars, gallstone ileus.

Anatomical classification
Small bowel obstruction
Duodenum
- Adults: carcinoma of pancreas or periampullary carcinoma, chronic peptic ulcer disease.
- Neonates: duodenal atresia, annular pancreas, congenital bands.

Jejunum/ileum
- Adults: adhesions, hernias, foreign body, tumours, Crohn's disease, Meckel's diverticulum.
- Neonates: meconium ileus, volvulus of malrotated gut, atresia, intussusception.

Large bowel obstruction
Colon
- Adults: tumours (usually left colon), diverticulitis, sigmoid volvulus, pseudo-obstruction.
- Neonates: Hirschsprung's disease, anal atresia.

Pathophysiology
- Bowel distal to obstruction collapses.
- Bowel proximal to obstruction distends and becomes hyperactive. Distension is due to swallowed air and accumulating intestinal secretions.
- The bowel wall becomes oedematous. Fluid and electrolytes accumulate in the wall and lumen (third space loss).
- Bacteria proliferate in the obstructed bowel.
- As the bowel distends, the intramural vessels become stretched and the blood supply is compromised, leading to ischaemia, necrosis and perforation.

Clinical features
- Vomiting, colicky abdominal pain, abdominal distension, absolute constipation (i.e. neither faeces nor flatus).
- Abdominal distension and increased bowel sounds.
- Dehydration and loss of skin turgor.
- Hypotension, tachycardia.
- Empty rectum on digital examination.
- Tenderness or rebound indicates peritonitis.

Investigations
- Hb, PCV: elevated due to dehydration.
- WCC: normal or slightly elevated.
- U+E: urea elevated, Na^+ and Cl^- low.
- Chest X-ray: elevated diaphragm due to abdominal distension.
- Abdominal supine X-ray:
  small bowel (central loops, non-anatomical distribution, valvulae conniventes shadows cross entire width of lumen like a ladder) or large bowel obstruction (peripheral distribution/haustral shadows do not cross entire width of bowel)
  look for cause (gallstone, characteristic patterns of volvulus, hernias)
  gas in the bowel wall (*pneumatosis intestinalis*) suggests gas-forming infection.
- Contrast CT scan – first investigation of choice for ALL suspected bowel obstruction – site and cause.
- Sigmoidoscopy – ?sigmoid volvulus (allows flatus tube passage).
- Single contrast large bowel enema – ?large bowel obstruction – site and cause ('bird-beak' deformity with volvulus, apple core with tumour).

> ### Essential management
> - Decompress the obstructed gut: pass nasogastric tube.
> - Replace fluid and electrolyte losses: give Ringer's lactate or NaCl with K^+ supplementation.
> - Give IV antibiotics if ischaemia is suspected.
> - Monitor the patient – fluid balance chart, urinary catheter, regular TPR chart, blood tests.
> - Request investigations appropriate to likely cause (contrast CT most helpful).
> - Relieve the obstruction surgically if:
>   underlying causes need surgical treatment (e.g. hernia, colonic carcinoma)
>   patient does not improve with conservative treatment (e.g. adhesion obstruction), or
>   there are signs of strangulation or peritonitis.

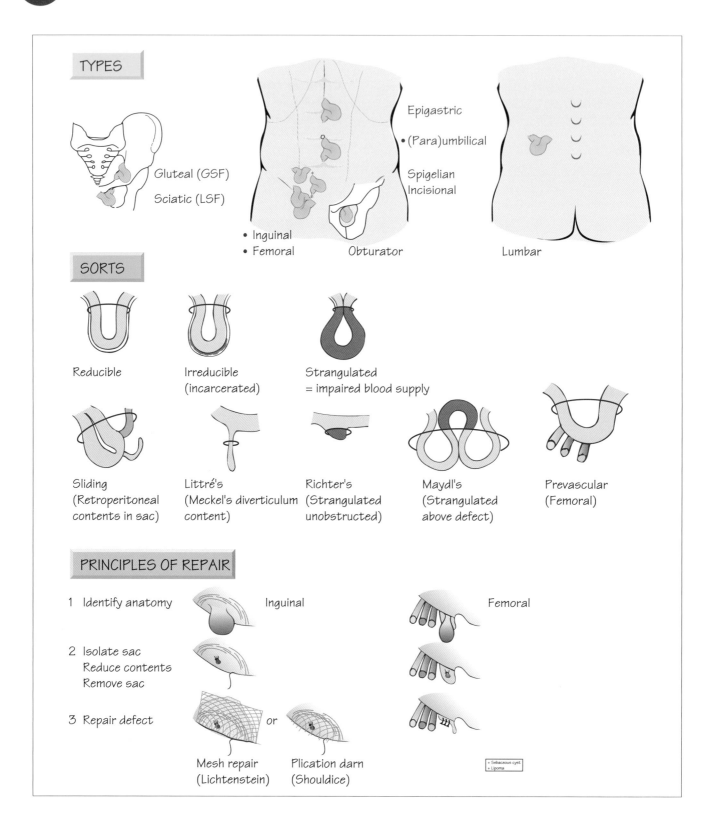

TYPES

Gluteal (GSF)
Sciatic (LSF)

Epigastric
• (Para)umbilical
Spigelian
Incisional

• Inguinal
• Femoral   Obturator   Lumbar

SORTS

Reducible

Irreducible
(incarcerated)

Strangulated
= impaired blood supply

Sliding
(Retroperitoneal
contents in sac)

Littré's
(Meckel's diverticulum
content)

Richter's
(Strangulated
unobstructed)

Maydl's
(Strangulated
above defect)

Prevascular
(Femoral)

PRINCIPLES OF REPAIR

1 Identify anatomy   Inguinal   Femoral

2 Isolate sac
   Reduce contents
   Remove sac

3 Repair defect   or

Mesh repair
(Lichtenstein)

Plication darn
(Shouldice)

+ Sebraceous cyst
+ Lipoma

Definitions

Hernia – the protrusion of a viscus or part of a viscus through an abnormal congenital or acquired opening in its coverings. An *abdominal wall hernia* is the protrusion of tissue (frequently peritoneum or fat) through an abnormal opening in the abdominal wall (frequently in the groin or umbilicus). The protruded peritoneum is the *hernial sac,* the point where the sac passes through the defect in the abdominal wall is the *neck*. The contents can be described as: *irreducible* – contents not reducible with manipulation; *incarcerated* – contents trapped with sac, irreducible and usually acutely symptomatic; *strangulated* – contents' blood supply is compromised with infarction likely.

Key points

- Abdominal wall hernias are common and cause many symptoms.
- Femoral hernias are more common in women than men but inguinal hernia is the most common hernia in women.
- All femoral hernias require prompt repair due to the risk of complications.
- Inguinal hernias may be repaired depending on symptoms.

Types

Common
- Umbilical/para-umbilical – common in adults and children.
- Inguinal (direct and indirect) – indirect common in infants.
- Femoral.
- Incisional.

Uncommon
- Epigastric.
- Spigelian, gluteal, lumbar, obturator, perineal.

Pathophysiology

- The defect in the abdominal wall may be congenital (e.g. umbilical hernia, femoral canal) or acquired (e.g. an incision) and is lined with peritoneum (the sac).
- Raised intra-abdominal pressure further weakens the defect allowing some of the intra-abdominal contents (e.g. omentum, small bowel loop) to migrate through the opening.
- Entrapment of the contents in the sac leads to incarceration (unable to reduce contents) and possibly strangulation (blood supply to incarcerated contents is compromised).

Clinical features

- Patient presents with a lump over the site of the hernia.
- Femoral hernias are below and lateral to the pubic tubercle, they usually flatten the groin crease and are 10 times more common in women than men. 50% present as a surgical emergency due to obstructed contents and 50% of these will require a small bowel resection. Femoral hernias are irreducible.
- Inguinal hernias start off above and medial to the pubic tubercle but may descend broadly when larger, they usually accentuate the groin crease. Most are benign and have a low risk of complications. Indirect inguinal hernias can be controlled by digital pressure over the internal inguinal ring, may be narrow-necked and are common in younger men (3% per annum present with complications). Direct inguinal hernias are poorly controlled by digital pressure, are often broad-necked and are more common in older men (0.3% per annum strangulate).
- Incisional hernias bulge, are usually broad-necked, poorly controlled by pressure and are accentuated by tensing the recti. Large, chronic, incisional hernias may contain much of the small bowel and may be irreducible/unrepairable due to the 'loss of the right of abode in the abdomen' of the contents.
- True umbilical hernias are present from birth and are symmetrical defects in the umbilicus. Most obliterate spontaneously by age 2–4 years. Only repair if persist after age 4 years.
- Para-umbilical hernias develop due to an acquired defect in the periumbilical fascia.

Essential management

- Assess the hernia for: severity of symptoms, risk of complications (type, size of neck), ease of repair (size, location), likelihood of success (size, loss of right of abode).
- Assess the patient for: fitness for surgery, impact of hernia on lifestyle (job, hobbies).
- Surgical repair is usually offered in suitable patients for:
  hernias at risk of complications whatever the symptoms
  hernias with previous symptoms of obstruction
  hernias at low risk of complications but symptoms interfering with lifestyle, etc.

Principles of hernia surgery

- Herniotomy: excision of the hernial sac alone for children.
- Herniorrhaphy: repairing the defect – mesh repair usual for inguinal hernias inserted via open or laparoscopic surgery.
- Incisional hernias may be repaired by open surgery or laparoscopically and usually require mesh to achieve satisfactory closure.

Complications of surgery

- Haematoma (wound or scrotal) or seroma.
- Acute urinary retention.
- Wound infection.
- Chronic pain.
- Testicular pain and swelling leading to testicular atrophy.
- Hernia recurrence (about 2%).

	Causes and symptoms	Cardinal symptoms and signs	Structure involved (diagnosis)		
			Gallbladder	CBD	Other
A	Presence of stone → Irritation → Contraction	Pain Nausea Vomiting Tender RUQ	Biliary colic ┊ May ↓	Biliary (ductal) colic ┊ May ↓	—
B	Obstruction of structure (simple)	As above + • Persistence of pain etc. • Mass RUQ (jaundice)	Mucocele ┊ May ↓	Obstructive jaundice ┊ May ↓	—
C	Obstruction of structure (+ infection)	As above + • Swinging fever • Tachycardia • Neutrophilia • Rigors	Empyema ┊ May ↓ perforate Biliary peritonitis	Cholangitis	—
D	Inflammation/ infection	As for A + • Fever • Tachycardia • Neutrophilia	Cholecystitis	(Cholangitis)	Pancreatitis

Other conditions associated with gallstones
• Gallstone ileus
• Adenocarcinoma gallbladder

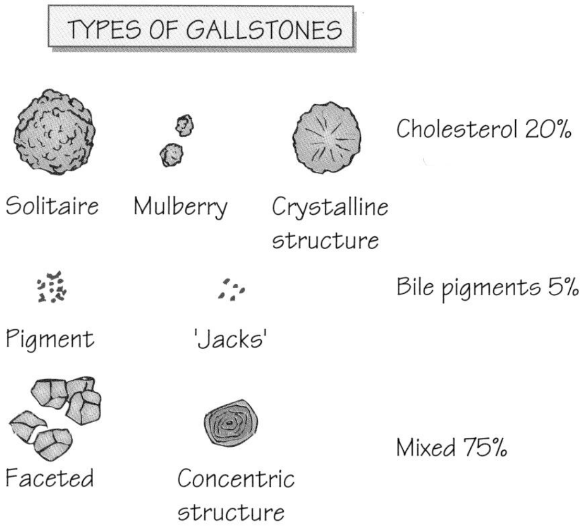

CAUSES

TYPES OF GALLSTONES

Solitaire   Mulberry   Crystalline structure   Cholesterol 20%

Pigment   'Jacks'   Bile pigments 5%

Faceted   Concentric structure   Mixed 75%

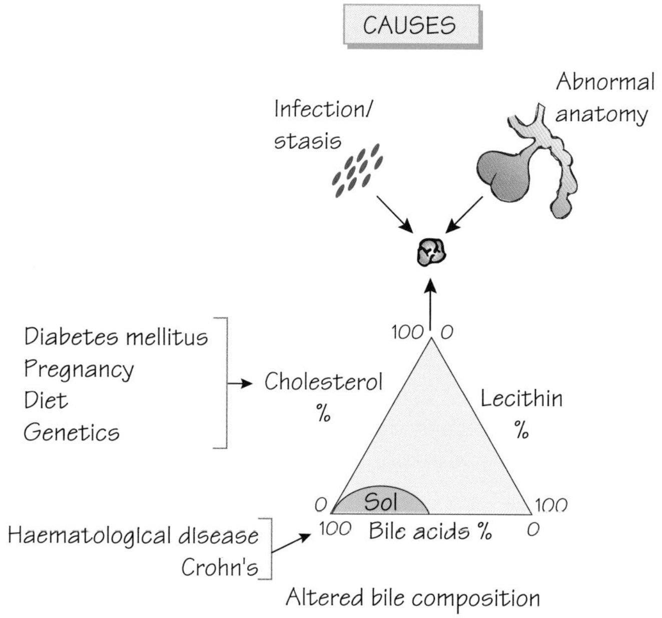

Infection/ stasis   Abnormal anatomy

Diabetes mellitus
Pregnancy
Diet
Genetics   → Cholesterol %   Lecithin %

100 ┊ 0

0   Sol   100

Haematological disease
Crohn's   → 100   Bile acids %   0

Altered bile composition

Definitions

Gallstones are round, oval or faceted concretions found in the biliary tract containing cholesterol, calcium carbonate, calcium bilirubinate or a mixture of these. *Microlithiasis* is the presence of small/microscopic solid elements within the bile.

Key points

- Gallstones are common, but they may not be the cause of the patient's symptoms.
- Incidentally found asymptomatic gallstones should not be treated.
- An attack of biliary colic/cholecystitis, acute pancreatitis, cholangitis or obstructive jaundice is an indication for prophylactic cholecystectomy.

Epidemiology

Male:female 1:2. Age 40 years onwards. High incidence of mixed stones in Western world. Pigment stones more common in the East.

Pathogenesis

- Cholesterol stones: imbalance in bile between cholesterol, bile salts and phospholipids, producing lithogenic bile. May be associated with inflammatory bowel disease.
- Mixed stones: associated with anatomical abnormalities, stasis, previous surgery, previous infections.
- Bilirubinate (pigment) stones: chronic haemolysis.
- Statins and coffee consumption appear to protect against gallstone formation.

Pathology

- Gallstones passing through the biliary system can cause biliary colic or pancreatitis.
- Stone obstruction at the gallbladder neck + infection leads to cholecystitis.
- Obstruction of the CBD + infection leads to septic cholangitis.
- Migration of a large stone via biliary-enteric fistula into the gut may cause intestinal obstruction (gallstone ileus).

Clinical features

- 90% of gallstones are (probably) asymptomatic.
- *Biliary colic*: severe upper abdominal pain radiating around the right costal margin ± vomiting. Often onset at night, spontaneously resolves after several hours.
- *Acute cholecystitis*: right hypochondrial pain, pyrexia, nausea, RUQ tenderness (positive Murphy's sign). Leucocytosis. Unresolved may lead to an empyema of the gallbladder.
- *'Chronic cholecystitis'*: uncertain diagnosis, vague, intermittent, right upper abdominal pain, abdominal distension, flatulence, fatty food intolerance.
- *Obstructive jaundice*: upper abdominal pain, pale/clay-like stools, dark brown urine, pruritus. May progress to *cholangitis* (Charcot's triad: abdominal pain, high fever/rigors, jaundice) if CBD remains obstructed.
- *Pancreatitis* (see Chapter 57): central/epigastric pain, back pain, fever, tachycardia, epigastric tenderness.
- *Gallstone ileus*: clinical features of small bowel obstruction. Elderly patients.

Gallstone disease/2

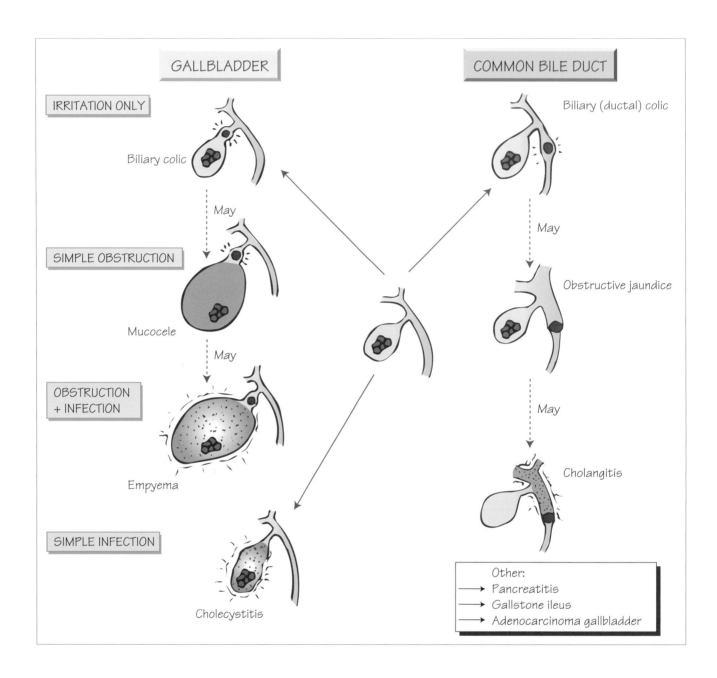

Surgery at a Glance, Fifth Edition. Pierce A. Grace and Neil R. Borley. © 2013 John Wiley & Sons, Ltd. Published 2013 by John Wiley & Sons, Ltd.

Investigations

- FBC: acute inflammatory complications, picture of haemolytic (microcytic) anaemia.
- U+E/creatinine: most important in jaundice to monitor renal function.
- LFTs: obstructive jaundice pattern.
- Plain X-ray of the abdomen shows only 10% of gallstones.
- Ultrasound: 90% of gallstones will be detected on ultrasound examination. Assesses CBD size and possible presence of CBD stones.
- MRCP is indicated for suspected CBD stones. If MRCP is positive then ERCP is indicated for CBD stone removal or stent placement.
- Endoluminal/transduodenal ultrasound – for the diagnosis of small ductal stones.
- OGD: to exclude PUD as a cause for uncomplicated disease symptoms.

Essential management

- Asymptomatic: no treatment required.
- Biliary colic: analgesia and elective laparoscopic cholecystectomy.
- Acute cholecystitis: analgesia, IV fluids, antibiotics + early or interval cholecystectomy.
- Chronic cholecystitis: elective laparoscopic cholecystectomy after other possible causes have been excluded.
- Empyema of gallbladder: early cholecystectomy or *cholecystostomy* i.e. drainage of gallbaldder (surgical or radiological) ± interval cholecystectomy.
- Ascending cholangitis: IV fluids, antibiotics, ductal drainage (now usually by ERCP, sphincterotomy and extraction of stones) + early laparoscopic cholecystectomy.
- Pancreatitis: early laparoscopic cholecystectomy once pancreatitis has resolved.
- Gallstone ileus: laparotomy removal of obstructing stone only – no Rx for biliary-enteric fistula. Mortality of 5–25% with gallstone ileus.

Complications of cholecystectomy

- Conversion: 5–10% of laparoscopic cholecystectomies are converted to an open operation.
- Leakage of bile from cystic duct or gallbladder bed. (Rx: ERCP and temporary CBD stent.)
- Jaundice due to retained ductal stones. (Rx: ERCP or if a T-tube is in place by extraction with a Dormia basket down the T-tube track (Burhenne manoeuvre).)
- Bleeding from cystic artery or gallbladder bed (may require re-operation).
- Injury to the CBD; requires major reconstructive surgery.

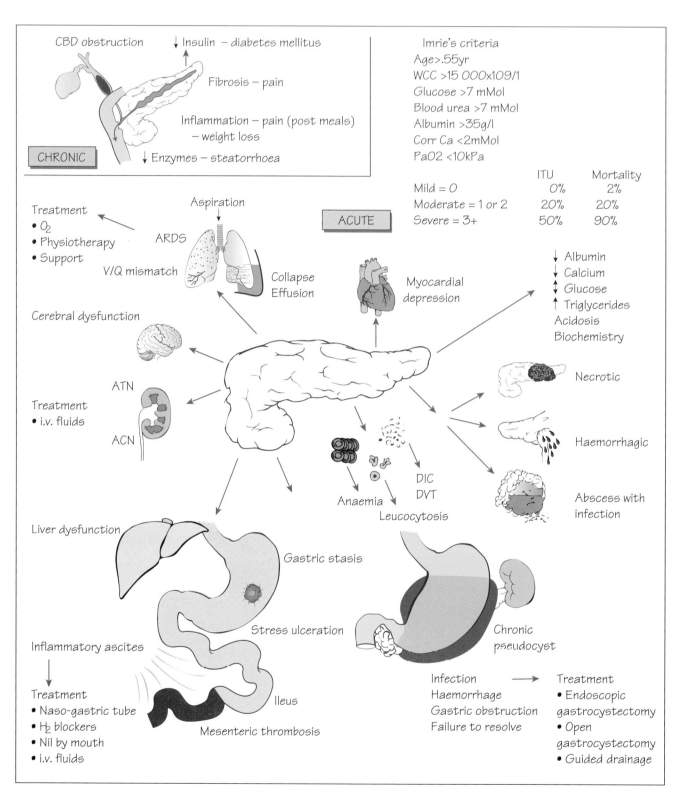

CBD obstruction ↓ Insulin – diabetes mellitus

Fibrosis – pain

Inflammation – pain (post meals)
– weight loss

CHRONIC ↓ Enzymes – steatorrhoea

Imrie's criterion
Age>.55yr
WCC >15 000x109/1
Glucose >7 mMol
Blood urea >7 mMol
Albumin >35g/l
Corr Ca <2mMol
PaO2 <10kPa

	ITU	Mortality
Mild = 0	0%	2%
Moderate = 1 or 2	20%	20%
Severe = 3+	50%	90%

Treatment
• O₂
• Physiotherapy
• Support

Aspiration

ARDS

V/Q mismatch

ACUTE

Collapse
Effusion

Myocardial
depression

↓ Albumin
↓ Calcium
↕ Glucose
↑ Triglycerides
Acidosis
Biochemistry

Cerebral dysfunction

ATN

Treatment
• i.v. fluids

ACN

Necrotic

Haemorrhagic

DIC
DVT

Anaemia

Leucocytosis

Abscess with
infection

Liver dysfunction

Gastric stasis

Stress ulceration

Chronic
pseudocyst

Inflammatory ascites

↓

Treatment
• Naso-gastric tube
• H₂ blockers
• Nil by mouth
• i.v. fluids

Ileus

Mesenteric thrombosis

Infection
Haemorrhage
Gastric obstruction
Failure to resolve

→

Treatment
• Endoscopic
gastrocystectomy
• Open
gastrocystectomy
• Guided drainage

Definition

Pancreatitis is an inflammatory condition of the exocrine pancreas that results from injury to the acinar cells. It may be acute or chronic. A *pancreatic pseudocyst* is a persisting accumulation of inflammatory fluid, usually in the lesser sac. It is called a *pseudo*cyst because it does not have an epithelial lining. *Necrotizing pancreatitis* is a severe form of pancreatitis with one or more diffuse or focal areas of non-viable pancreatic parenchyma. *Chronic pancreatitis* is a continuing inflammation of the pancreas leading to an atrophic pancreas, chronic abdominal pain and impaired endocrine/exocrine function.

Key points

- Most pancreatitis (>80%) is mild and spontaneously resolves.
- All patients should have a cause sought by imaging and the severity assessed by recognized criteria.
- A normal or mildly elevated serum amylase does not exclude pancreatitis.
- Severe or complicated pancreatitis may worsen rapidly and require ICU support.
- Surgery has little place other than to treat severe complications.

Aetiology

- Gallstones and alcohol account for 95% of cases of acute pancreatitis.
- Other causes include: drugs, idiopathic, hypercalcaemia, hyperlipidaemia, congenital structural abnormalities, viral infections, hypothermia and trauma.

Pathology

Acute

- Mild injury: acinar (exocrine) cell damage with enzymatic spillage, inflammatory cascade activation and localized oedema. Local exudate may also lead to increased serum levels of pancreatic enzymes (amylase, lipase, colipase).
- Moderate injury: increasing local inflammation leads to intrapancreatic bleeding, fluid collections and spreading local oedema involving the mesentery and retroperitoneum. Activation of the systemic inflammatory response leads to progressive involvement of other organs.
- Severe injury: progressive pancreatic destruction leads to necrosis, profound localized bleeding and fluid collections around the pancreas. Spread to local structures and the peritoneal cavity may result in mesenteric infarction, peritonitis and intra-abdominal fat 'saponification'.

Chronic

Recurrent episodes of acute inflammation lead to progressive destruction of acinar cells with healing by fibrosis. Incidental islet cell damage may lead to endocrine gland failure.

Clinical features

- Mild/moderate pancreatitis: constant upper abdominal pain radiating to back, nausea, vomiting, pyrexia, tachycardia ± jaundice.
- Severe/necrotizing pancreatitis: severe upper abdominal pain, signs of hypovolaemic shock, respiratory and renal impairment, silent abdomen, retroperitoneal bleeding with flank and umbilical bruising (Grey Turner's and Cullen's signs).

Essential management

- Attempt to confirm diagnosis (serum amylase >1000 iu diagnostic – may be clinical diagnosis).
- Assess disease severity (Imrie criteria): severe is 3+ of the following:
  age > 55 years
  WBC >15 × 10⁹/L
  PaO_2 < 10 kPa
  blood glucose > 7 mmol/L
  albumin < 35 g/L
  urea > 7 mmol/L
  Ca^{2+} < 2.0 mmol/L.
- Resuscitate the patient:
  mild/moderate disease: IV fluids, analgesia, monitor progress with pulse, BP, temperature
  severe pancreatitis: full resuscitation in ICU with invasive monitoring.
- Establish the cause: ultrasound to look for gallstones, MRCP if choledocholithiasis suspected, CT to assess state of pancreas.

Further management

- No proven use for routine nasogastric tube or antibiotics.
- ?Vitamin supplements and sedatives if alcoholic cause.
- Proven CBD gallstones may require urgent ERCP and biliary drainage.
- Proven gallstones should be treated by cholecystectomy during the same admission if attack mild.
- Failure to respond to treatment or uncertain diagnosis warrants abdominal CT scan (the most reliable imaging modality in diagnosis of acute pancreatitis).
- Suspected/proven (by CT-guided aspiration) infection of necrotic pancreas – antibiotics ± radiological drainage of abscesses, laparoscopic or open surgical débridement of pancreas.

Complications – acute pancreatitis

Acute

- Pancreatic abscess: usually necrotic pancreas present.
- Intra-abdominal sepsis.
- Necrosis of the transverse colon.
- Respiratory (ARDS) or renal (ATN) failure.
- Pancreatic haemorrhage.

Subacute/chronic

- Pseudocyst formation: may need to be drained internally (endoscopically or surgically) or externally (radiological).
- Chronic pancreatitis.

Chronic pancreatitis

- Usually caused by chronic alcohol abuse.
- Presents with intractable abdominal pain and evidence of exocrine (steatorrhoea) and endocrine (diabetes mellitus) pancreatic failure.
- Medical treatment is with analgesia, exocrine pancreatic enzyme replacement and treatment of diabetes. Surgical treatment is by drainage of dilated pancreatic ducts or excision of the pancreas in some cases.

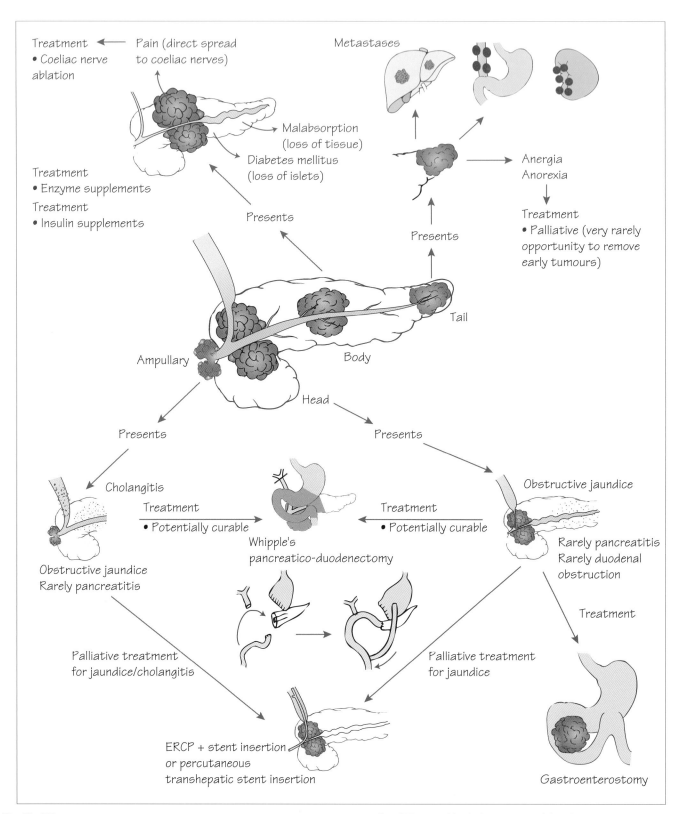

Treatment
• Coeliac nerve ablation ← Pain (direct spread to coeliac nerves)

Metastases

Treatment
• Enzyme supplements

Treatment
• Insulin supplements

Malabsorption (loss of tissue)
Diabetes mellitus (loss of islets)

Presents

Anergia
Anorexia

Treatment
• Palliative (very rarely opportunity to remove early tumours)

Presents

Tail

Ampullary

Body

Head

Presents

Presents

Cholangitis

Treatment
• Potentially curable

Obstructive jaundice

Treatment
• Potentially curable

Whipple's pancreatico-duodenectomy

Rarely pancreatitis
Rarely duodenal obstruction

Obstructive jaundice
Rarely pancreatitis

Treatment

Palliative treatment for jaundice/cholangitis

Palliative treatment for jaundice

ERCP + stent insertion or percutaneous transhepatic stent insertion

Gastroenterostomy

Definitions

Pancreatic adenocarcinoma is a malignant lesion of the head, body or tail of the pancreas. *Periampullary carcinomas* arise around the ampulla of Vater and include tumours arising from the pancreas, duodenum, distal bile duct and the ampulla itself. *Neuroendocrine tumours*

of the pancreas cause a variety of syndromes secondary to the secretion of active peptides.

> ## Key points
>
> - Most pancreatic cancer is not surgically curable. Overall 5-year survival is only 5%.
> - New, chronic back pain and vague symptoms may be the only presenting feature.
> - The best prognosis is for true periampullary cancers.
> - Good palliation of jaundice is possible without surgery.

Epidemiology
Male: female 2:1, peak incidence 50–70 years. Incidence of pancreatic carcinoma is increasing in the Western world.

Aetiology
Predisposing factors: smoking, diabetes, chronic pancreatitis.

Pathology
- Site: 55% involve head of pancreas, 25% body, 15% tail, 5% periampullary region.
- Macroscopic: growth is hard and infiltrating.
- Histology: 90% ductal carcinoma, 7% acinar cell carcinoma, 2% cystic carcinoma, 1% connective tissue origins.
- Spread:
  local into vital structures (portal vein, superior mesenteric vessels)
  lymphatics to peritoneum and regional nodes
  via bloodstream to liver and lung – metastases often present at time of diagnosis.

Clinical features
- Jaundice, abdominal pain and weight loss, 50% have one of these symptoms.
- Head or periampullary: painless, progressive jaundice with a palpable gallbladder (Courvoisier's law: a palpable gallbladder in the presence of jaundice is unlikely to be due to gallstones).
- Occasionally, duodenal obstruction causing vomiting.
- Body: back pain, anorexia, weight loss, steatorrhoea.
- Tail: often presents with metastases, malignant ascites or unexplained anaemia.
- New onset diabetes may be first presentation in up to 10% of patients

Investigations
- Ultrasound: may see mass in head of pancreas and distended biliary tree.
- Spiral CT scan: demonstrates tumour mass, facilitates biopsy, assess involvement of surrounding structures and local lymph node spread. Best method for staging.
- EUS ± fine needle biopsy: staging, vascular involvement, tissue diagnosis.
- MRCP/ERCP: very accurate in making diagnosis; obtain specimen or shed cells for cytology and stent may be placed to relieve jaundice.
- (Barium meal: widening of the duodenal loop with medial filling defect, the reversed '3' sign. Not used very much anymore.)
- Tumour marker (CA19.9) not diagnostic but useful to monitor treatment response.

> ## Essential management
> ### Palliation
> - Pancreatic adenocarcinoma is usually incurable at time of diagnosis.
> - Jaundice can be relieved by placing a stent through the tumour endoscopically (at ERCP).
> - Duodenal obstruction (10%) may be relieved by gastrojejunostomy.
> - Pain should be treated with opioids ± percutaneous cellacoplexus block.
>
> ### Curative treatment
> Rarely (<20%), radical surgical resection (Whipple's procedure) of small tumours of the head of the pancreas is curative if lymph nodes are not involved. Only indicated for Stage I disease (T1 or T2/N0/M0).

Prognosis
- 90% of patients with pancreatic adenocarcinoma are dead within 12 months of diagnosis.
- 5-year survival following radical resection is only 10%.
- It is important to obtain histology from tumours around the head of the pancreas as the prognosis from non-pancreatic periampullary cancers is considerably better (50% 5-year survival) following resection.

> ## 2-week wait referral criteria for suspected upper GI cancer
>
> - New-onset dysphagia (any age).
> - Dyspepsia + weight loss/anaemia/vomiting.
> - Dyspepsia + FHx/Barrett's oesophagus/previous peptic ulcer surgery/atrophic gastritis/pernicious anaemia.
> - New dyspepsia >55 years.
> - Jaundice.
> - Upper abdominal mass.

Neuroendocrine tumours of the pancreas
- Rare (4–12 per million population), any age, male: female 1:1.
- Classified into *non-functioning* (50%) and *functioning* (insulinomas (25%), gastrinomas (15%), VIP-omas, glucagonomas and somatostatinomas (15%)).
- 15–30% of patients with pancreatic endocrine tumours have MEN type 1: (3 P's) parathyroid (hyperparathyroidism), pancreas (gastrinoma), pituitary (prolactinoma).
- Presentation: non-functioning may be found incidentally. Functioning present with symptoms due to excess production of specific hormone produced, e.g. hypoglycaemia with insulinoma, peptic ulcer with gastrinoma.
- Diagnosis:
  imaging – ultrasound, EUS, CT, MRI, MRA, SRS
  biochemistry – chromogranin A (general tumour marker increased in most endocrine tumours), hormone levels.
- Treatment: surgery, chemotherapy.
- Prognosis: 5-year survival – local disease 60–100%, regional disease 40%, distant metastases 30%.

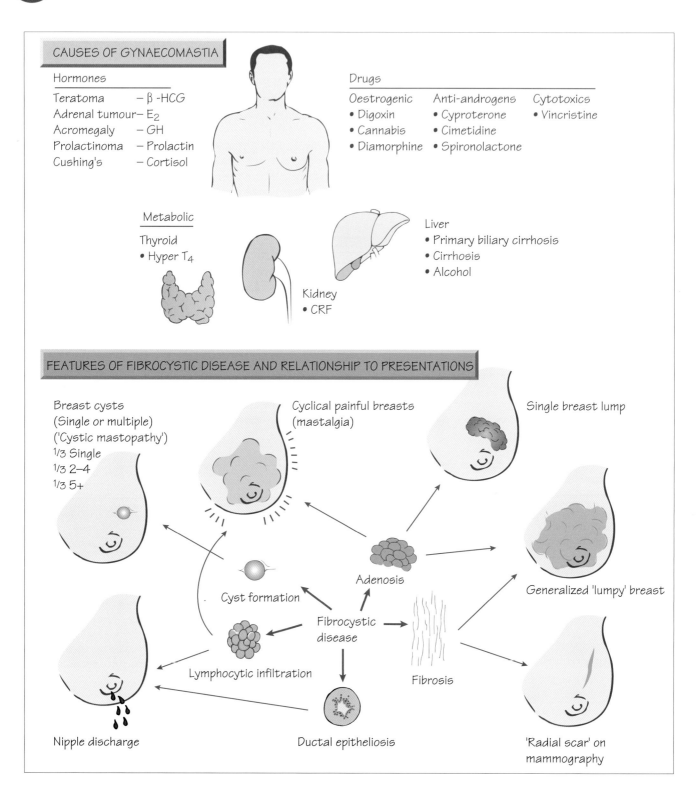

CAUSES OF GYNAECOMASTIA

Hormones

Teratoma	$-\beta$-HCG
Adrenal tumour	$-E_2$
Acromegaly	$-GH$
Prolactinoma	$-Prolactin$
Cushing's	$-Cortisol$

Drugs

Oestrogenic	Anti-androgens	Cytotoxics
• Digoxin	• Cyproterone	• Vincristine
• Cannabis	• Cimetidine	
• Diamorphine	• Spironolactone	

Metabolic

Thyroid
• Hyper T_4

Kidney
• CRF

Liver
• Primary biliary cirrhosis
• Cirrhosis
• Alcohol

FEATURES OF FIBROCYSTIC DISEASE AND RELATIONSHIP TO PRESENTATIONS

Breast cysts
(Single or multiple)
('Cystic mastopathy')
1/3 Single
1/3 2–4
1/3 5+

Cyclical painful breasts
(mastalgia)

Single breast lump

Cyst formation

Adenosis

Generalized 'lumpy' breast

Fibrocystic
disease

Fibrosis

Lymphocytic infiltration

Nipple discharge

Ductal epitheliosis

'Radial scar' on
mammography

Definition

Abnormalities of **N**ormal **D**evelopment and **I**nvolution of the breast (ANDI) is a broad term covering benign conditions with overlapping features including fibroadenoma, fibrocystic disease, mastalgia, breast infections and nipple disorders.

Key points

- *Any* breast lump should be evaluated by triple assessment for risk of malignancy.
- Triple assessment comprises: (1) clinical examination, (2) imaging (mammography for women aged 35 or over and ultra-sonography for women aged under 35) and (3) FNAC.
- ANDI disorders are common in younger, premenopausal women and often cause considerable anxiety.
- Gynaecomastia is usually physiological but may need to be investigated for hormonal causes.

Abnormalities of development
Fibroadenoma

- Benign breast lump caused by overgrowth of single breast lobule. Manifests as one or more firm, mobile, painless lumps usually in women <30 years.
- Investigation: 'triple assessment' (clinical/radiological/cytological).
- Treatment:
  age <30 years: either observe or excise if worried
  age >30 years: consider excision to exclude malignancy.

Abnormalities of cycles
Fibrocystic disease

- Usually presents age 25–45 years. May present as breast pain (*mastalgia*), tenderness, breast lump(s), breast cyst(s), especially during the second half of the menstrual cycle.
- Investigation: 'triple assessment' of all lumps.
- Treatment: patient reassurance, analgesics, γ-linoleic acid, hormone manipulation (e.g. danazol inhibits FSH and LH in pituitary, bromocriptine reduces prolactin secretion), cyst aspiration, excision of persistent localized masses after aspiration. Avoid xanthine-containing substances (coffee).

Abnormalities of involution
Breast cyst

- May be single or multiple. Firm, round, discrete lump(s).
- Investigation: aspiration ± mammography. Triple assessment for any associated lumps.
- Treatment: reassurance, aspiration (repeated), hormone manipulation.

Other benign conditions
Breast abscess

- Usually infection of the lactating or pregnant breast with *Staphylococcus aureus*. Acute abscess: redness, swelling, heat and pain in the breast. Chronic/recurrent sepsis associated with smoking and ductal ectasia with mixed anaerobic infection.
- Treatment: Acute abscess: antibiotics (flucloxacillin) + repeated aspiration (occasionally I&D will be required). Lactation/breastfeeding does not need to be suppressed while the abscess is being treated. Chronic sepsis: metronidazole and recurrent aspirations if necessary.

Mammary duct ectasia

- Dilated subareolar ducts are filled with cellular debris which causes a periductal inflammatory response. Associated with smoking and recurrent non-lactational abscesses. The usual presentation is a green, multifocal, ductal nipple discharge and a subareolar lump.
- Treatment is by subareolar excision of the involved ducts if troublesome symptoms persist or the diagnosis is unsure.

Duct papilloma

- Small papillomas arise in the major breast ducts. They cause a bloody or serous nipple discharge usually from one duct.
- Treatment is usually by excision of the affected duct by microdochectomy if the symptoms persist.

Fat necrosis

- A fibrous scar in the breast tissue caused by injury, haematoma and necrosis of breast fat with subsequent scarring. History of trauma to the breast in 50% of cases ± superficial ecchymoses. Histology: periductal cellular infiltrate and fibrosis.
- Investigation: triple assessment.
- Treatment: surgical excision if mass fails to resolve or there is concern to exclude malignancy.

Cystosarcoma phylloides

- Large, predominantly benign (90%), fleshy, non-epithelial tumour of the breast presenting in middle age. Accounts for 1% of all breast tumours.
- Incisional or excisional biopsy is required to make a firm diagnosis.
- Wide local excision is the treatment of choice.
- Local recurrence is high with inadequate excision.
- Malignant lesions frequently metastasize to the lungs – prognosis is poor.

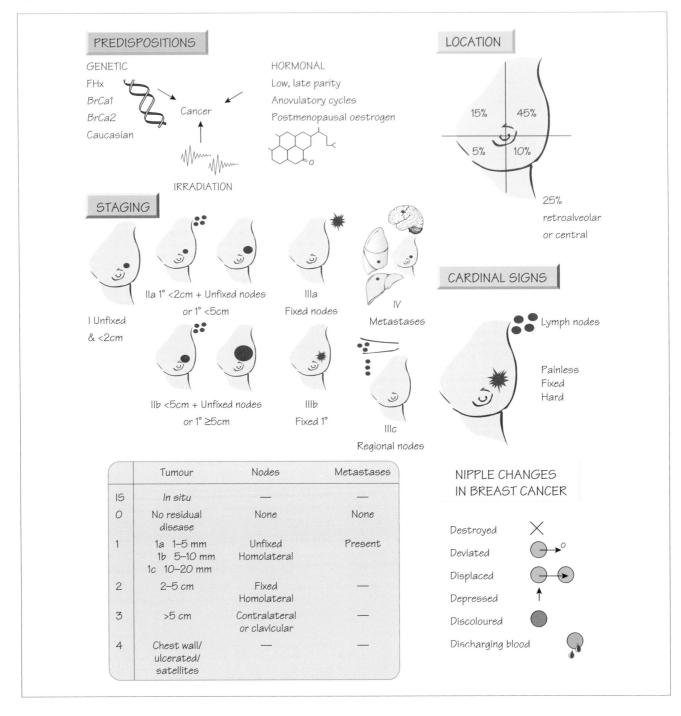

PREDISPOSITIONS

GENETIC
FHx
BrCa1
BrCa2
Caucasian

Cancer

HORMONAL
Low, late parity
Anovulatory cycles
Postmenopausal oestrogen

IRRADIATION

LOCATION

15%   45%
5%   10%

25%
retroalveolar
or central

STAGING

I Unfixed
& <2cm

IIa 1° <2cm + Unfixed nodes
or 1° <5cm

IIb <5cm + Unfixed nodes
or 1° ≥5cm

IIIa
Fixed nodes

IIIb
Fixed 1°

IIIc
Regional nodes

IV
Metastases

CARDINAL SIGNS

Lymph nodes

Painless
Fixed
Hard

	Tumour	Nodes	Metastases
IS	In situ	—	—
0	No residual disease	None	None
1	1a 1–5 mm 1b 5–10 mm 1c 10–20 mm	Unfixed Homolateral	Present
2	2–5 cm	Fixed Homolateral	—
3	>5 cm	Contralateral or clavicular	—
4	Chest wall/ulcerated/satellites	—	—

NIPPLE CHANGES IN BREAST CANCER

Destroyed
Deviated
Displaced
Depressed
Discoloured
Discharging blood

Definition

Malignant lesion of (predominantly) the female breast.

Key points
- Breast lump: triple assessment, clinical, radiology, cytology.
- Early breast cancer treatment intent is *curative*.
- Late breast cancer treatment intent is *palliative*.
- HER2+ tumours to be treated with *trastuzumab* (Herceptin®).

Epidemiology

M : F 1:100. >30 years. 1 in 9 women develop breast cancer in their lifetime.

Aetiology

- Female gender, advanced age, personal or family history of breast cancer (genetic factors – *BRCA1* or *BRCA2* gene mutations).
- Early menarche and late menopause, nulliparity, HRT.
- Smoking, alcohol, fat consumption, lack of exercise and obesity.
- Higher socioecomnomic groups, developed world.

Pathology

- Histology: adenocarcinomas (glandular epithelium). Common types are invasive ductal (80%) or lobular (15%) carcinoma. *Paget's disease* is ductal carcinoma-in-situ involving the nipple.
- Spread: lymphatics, direct, haematogenous (lung, liver, bone, brain, adrenal, ovary).
- Staging: TNM classification – important for treatment and prognosis. Also ductal carcinoma-in-situ (DCIS) and stages 0, I, IIA, IIB, IIIA, IIIB and IV (AJCC).
- Molecular subtypes: *Luminal A* (ER+/PR+/HER2–, low Ki67), *Luminal B* (ER+/PR+/HER2+ or HER2– high Ki67), *Triple negative/ basal-like* (RE–/PR–/HER2–), *HER2 type* (ER–/PR–/HER2+).

Screening

- Women aged 50–70 years should be screened for breast cancer every 3 years by two-view (craniocaudal and mediolateral) mammography. Screening from 40 years in high risk groups.
- Participation in national screening programmes reduces breast cancer mortality by 35%.

Clinical features

- Palpable, hard, irregular, fixed breast lump, usually painless.
- Nipple retraction and skin dimpling.
- Nipple eczema in Paget's disease.
- *Peau d'orange* (cutaneous oedema 2° lymphatic obstruction).
- Palpable axillary nodes.

Investigations

- Triple assessment: clinical examination/imaging/cytology.
- Imaging: *mammography:* mass (irregular, spiculated), asymmetry, microcalcification, distortion. Not used <35 years unless strong clinical suspicion of carcinoma.
  ultrasound: women <35 years or part of triple therapy
  MRI: helpful when U/S not diagnostic. Indicated for axillary disease without obvious primary source and for lobular carcinoma.
- Cytological assessment: FNAC or core biopsy.
- Breast biopsy: excision biopsy rarely required for diagnosis.
- Staging investigations for proven carcinoma: *All:* CXR, FBC, serum alkaline phosphatase, γ-GT and calcium. *If metastases clinically suspected:* isotope bone scan, brain, thorax and abdomen CT scan.
- Breast tissue for receptor status (*Estrogen Receptor/Progesterone receptor* (ER/PR) + or –, *Human Epidermal Growth Factor Receptor 2* (HER2) + or –). Important for treatment and prognosis. Tumour *Urokinase plasminogen activator* (uPA) and *plasminogen activator inhibitor-1* (PAI-1) may help in deciding about adjuvant chemotherapy in some ER/PR+ patients). *Ki-67*, a cancer antigen found in growing, dividing cells but is absent in the resting phase of cell growth may help in predicting prognosis.

- Management of axillary lymph nodes (for staging, prognosis and treatment):
  clinically negative nodes: sentinel node biopsy reliably confirms negativity. Completion axillary lymph node dissection (ALND) is **not** required
  clinically positive nodes: axillary ultrasound + FNA *or* biopsy to confirm positivity. Proceed to ALND (level 1 or 2) *or* axillary radiation.
  Lymphoedema may occur as a complication in up to 25% of patients.
- Prognosis depends on lymph nodes status, tumour size, histological grade and receptor status. 10-year survival rates: Stage I 85%, Stage II 60%, overall 80%.

Adjuvant systemic therapy: all HER2+ cancers should receive the monoclonal antibody *trastuzumab* (Herceptin).

Receptor	Tumour size	Axillary node negative	Axillary node positive
Pre M ER/PR+	≤0.5 cm	±EM	±EM
Pre M ER/PR+	0.6–1.0 cm	EM ± chemotherapy	EM + chemotherapy
Pre M ER/PR+	>1.0 cm	EM + chemotherapy	EM + chemotherapy
Pre M ER/PR–	≤0.5 cm	no adjuvant Rx	±chemotherapy
Pre M ER/PR–	0.6–1.0 cm	±chemotherapy	chemotherapy
Pre M ER/PR–	≥1.0 cm	chemotherapy	chemotherapy
Post M ER/PR+	<1.0 cm	EM *or* no adjuvant Rx	EM + chemotherapy
Post M ER/PR+	≥1.0 cm	EM ± chemotherapy (gene expression analysis)	EM + chemotherapy
Post M ER/PR–	any size	chemotherapy	chemotherapy

M, menopause; **ER/PR**, estrogen receptor/progesterone receptor; **EM**, endocrine manipulation (tamoxifen, aromatase inhibitors, LH-RH analogues – for ovarian ablation/supression); **chemotherapy** (e.g. **CMF**, cyclophosphamide, methotrexate, 5-FU; **CAF**, cyclophosphamide, adriamycin, 5-FU; **ACT**, adriamycin, cyclophosphamide, Taxol. **Gene expression analysis** of individual tumours may allow for individual customized adjuvant therapy (e.g. Oncotype DX®: 21-gene assay that provides and individual recurrence score).

Advanced breast cancer (T3–4, N2–3, M0–1)
(Distant spread at time of diagnosis – Rx is palliative.)
- Local treatment is directed at controlling locally advanced disease or local recurrence: lumpectomy/mastectomy/radiotherapy. Neoadjuvant chemotherapy therapy is used to induce a tumour response to facilitate local control by surgery or radiotherapy.
- Distant metastases: radiotherapy for pain relief from bony metastases; EM if ER/PR+. Chemo Rx (anthracylines (doxorubicin, epirubicin) or Taxol) or targeted Rx (Trastuzumab for all HER2+ cancers). Bisphosphonates for symptomatic bone metastases.
- Prognosis: 10-year survival rates: Stage III 40%; Stage IV 10%

Essential management

Early breast cancer (T1–2, N0–1)
(No evidence of distant spread at diagnosis – Rx is curative.)
Local treatment is usually either:
- Breast conservation surgery (lumpectomy) + radiotherapy to breast *or* simple mastectomy ± breast reconstruction. (Neoadjuvant systemic therapy is used in some patients to reduce tumour size to facilitate breast conservation.)

2-week wait referral criteria for suspected breast cancer
- Discrete lump in breast or axilla >35 years.
- Breast ulceration/breast skin nodules/breast skin distortion.
- Nipple eczema.
- Recent nipple retraction/distortion.
- Bloody nipple discharge.

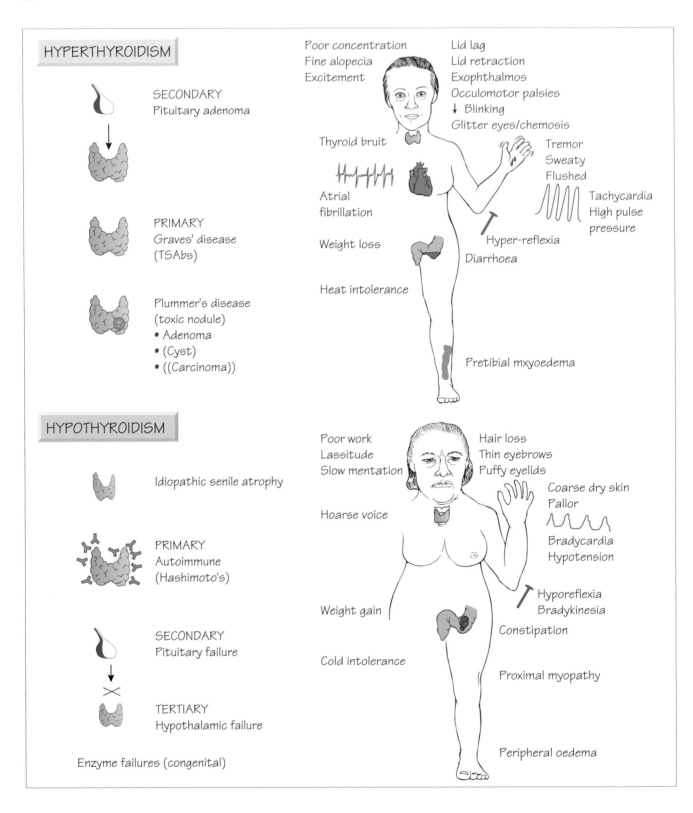

HYPERTHYROIDISM

SECONDARY
Pituitary adenoma

PRIMARY
Graves' disease
(TSAbs)

Plummer's disease
(toxic nodule)
• Adenoma
• (Cyst)
• ((Carcinoma))

Poor concentration
Fine alopecia
Excitement

Lid lag
Lid retraction
Exophthalmos
Occulomotor palsies
↓ Blinking
Glitter eyes/chemosis

Thyroid bruit

Atrial
fibrillation

Weight loss

Heat intolerance

Tremor
Sweaty
Flushed

Tachycardia
High pulse
pressure

Hyper-reflexia

Diarrhoea

Pretibial mxyoedema

HYPOTHYROIDISM

Idiopathic senile atrophy

PRIMARY
Autoimmune
(Hashimoto's)

SECONDARY
Pituitary failure

TERTIARY
Hypothalamic failure

Enzyme failures (congenital)

Poor work
Lassitude
Slow mentation

Hair loss
Thin eyebrows
Puffy eyelids

Hoarse voice

Coarse dry skin
Pallor

Bradycardia
Hypotension

Weight gain

Hyporeflexia
Bradykinesia

Constipation

Cold intolerance

Proximal myopathy

Peripheral oedema

Definition

A *goitre* is an enlargement of the thyroid gland from any cause.

Key points

- Toxic goitres are rarely malignant.
- In hyperthyroidism serum TSH is low and serum T4 and T3 are high.
- In hypothyroidism TSH is high and T4 is low.
- All solitary nodules should have U/S, radionuclide imaging, FNAC) to exclude carcinoma.
- Surgery is rarely necessary in autoimmune or inflammatory thyroid disease.

Common causes

- Physiological: gland increases in size as a result of increased demand for thyroid hormone at puberty and during pregnancy.
- Iodine deficiency (endemic): deficiency of iodine results in decreased T_4 levels and increased TSH stimulation leading to a diffuse goitre.
- Primary hyperthyroidism (Graves' disease): goitre and thyrotoxicosis due to circulating immunoglobulin LATS.
- Adenomatous (nodular) goitre: benign hyperplasia of the thyroid gland.
- Thyroiditis: autoimmune (Hashimoto's); subacute (de Quervain's); Riedel's (struma).
- Thyroid malignancies.

Clinical features
Hyperthyroidism
Symptoms

- Heat intolerance and excessive sweating.
- Increased appetite, weight loss, diarrhoea.
- Anxiety, tiredness, palpitations.
- Oligomenorrhoea.

Signs

- Goitre.
- Exophthalmos, lid lag and retraction.
- Warm moist palms, tremor.
- Atrial fibrillation.
- Pretibial myxoedema.

Hypothyroidism
Symptoms

- Cold intolerance, decreased sweating.
- Hoarseness.
- Weight increase, constipation.
- Slow cerebration, tiredness.
- Muscle pains.

Signs

- Pale/yellow skin, dry, thickened skin, thin hair.
- Periorbital puffiness, loss of outer third of eyebrow.
- Dementia, nerve deafness, hyporeflexia.
- Slow pulse, large tongue, peripheral oedema.

Investigations and essential management

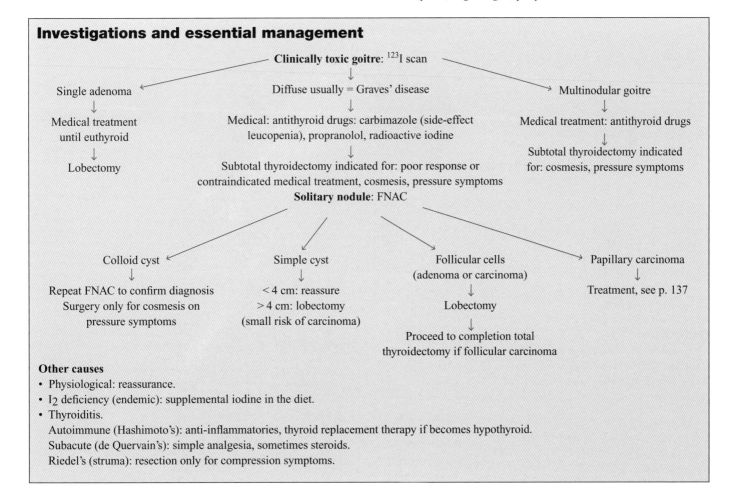

Other causes
- Physiological: reassurance.
- I_2 deficiency (endemic): supplemental iodine in the diet.
- Thyroiditis.
  Autoimmune (Hashimoto's): anti-inflammatories, thyroid replacement therapy if becomes hypothyroid.
  Subacute (de Quervain's): simple analgesia, sometimes steroids.
  Riedel's (struma): resection only for compression symptoms.

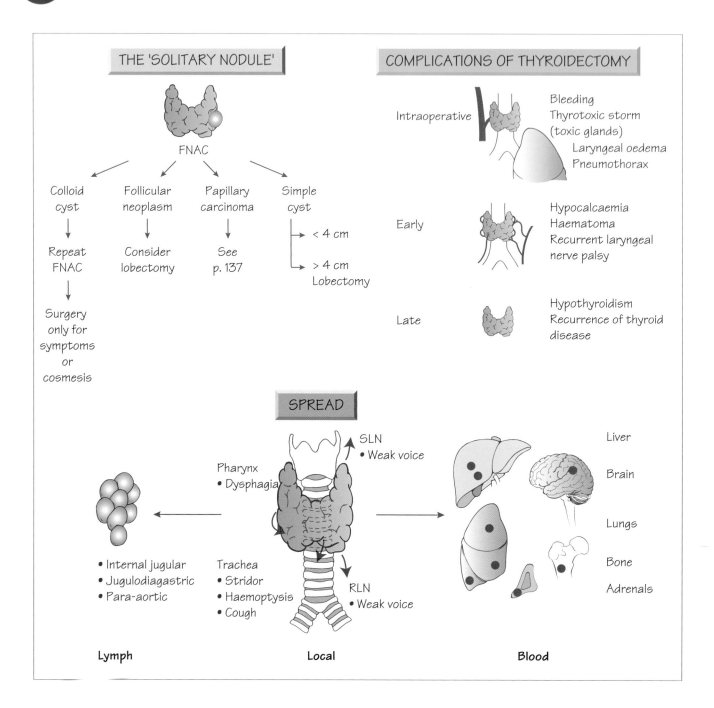

Definition

Malignant lesions of the thyroid gland. Papillary and follicular are known as differentiated carcinomas. Anaplastic and medullary are poorly or undifferentiated carcinomas.

Key points

- Many thyroid cancers found in young adults. Occasionally occur in childhood.
- Isolated thyroid lumps should always be investigated to confirm a cause.
- The prognosis is often good with surgical resection and medical adjuvant treatment.
- All patients should be managed by an MDT.

Epidemiology

Male:female 1:2. Peak incidence depends on histology (papillary, young adults; follicular, middle age; anaplastic, elderly; medullary, any age).

Pathology

Histology of thyroid malignancies.

Type	(%)	Cell of origin	Differentiation	Spread
Papillary	(60%)	Epithelial	Well	Lymphatic
Follicular	(25%)	Epithelial	Well	Haematogenous
Anaplastic	(10%)	Epithelial	Poor	Direct, lymphatic and haematogenous
Medullary	(5%)	Parafollicular	Moderate	Lymphatic and haematogenous

Aetiology

Predisposing factors:
- Pre-existing goitre.
- Previous radiation of the neck.
- Thyroid cancer in first degree relative.

Clinical features

- Papillary: solitary thyroid nodule.
- Follicular: slow-growing thyroid mass, symptoms from distant metastases.
- Anaplastic: rapidly growing thyroid mass causing tracheal and oesophageal compression.
- Medullary: thyroid lump, may have *MEN IIA* (medullary thyroid carcinoma, phaeochromocytoma, hyperparathyroidism) or *MEN IIB* (medullary thyroid carcinoma, phaeochromocytoma, multiple mucosal neuromas, Marfanoid habitus) syndrome or *familial medullary thyroid cancer* (FMTC).

Essential management

Papillary
- Surgery: total thyroidectomy and removal of involved lymph nodes.
- Adjunctive treatment: ^{131}I ablation and TSH suppression (T_4 therapy) (rationale: TSH production stimulates papillary tumour growth).
- Prognosis: no metastases, 97% 5-year survival; metastases, 50% 5-year survival.

Follicular
- Surgery: thyroid lobectomy and removal of involved nodes for tumours <1 cm or total thyroidectomy and removal of involved nodes for tumours >1 cm or if metastases or local spread are present.
- Adjunctive treatment: TSH suppression (T_4 therapy) for all tumours. ^{131}I ablation and TSH suppression for tumours treated by total thyroidectomy.
- Prognosis: no metastases, 90% 5-year survival; metastases, 50% 5-year survival.

Anaplastic
- Surgery: only to relieve pressure symptoms.
- Adjunctive treatment: neither radiotherapy nor chemotherapy is effective. Some response to doxorubicin ± cisplatin.
- Prognosis: dismal – most patients will be dead within 12 months of diagnosis.

Medullary
- Exclude phaeochromocytoma before treating (MEN II).
- Surgery: total thyroidectomy and excision of regional lymph nodes.
- Adjuvant radiotherapy and chemotherapy ineffective.
- Prognosis: overall 85% 5-year survival.

Investigations
- Ultrasound of the thyroid gland.
- FNAC: may give histological diagnosis.
- Bone scan and radiographs of bones for secondary deposits.
- Calcitonin levels as a marker for medullary carcinoma.
- Serum thyroglobulin is an excellent tumour marker in patients who have had total thyroidectomy and ^{131}I ablation.

Complications of thyroid surgery
- Postoperative bleeding: an expanding haematoma can cause laryngeal oedema and airway obstruction. Rx – relieve haematoma, intubate.
- Voice dysfunction: damage to recurrent or external laryngeal nerves (only 1% have permanent injury and few require treatment). Vocal cords should checked by laryngoscopy pre-operatively.
- Hypocalcaemia: damage to parathyroid glands. Rx: 500 mg elemental calcium t.d.s. ± vitamin D (alfacalcidol or calcitrol). If severe symptoms give calcium gluconate IV slowly.
- Hypothyroidism: expected consequence of total thyroidectomy. Measure TSH levels and replace with T_4 (or T_3).
- Thyrotoxic storm: rare now. May occur during or after surgery for Graves' disease. Rx: beta-blockade, steroids, iodine and propylthiouracil.

2-week wait referral criteria for suspected head and neck cancer

- Horseness >6 weeks.
- Oral ulceration >3 weeks.
- Oral swellings >3 weeks.
- Dysphagia >3 weeks.
- Neck mass >3 weeks.
- Cranial neuropathies.
- Rapidly developed thyroid lump.

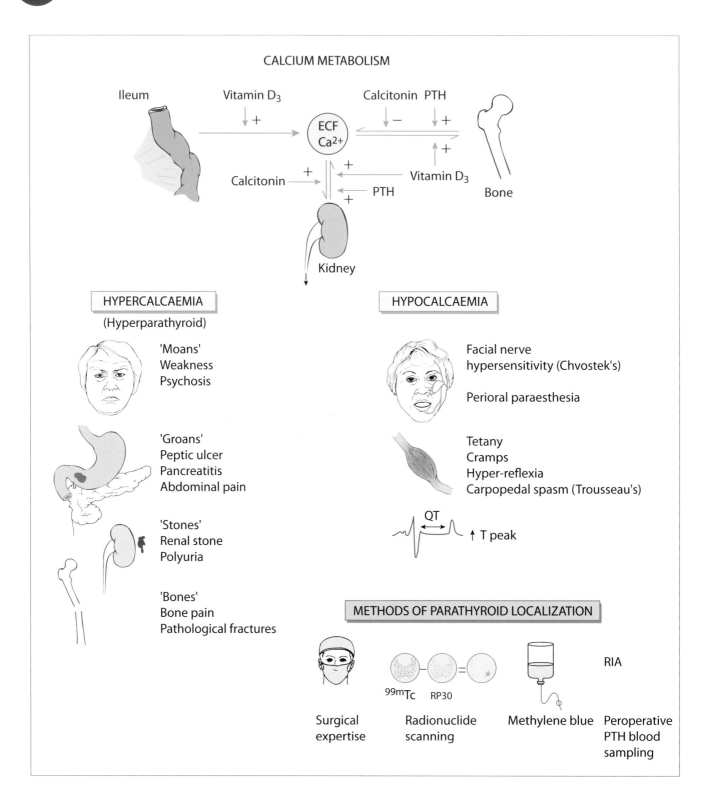

CALCIUM METABOLISM

Ileum — Vitamin D₃ + → ECF Ca²⁺ ← Calcitonin (−) PTH (+) → Bone

HYPERCALCAEMIA
(Hyperparathyroid)

'Moans'
Weakness
Psychosis

'Groans'
Peptic ulcer
Pancreatitis
Abdominal pain

'Stones'
Renal stone
Polyuria

'Bones'
Bone pain
Pathological fractures

HYPOCALCAEMIA

Facial nerve
hypersensitivity (Chvostek's)

Perioral paraesthesia

Tetany
Cramps
Hyper-reflexia
Carpopedal spasm (Trousseau's)

QT
↑ T peak

METHODS OF PARATHYROID LOCALIZATION

Surgical expertise

Radionuclide scanning
⁹⁹ᵐTc RP30

Methylene blue

RIA
Peroperative PTH blood sampling

Hyperparathyroidism

Definition

Hyperparathyroidism is a condition characterized by hypercalcaemia caused by excess production of parathyroid hormone (PTH).

Key points

- Hyperparathyroidism often presents with vague symptoms to many different specialists.
- Asymptomatic hypercalcemia is most common clinical presentation of primary hyperparathyroidism.
- Surgery is the treatment of choice for primary hyperparathyroidism.
- Hypoparathyroidism post surgery is rare and mostly transient.

Causes

- *Primary* hyperparathyroidism (PHPT) is usually due to a parathyroid benign adenoma (75%) or parathyroid hyperplasia (20%). 1.0% have parathyroid carcinoma.
- *Secondary* hyperparathyroidism is hyperplasia of the gland in response to hypocalcaemia (e.g. in chronic renal failure).
- In *tertiary* hyperparathyroidism, autonomous secretion of parathormone occurs when the secondary stimulus has been removed (e.g. after renal transplantation).
- *MEN syndromes* (type I (parathyroid adenoma, pancreatic islet cell tumours, pituitary adenoma) and type II (parathyroid adenoma, medullary thyroid cancer, phaeochromocytoma) and *ectopic* parathormone production (e.g. from small cell lung cancer).

Pathology

Parathormone mobilizes calcium from bone, enhances renal tubular absorption and, with vitamin D, intestinal absorption of calcium. The net result is *hypercalcaemia*.

Clinical features

- Older women, >40 years of age.
- Renal calculi or renal calcification – occurs in 20% of patients, polyuria ('renal stones').
- Bone pain or deformity, osteitis fibrosa cystica, pathological fractures ('painful bones').
- Muscle weakness, anorexia, intestinal atony, psychosis ('psychic moans').
- Peptic ulceration and pancreatitis ('abdominal groans').

Diagnosis

Laboratory

- Elevated PTH in the setting of hypercalcaemia.
- Serum calcium (specimen taken on three occasions with patient fasting, at rest and without a tourniquet). Normal range 2.2–2.6 mmol/L. Calcium is bound to albumin and the level has to be 'corrected' when albumin levels are abnormal.
- May be decreased serum phosphate and elevated alkaline phosphatase.

Imaging

- High-resolution ultrasound.
- ^{99m}Tc sestamibi scintigraphy ± sestamibi-single photon emission computed tomography (SPECT).
- CT and MRI scanning.
- DXA scans for bone density measurement in all patients with hyperparathyroidism.
- Selective vein catheterization and digital subtraction angiography in patients in whom exploration has been unsuccessful.

Essential management

- Treat hypercalcaemia if calcium levels very high (>2.88 mmol/L).
- Patients with symptomatic PHPT are candidates for surgery: excise adenoma if present, remove 3.5 of 4 glands for hyperplasia. Intraoperative rapid PTH assay facilitates minimally invasive parathyroidectomy under LA with >95% success rate, i.e. return to normocalcaemia.
- Asymptomatic or patients refuse or unfit for surgery: bisphosphonates (inhibit bone resorption), calcimimetics (cinacalcet inhibits PTH secretion), oestrogen-progestin in postmenopausal women, maintain moderate vitamin D and calcium intake and encourage hydration (8 glasses of water/day).

Hypoparathyroidism

Definition

Hypoparathyroidism is a rare condition characterized by hypocalcaemia due to reduced production of parathormone.

Causes

- Post-thyroid or parathyroid surgery ('hungry bone syndrome') or neck irradiation.
- Idiopathic (often autoimmune and presents in children or young adults).
- Congenital enzymatic deficiencies (numerous syndromes).
- Metal overload (e.g. iron (haemochromatosis or thalassaemia), copper (Wilson's disease), magnesium).
- Pseudohypoparathyroidism (reduced sensitivity to parathormone).

Pathology

Reduced serum calcium increases neuromuscular excitability.

Clinical features

- Perioral paraesthesia, cramps, tetany.
- *Chvostek's sign*: tapping over facial nerve induces facial muscle contractions.
- *Trousseau's sign*: inflating BP cuff to above systolic pressure induces typical *main d'accoucheur* carpal spasm.
- Prolonged QT interval on ECG.

Diagnosis

Calcium and parathormone levels decreased. Also measure vitamin D and magnesium.

Essential management

Calcium and vitamin D.

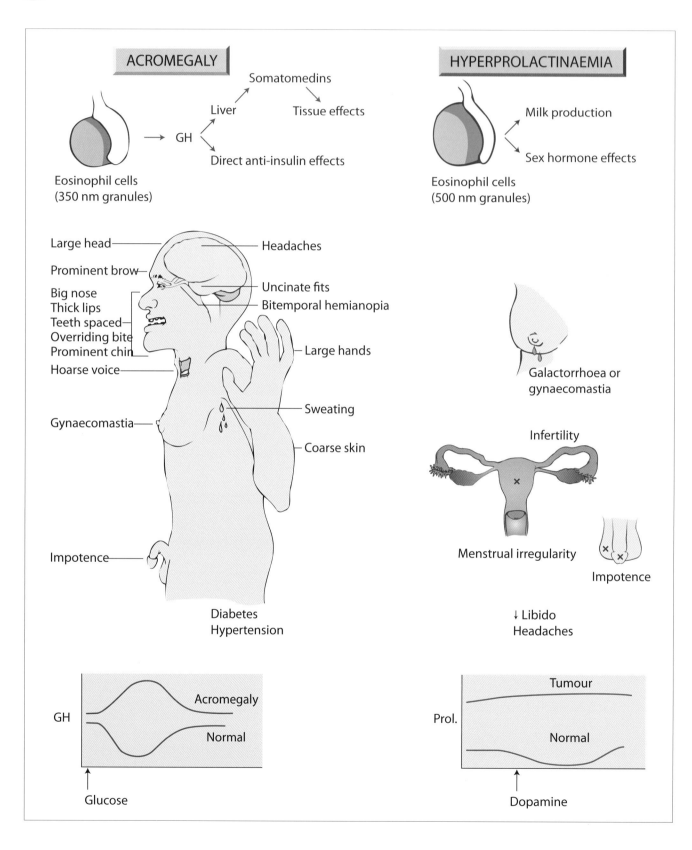

ACROMEGALY

Somatomedins

Liver → Tissue effects

GH → Direct anti-insulin effects

Eosinophil cells
(350 nm granules)

Large head — Headaches
Prominent brow
Big nose — Uncinate fits
Thick lips — Bitemporal hemianopia
Teeth spaced
Overriding bite
Prominent chin
Hoarse voice — Large hands

Gynaecomastia — Sweating

— Coarse skin

Impotence

Diabetes
Hypertension

GH — Acromegaly / Normal

Glucose

HYPERPROLACTINAEMIA

Milk production

Sex hormone effects

Eosinophil cells
(500 nm granules)

Galactorrhoea or
gynaecomastia

Infertility

Menstrual irregularity

Impotence

↓ Libido
Headaches

Prol. — Tumour / Normal

Dopamine

Definition

Pituitary disorders are characterized either by a *failure of secretion* of pituitary hormones or by tumours, which cause *local pressure effects* or specific syndromes due to *hormone overproduction.*

Key points

- Acromegaly is often insidious in onset and slow to be diagnosed.
- Deficiencies of pituitary function are generally tested for by stimulation tests and overactivity by suppressions tests. Direct serum hormone levels may also be measured.
- Imaging the pituitary gland is best done by MRI.

Common causes

- Primary failure of *anterior* pituitary secretion (GH, gonadotrophins, TSH and ACTH) causes pan-hypopituitarism (Simmonds' disease):

  pressure from a tumour – adenoma or craniopharyngioma

  infarction or ischaemia – haemorrhagic shock, especially postpartum (Sheehan's syndrome)

  inflammatory – meningitis, pituitary abscess, sarcoidosis

  infiltrative – haemochromatosis

  iatrogenic – surgery, radiotherapy.

- Secondary *anterior* pituitary secretion failure from hypothalamic causes.
- Failure of ADH production from the *posterior* pituitary gland leads to central diabetes insipidus (CDI). Nephrogenic diabetes insipidus (NDI) results from renal resistance to ADH. Causes of CDI are:

  idiopathic – some genetic (abnormality of ADH gene on chromosome 20)

  trauma – especially skull base fractures

  tumours – sellar and suprasellar, e.g. craniopharyngioma

  granulomas – TB or sarcoidosis

  vascular – aneurysm or thrombosis.

Clinical features

- Pan-hypopituitarism: pallor (MSH), hypothyroidism (TSH), failure of lactation (PL), chronic adrenal insufficiency (ACTH), delayed puberty, ovarian failure and amenorrhoea (FSH, LH). GH loss in adults is usually asymptomatic or may lead to loss of energy.
- Diabetes insipidus (ADH): insidious or abrupt onset of *polyuria* (5–20 L/day) and *polydipsia.*

- Tumours: clinical features of a mass lesion: (headache, bitemporal hemianopia, altered appetite, thirst).
- Hyperpituitarism is virtually always selective:

  acromegaly/gigantism (excess GH): thickened skin, increased skull size, prognathism, enlarged tongue, goitre, osteoporosis, organomegaly, spade-like hands and feet

  Cushing's disease (excess ACTH): malaise, muscle weakness, weight gain, bruising, moon facies, buffalo hump, hirsutism, amenorrhoea, impotence, polyuria, diabetes, emotional instability

  galactorrhoea (excess PL): spontaneous flow of milk from the nipple at any time other than during breastfeeding.

Investigations

- Pan-hypopituitarism: serum assay of pituitary and target gland hormones, dynamic tests of pituitary function.
- CDI: very low urinary specific gravity (<1.005 and osmolality <200 mOsm/L) which does not increase with a *water deprivation test.*
- Tumours: visual field measurements, hormone assay, MRI or CT scanning. CTA may be useful in planning surgery.

Essential management

- Pan-hypopituitarism: replacement therapy – cyclical oestrogen – progesterone, hydrocortisone, thyroxine.
- Diabetes insipidus: vasopressin analogue, desmopressin, administered as nasal spray.
- Tumours: bromocriptine suppresses PL release from prolactinomas, ^{90}Y implant for pituitary ablation, surgery (hypophysectomy via nasal or transcranial route).

Tumours (% of total)	Cell type
Endocrinologically active (75%)	
Prolactinomas (35%)	Acidophil
GH-secreting tumours (20%)	Acidophil
Mixed PL and GH (10%)	Acidophil
ACTH-secreting tumours (10%)	Basophil
Endocrinologically inactive (25%)	Chromophobe
Craniopharyngioma (Rathke's pouch tumour)	Odontogenic epithelium

65 Adrenal disorders

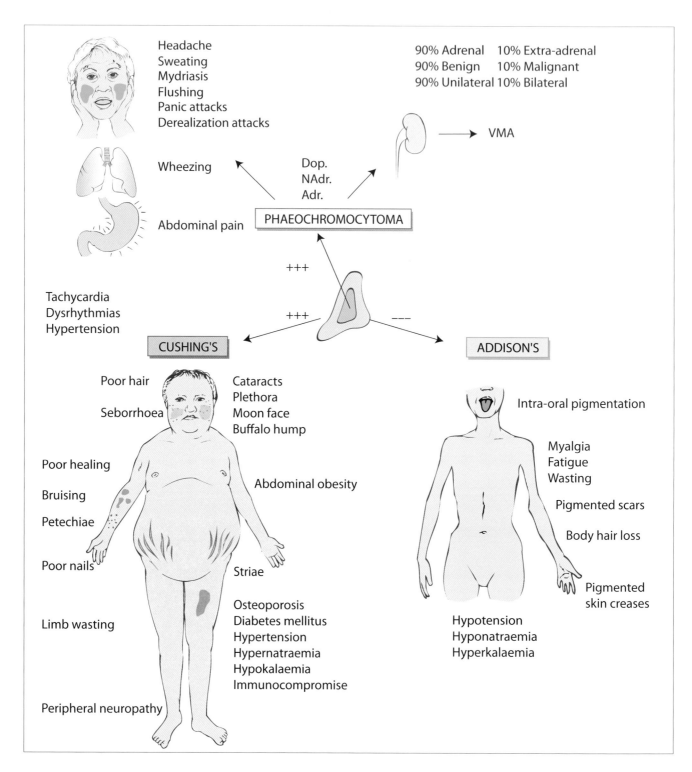

Definitions

Adrenal gland disorders are characterized by clinical syndromes resulting from either a *failure of secretion* or *excessive secretion* of adrenal cortical hormones (glucocorticoids (cortisol), mineralocorticoids (aldosterone), and androgens (DHEA)) or medullary hormones (mostly adrenaline (epinephrine)). *Cushing's syndrome* describes the clinical features irrespective of the cause; *Cushing's disease* refers to a pituitary adenoma with secondary adrenal hyperplasia. A small number of patients have non-functioning adrenal adenomas discovered incidentally.

Common causes

Failure of secretion

Addison's disease or *adrenal insufficiency*: idiopathic atrophy, autoimmune, bilateral adrenal haemorrhage in sepsis (Waterhouse–Friderichsen syndrome), TB, pituitary insufficiency, metastatic deposits.

Excessive secretion

- Cushing's syndrome: *excess corticosteroid* due to steroid therapy, ACTH-producing pituitary tumour, adenoma or carcinoma of the adrenal cortex, ectopic ACTH production, e.g. oat cell carcinoma of lung.
- Conn's syndrome (primary hyperaldosteronism): *excess aldosterone* due to adenoma or carcinoma of adrenal cortex, bilateral cortical hyperplasia.
- Congenital adrenal hyperplasia (adrenogenital syndrome): caused by *excess androgen* production from adrenal cortical hyperplasia or a cortical tumour.
- Phaeochromocytoma: *excess catecholamines* due to adrenal medullary tumours, 95% are benign.

Clinical features

- Addison's disease: see opposite. Addisonian crisis: an acute collapse which may mimic an abdominal emergency.
- Cushing's syndrome: see opposite (moon face, buffalo hump, striae).
- Conn's syndrome, primary hyperaldosteronism: muscle weakness, paraesthesias, transient paralysis, tetany, polyuria, polydipsia, hypertension, hypokalaemia.
- Congenital adrenal hyperplasia: virilization in female children, ambiguous genitalia, precocious puberty, hirsuitism, baldness, acne.
- Phaeochromocytoma: see opposite.

Investigations

Basic principles

- Establish the 'endocrine' diagnosis by serum levels or suppressions/stimulation tests.
- Correct the endocrine abnormalities.
- Localize the cause by investigation and imaging.
- Consider whether definitive (surgical) treatment is necessary.

Addison's disease

U+E ($\downarrow$ Na$^+$ <135 mmol/L, $\uparrow$ K$^+$ >5.0 mmol/L), fasting plasma glucose <2.78 mmol/L) and low plasma cortisol (<138 nmol/L). ACTH measurement and short Synacthen test to confirm diagnosis. Long Synacthen test to differentiate primary (adrenal) from secondary (pituitary) insufficiency.

Cushing's syndrome

- Elevated plasma or salivary cortisol (taken at 24.00 hours) and loss of diurnal variation.
- Low-dose dexamethasone suppression test to confirm diagnosis.
- High-dose test to distinguish adrenal from pituitary disease.
- Serum ACTH to identify secondary cause.

Conn's syndrome

- U+E ($\downarrow$ K$^+$, normal or $\uparrow$ Na$^+$).
- $\uparrow$ 24-hour urine aldosterone and $\downarrow$ renin levels. Aldosterone/renin ratio $\uparrow$.
- Metabolic alkalosis.

Congenital adrenal hyperplasia

$\uparrow$ plasma DHEA-sulphate, 17-OH progesterone, testosterone and androstenedione. Increase in 17-OH after Synacthen suggests adrenal hyperplasia. Failure of suppression of androgens production following dexamethasone suggests presence of androgen-secreting tumour.

Phaeochromocytoma

Plasma-free metanephrines is 99% sensitive. 24-hour urinary VMA and HVA may be used. (Consider MEN type II (parathyroid adenoma, medullary thyroid cancer, phaeochromocytoma).)

Localization imaging

- Helical CT and MRI: excellent for adrenal gland, retroperitoneum.
- ^{123}I-MIBG scan: neuroendocrine tumours (phaeochromocytoma).
- Arteriography and venous sampling: occasionally required.

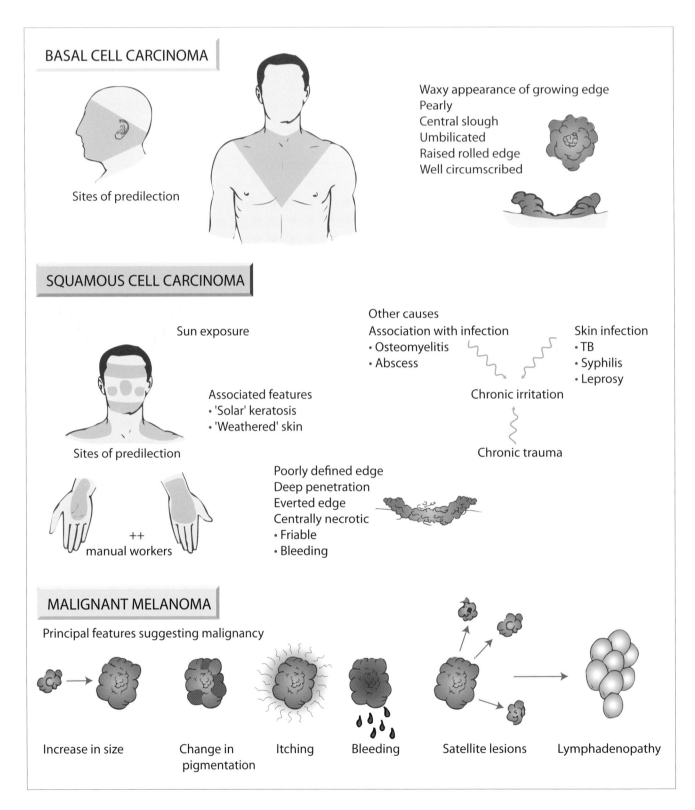

BASAL CELL CARCINOMA

Sites of predilection

Waxy appearance of growing edge
Pearly
Central slough
Umbilicated
Raised rolled edge
Well circumscribed

SQUAMOUS CELL CARCINOMA

Sun exposure

Other causes
Association with infection
• Osteomyelitis
• Abscess

Skin infection
• TB
• Syphilis
• Leprosy

Associated features
• 'Solar' keratosis
• 'Weathered' skin

Chronic irritation

Sites of predilection

Chronic trauma

++
manual workers

Poorly defined edge
Deep penetration
Everted edge
Centrally necrotic
• Friable
• Bleeding

MALIGNANT MELANOMA

Principal features suggesting malignancy

Increase in size   Change in pigmentation   Itching   Bleeding   Satellite lesions   Lymphadenopathy

Definition

Malignant lesions of skin epidermis comprising *basal cell carcinoma* (BCC), *squamous cell carcinoma* (SCC) and *malignant melanoma* (MM).

> ## Key points
>
> - Protection from sun exposure (especially UV-B radiation) reduces risk of all skin cancers ('*slip* on a shirt, *slop* on sunscreen, and *slap* on a hat').
> - Not all MMs are pigmented.
> - All pigmented lesions with suspicious features should be excision biopsied.
> - The prognosis from early MM is excellent with surgery but poor with advanced disease.
> - SCC is often good prognosis especially in the elderly.

Epidemiology

Male:female 2:1 for BCC and SCC. Elderly males. Equal sex distribution and all adults for MM. Most common in fair skinned peoples (Irish, Scottish). All tumours common in areas of high annual sunshine (e.g. Australia, southern USA). BCC is the most common human cancer.

Malignant melanoma

Aetiology/predisposing factors

- Exposure to sunlight – both UV-A (wave length 320–400 nm) and especially UV-B (290–320 nm) radiation damage skin. (UV-C (200–290 nm) does not penetrate the ozone layer.)
- Naevi (50% of MM arise in pre-existing benign pigmented lesions).
- *CDKN2A* (*p16*) tumour suppressor gene mutation.

Pathology

- Arises from the melanocytes often in pre-existing naevi.
- Superficial spreading (70%), nodular types (10–15%) and lentigo maligna (10–15%) acral lentiginous (5%).
- Radial and vertical growth phases. Lymphatic spread is to regional lymph nodes and haematogenous spread to liver, bone and brain.
- Immunohistochemistry helpful in diagnosing nodal metastases.

Clinical features

Pigmented lesions (occasionally not pigmented – amelanotic), 1 cm in diameter on lower limbs, feet, head and neck. (Also eyes, GI tract and oral and genital mucus membranes.) Usually present as a change in a pigmented lesion: increasing size or pigmentation/bleeding/pain or itching/ulceration/satellite lesions.

Squamous cell carcinoma

Aetiology/predisposing factors

- Exposure to sunlight
- Immunosuppression (high incidence after renal transplant).
- Radiation exposure (radiotherapy, among radiologists).
- Chemical carcinogens (hydrocarbons, arsenic, coal tar).
- Inherited disorders (albinism, xeroderma pigmentosum).
- Leukoplakia (clinical term to describe a white patch usually seen in the mouth).
- Chronic irritation: old burns, scars sites of radiotherapy, chronic ulcers (Marjolin's ulcer).
- Bowen's disease and erythroplasia of Queyrat.
- HPV infection and intraepithelial neoplasia (especially SCC perianal and perineal skin).

Pathology

- Arises from keratinocytes in the epidermis. *Bowen's disease* = SCC *in situ*, *Erythroplasia of Queyrat* = SCC *in situ* of the penis.
- Spreads by local invasion, lymphatic spread and metastases. Large lesions (>2 cm) or deep lesions (>4 mm) may metastasize in 1–5% of cases.

Clinical features

Lesions (erythematous papules, nodules, ulcers) usually on sun-exposed areas of the body.

Actinic keratoses or chronic ulcers may progress to SCC.

Basal cell carcinoma

Aetiology/predisposing factors

- Exposure to sunlight.
- Immunosuppression (high incidence after renal transplant).
- Radiation exposure (radiotherapy, among radiologists).

Pathology

- Arises from basal cells of epidermis.
- Spreads by local invasion with tendency to recur if incompletely excised, distant metastases uncommon.

Clinical features

Recurring, ulcerated, umbilicated skin lesion on forehead or face (70%). Ulcer has a raised, pearl-coloured edge. Untreated, large areas of the face may be eroded (rodent ulcer).

Staging

- SCC: TNM (Stages I–IV).
- MM: TNM (Stages I–IV) has replaced Clarke's levels I–V and Breslow's tumour thickness.

Investigations

- Biopsy (usually excisional) of the lesion unless clinically certain (definitive surgery).
- For MM – helical CT scan for ?involved draining nodes, FNAC for palpable draining nodes, ?peroperative sentinel node biopsy using dye injection mapping.

Essential management

Basal cell carcinoma

- Curettage/cautery/cryotherapy/photodynamic therapy/topical chemotherapy (5-FU, imiquimod). These treatments may be suitable for small lesions.
- Surgical excision/radiotherapy – most effective treatments. Mohs' micrographic surgery (the tumour is removed layer by layer until completely gone as determined histologically) is the most effective treatment for high-risk facial BCC.

Squamous cell carcinoma

- Surgical excision/radiotherapy/cryosurgery for small lesions/ Mohs' micrographic surgery.
- Topical 5-FU is not recommended for SCC.

Malignant melanoma

- Excisional biopsy. If positive re-excision with margins depending on depth of tumour:
  <1 mm thickness (T1) – 1 cm margin
  1–4 mm thickness (T2–T3) – 2 cm margin
  >4 mm thickness (T4) – at least 2 cm margin
- Lymph node dissection if CT, FNAC or sentinel node biopsy positive for metastases with no systemic disease.
- Adjuvant therapy may be indicated for patients with deep primary disease (>4 mm) or advanced disease. Immunotherapy (interferon-α2b), chemotherapy (dacarbazine) or combinations of these therapies.

Prognosis

- BCC, SCC prognosis is usually excellent – SCC should be followed for 5 years.
- MM prognosis depends on TNM staging (based on primary tumour thickness (T1 = ≤1.0 mm, T2 = 1.01–2.0 mm, T3 = 2.01–4.0 mm, T4 = >4.00 mm) and ulceration, nodal involvement and metastases. See http://www.melanomaprognosis.org/ for prognostic calculator.

Stage	Treatment	5-year survival
I	Wide local excision	>90%
II	Wide local excision	45–77%
III	Wide local excison + lymph node dissection	27–50%
IV	Local excision and adjuvant Rx	<20%

2-week wait referral criteria for suspected skin cancer

- Pigmented lesion + increased size/changed shape/changed colour/mixed colour/irregular/ulceration.
- Non-healing skin lesion.
- Biopsy-proven squamous carcinoma.
- New skin lesion in immunosuppressed.

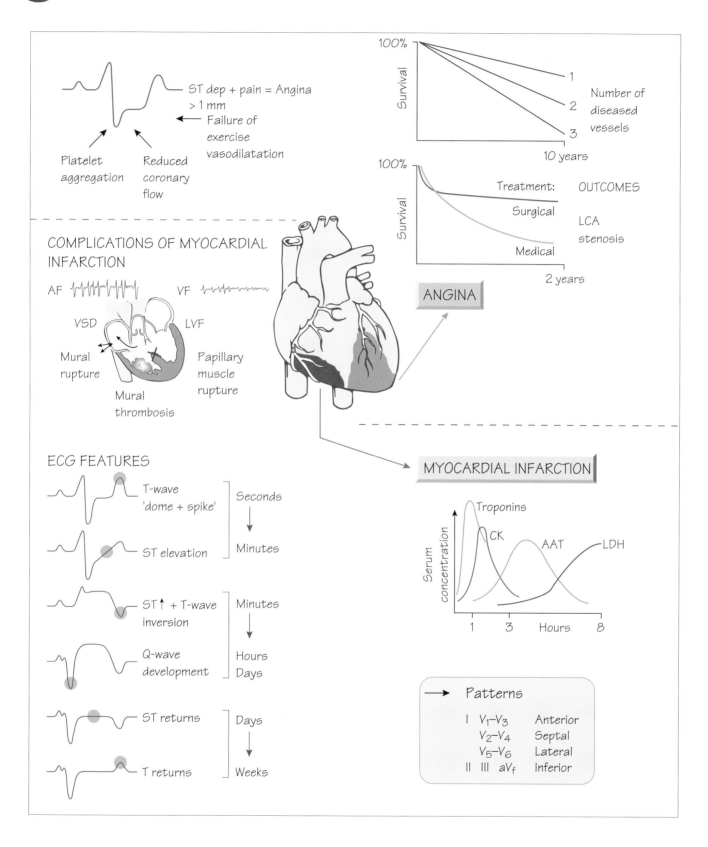

Definition

Ischaemic heart disease is caused by acute or chronic interruption of the blood supply to the myocardium, usually due to atherosclerosis of the coronary arteries (*coronary artery disease* [CAD]). *Angina pectoris* (AP) is ischaemic chest pain induced by exercise and relieved by rest or GTN. *Myocardial infarction* (MI) is ischaemic death of heart muscle with (*STEMI*) or without (*NSTEMI*) ST-elevation on ECG. Acute coronary syndrome (*ACS*) is any acute ischaemic symptoms attributable to the coronary circulation.

Key points

- Mortality from CAD is declining. Up to 20% of patients with an acute MI will die.
- Serum troponins are highly sensitive and very specific for myocardial injury.
- Urgent treatment (PCI, fibrinolysis, CABG) reduces the risk of death from MI.

Epidemiology

Male > female before 65 years. Increasing risk with increasing age up to 80 years. Most common cause of death in the Western world. Lower incidence of CAD in countries with Mediterranean diet (French paradox).

Aetiology

- Atherosclerosis and thrombosis.
- Thromboemboli (especially plaque rupture).
- Arteritis (e.g. periarteritis nodosa).
- Coronary artery spasm.
- Extension of aortic dissection/syphilitic aortitis.

Risk factors

- Family history.
- Hypertension.
- Diabetes mellitus.
- Metabolic syndrome.
- Hyperhomocysteinaemia.
- Cigarette smoking.
- Poor lipid profile (especially high LDL).
- Obesity.
- Type A personality.

Pathology

- Atherosclerosis is initiated by vascular endothelial injury caused by altered haemodynamics, hyperglycaemia, dyslipidaemia, cigarette smoking, infection (*Chlamydia pneumoniae, Helicobacter pylori, herpes simplex virus*).
- Reduction in coronary blood flow is critical when the lumen is decreased by 90%.
- Plaque rupture in non-critically stenosed arteries (<50% occlusion), precipitating local thrombosis and vessel occlusion, frequently causes of acute ischaemia.

- The heart muscle in the territory of the occluded vessel becomes ischaemic.
- Angina pectoris results when the supply of O_2 to the heart muscle is unable to meet increased demands, e.g. during exercise, cold, after a meal.

Clinical features

Spectrum of presentations: non-acute (stable angina) – acute coronary syndromes (unstable angina, NSTEMI, STEMI) – cardiac arrest – CCF – arrythmias.

Non-acute coronary artery disease

- Central chest pain on exertion, especially in cold weather, lasts 1–15 minutes.
- Radiates to neck, jaw, arms.
- Relieved by GTN.
- Usually no signs.

Acute coronary artery disease

- Severe central chest pain for >30 minutes' duration.
- Radiates to neck, jaw, arms.
- Not relieved by GTN.
- Cardiogenic shock (sweating, dyspnoea, tachycardia, hypotension ± CCF, murmurs).
- Arrhythmias.

Investigations
Non-acute coronary artery disease

- FBC and baseline chemistry.
- Lipid profile (total cholesterol, LDL, HDL, triglycerides).
- Inflammatory markers (CRP – in combination with LDL and HDL – identifies patients at risk of acute coronary syndromes).
- Thyroid function tests.
- Homocysteine levels.
- Chest X-ray: heart size.
- 12-lead ECG – ST segment changes.
- Exercise ECG and 24-hour ambulatory ECG monitoring.
- Myocardial perfusion nuclear (± stress) imaging – detects reversible myocardial perfusion defects.
- Coronary angiography, measurement of flow reserve and intravascular ultrasound assessment of atheromatous lesions.

Acute coronary syndromes

- FBC, platelets, baseline chemistry (K^+ and Mg^{2+}) and creatinine, CRP.
- Serial ECG: Q waves, ST segment and T-wave changes.
- Serial serum markers: troponins (I and T), creatine kinase – myocardial band (CPK-MB), ischaemia-modified albumin, B-type natriuretic peptide.
- Chest X-ray: heart size, evidence of pulmonary oedema.
- Echocardiography (transthoracic for LV and valve function, transoesophageal for ?aortic dissection) ± stress echo (exercise or pharmacological).
- Angiography:
  non-invasive – MRA, multidetector CT angiography
  invasive – transluminal coronary angiography (cardiac catherization).

Essential management

Non-acute coronary artery disease (stable angina)

Aim of Rx: relieve symptoms, prevent ACS and sudden cardiac death.

Relieve symptoms:
- Nitrates and beta-blockers; calcium-channel blockers; ranolazine

Prolong survival:
- Lifestyle modification: stop smoking, lose weight, exercise.
- Antiplatelet agents (aspirin/clopidogrel), statins, beta-blockers, nitrates.
- Treatment of hypertension and hyperlipidaemia.
- ± Revascularization: percutaneous coronary intervention (PCI) or CABG.

Acute coronary syndromes (ACS) (unstable angina, STEMI, NSTEMI)

Aim of treatment is to relieve symptoms, restore myocardial perfusion, prevent/treat complications and future cardiac events.
- Relieve symptoms: admit to CCU, bed rest, O_2, morphine, nitrates
- Restore myocardial perfusion:
  percutaneous coronary intervention (PCI) – angioplasty ± stent
  fibrinolysis (tPA) – indicated within 90 mins in patients with STEMI
  emergency/urgent CABG (rarely).
- Prevent/treat complications:
  beta-blockers – give to all MIs unless contraindicated
  ACE inhibitors (or angiotensin receptor blocker [ARB]) improves outcome
  treat arrhythmias and heart failure.
- Long-term management as for non-acute coronary syndromes.

Indications for CABG
- Left main brainstem disease.
- Three-vessel disease.
- Two-vessel disease involving LAD.
- Chronic ischaemia + LV dysfunction.

Complications of MI
- Arrhythmias.
- Cardiogenic shock.
- Myocardial rupture.
- Papillary muscle rupture causing mitral incompetence.
- Ventricular aneurysm.
- Pericarditis.
- Mural thrombosis and peripheral embolism.

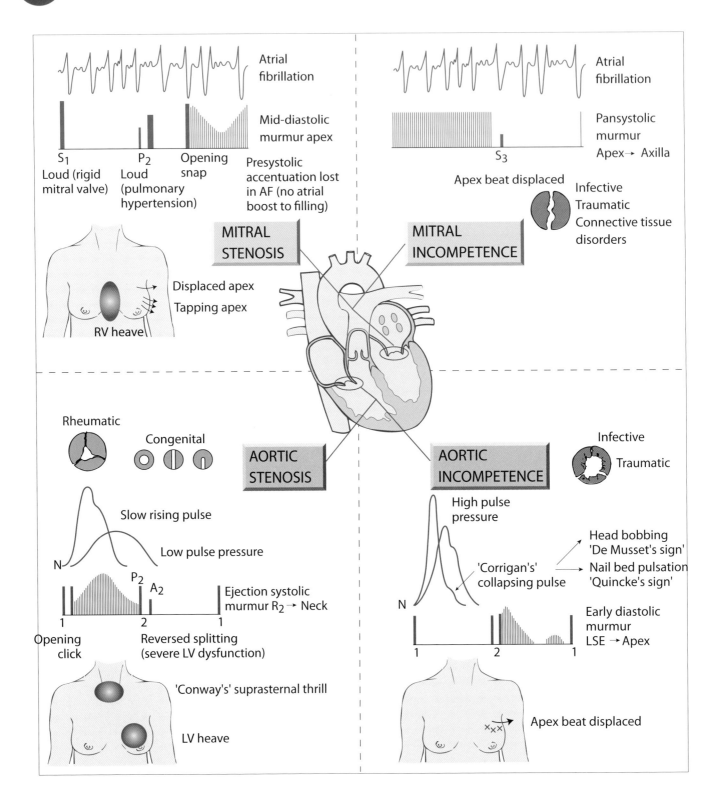

Atrial fibrillation

Mid-diastolic murmur apex

S₁ — Loud (rigid mitral valve)
P₂ — Loud (pulmonary hypertension)
Opening snap

Presystolic accentuation lost in AF (no atrial boost to filling)

MITRAL STENOSIS

Displaced apex
Tapping apex
RV heave

Atrial fibrillation

Pansystolic murmur
Apex → Axilla

S₃

Apex beat displaced

Infective
Traumatic
Connective tissue disorders

MITRAL INCOMPETENCE

Rheumatic
Congenital

AORTIC STENOSIS

Slow rising pulse
Low pulse pressure

P₂ A₂

1   2   1

Opening click
Reversed splitting (severe LV dysfunction)

Ejection systolic murmur R₂ → Neck

'Conway's' suprasternal thrill
LV heave

AORTIC INCOMPETENCE

Infective
Traumatic

High pulse pressure

'Corrigan's' collapsing pulse

Head bobbing 'De Musset's sign'
Nail bed pulsation 'Quincke's sign'

N

1   2   1

Early diastolic murmur
LSE → Apex

Apex beat displaced

Definition

Valvular heart disease comprises a group of congenital or acquired conditions characterized by damage to the heart valve(s), resulting in deranged blood flow through the heart chambers.

Key points

- Valve replacements are uncommon but prognosis is very good.
- Biological valves tend to degenerate after 10–15 years.

Epidemiology

Rheumatic fever is still a major problem in developing countries, while congenital heart disease occurs in 8–10 cases per 1000 live births worldwide.

Aetiology

- Congenital valve abnormalities.
- Rheumatic fever.
- Infective endocarditis.
- Degenerative valve disease.
- Drug induced (ergot, dopamine agonists).

Pathology

- Rheumatic fever: *immune-mediated acute inflammation* of heart valves due to a cross-reaction between group A α-haemolytic *Streptococcus* antigens and cardiac proteins.
- Disease may narrow valve orifice (*stenosis*) or make it *incompetent* (*regurgitation*) or both.
- Stenosis causes a *pressure load* while regurgitation causes a *volume load* on the heart chamber immediately proximal to it with upstream and downstream effects.

Clinical features

Aortic stenosis
(Senile degeneration most common cause.)
- Angina pectoris.
- Dizziness, syncope.
- Left heart failure.
- Slow upstroke arterial pulse.
- Precordial systolic thrill (second right ICS).
- Harsh midsystolic ejection murmur (second right ICS).

Aortic regurgitation
(Congenital, rheumatic, infective endocarditis most common causes.)
- Dyspnoea, palpitations.
- Congestive cardiac failure.
- Wide pulse pressure.
- Water-hammer pulse.
- Decrescendo diastolic murmur (lower LSE).

Mitral stenosis
(Rheumatic and congenital most common causes.)
- Pulmonary hypertension.
- Paroxysmal nocturnal dyspnoea.
- Atrial fibrillation.
- Malar flush

- Loud first heart sound and opening snap.
- Low-pitched diastolic murmur with presystolic accentuation at the apex.

Mitral regurgitation
(Functional, degenerative, rheumatic, infective carditis most common causes.)
- Dyspnoea, chronic fatigue, palpitations.
- Pulmonary oedema.
- Apex laterally displaced, hyperdynamic praecordium.
- Apical pansystolic murmur radiating to axilla.

Tricuspid stenosis
(Rheumatic most common cause – usually aortic or mitral disease as well.)
- Fatigue.
- Peripheral oedema.
- Liver enlargement/ascites.
- Prominent JVP with large a waves.
- Lung fields are clear.
- Rumbling diastolic murmur (lower left sternal border).

Tricuspid regurgitation
(Functional, rheumatic, infective carditis most common causes.)
- Chronic fatigue.
- Hepatomegaly/ascites.
- Peripheral oedema.
- Right ventricular heave.
- Prominent JVP with large v waves.
- Pansystolic murmur (subxiphoid area).

Investigations
- ECG.
- Chest X-ray.
- Echocardiography and colour Doppler techniques.
- Cardiac catheterization with measurement of transvalvular gradients.

Essential managemenet

Medical

Treat cardiac failure, diuretics, restrict salt intake, reduce exercise, digitalis for rapid atrial fibrillation and anticoagulation for peripheral embolization. Secondary prophylaxis (penicillin) against further streptococcal infection.

Surgical/interventional

Repair (valvotomy or valvuoplasty) (possible in mitral and tricuspid valve only). Replacement – may be transluminal or open surgical (requires cardiopulmonary bypass). *Mechanical* valves (synthetic materials and lifelong anticoagulation) or *biological valves* (*autograft* (patient's own tissues), *xenograft* (pig or cow) or *homograft* (cadaver)). Biological valves last 10–15 years before they begin to fail due to tissue degeneration but do not require lifelong anticoagulation.

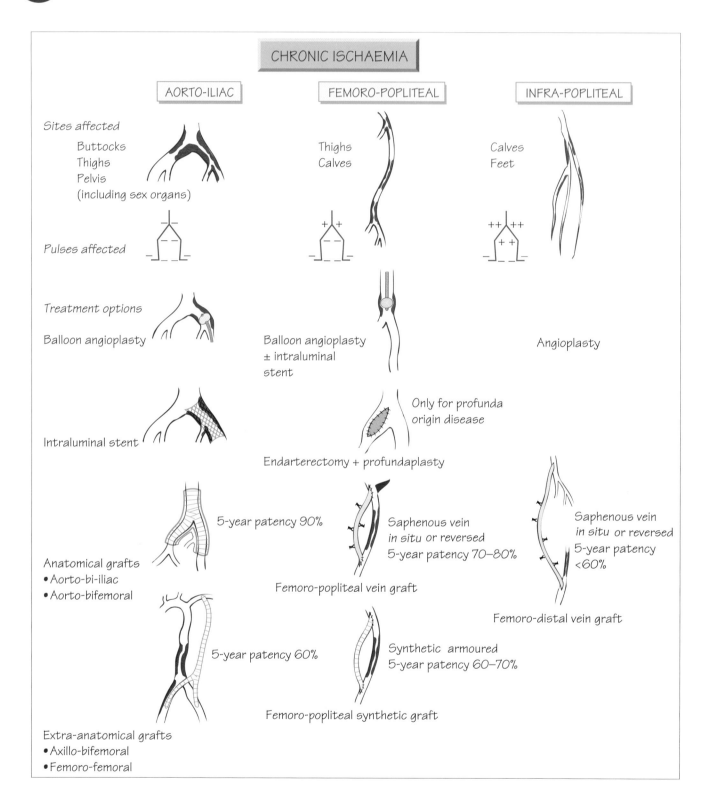

CHRONIC ISCHAEMIA

AORTO-ILIAC | **FEMORO-POPLITEAL** | **INFRA-POPLITEAL**

Sites affected
- Buttocks
- Thighs
- Pelvis
(including sex organs)

Thighs
Calves

Calves
Feet

Pulses affected

Treatment options

Balloon angioplasty

Balloon angioplasty
± intraluminal
stent

Angioplasty

Intraluminal stent

Only for profunda
origin disease

Endarterectomy + profundaplasty

Anatomical grafts
• Aorto-bi-iliac
• Aorto-bifemoral

5-year patency 90%

Saphenous vein
in situ or reversed
5-year patency 70–80%

Femoro-popliteal vein graft

Saphenous vein
in situ or reversed
5-year patency
<60%

Femoro-distal vein graft

5-year patency 60%

Synthetic armoured
5-year patency 60–70%

Femoro-popliteal synthetic graft

Extra-anatomical grafts
• Axillo-bifemoral
• Femoro-femoral

Definition

Peripheral arterial disease (PAD) (*peripheral arterial occlusive disease, peripheral occlusive vascular disease*) is a common disorder caused by acute or chronic interruption of blood supply to the limbs, usually due to atherosclerosis.

Epidemiology

Male > female before 65 years. Increased risk with increased age. Affects 10% of population >65 years in Western world.

Aetiology

- Atherosclerosis and thrombosis.
- Embolism (80% cardiac in origin, microemboli cause 'blue toe syndrome').
- Vascular trauma.
- Vasculitis (e.g. Buerger's disease).

Risk factors

Cigarette smoking, hypertension, hyperlipidaemia, diabetes mellitus, elevated homocysteine, family history.

Pathology

Reduction in blood flow to the peripheral tissues results in ischaemia which may be acute or chronic. Critical ischaemia is present when tissue viability cannot be sustained (i.e., tissue loss, rest pain for 2 weeks, ankle pressure ≤50 mmHg).

Clinical features

Fontaine classification

- Stage I, asymptomatic.
- Stage II, intermitent claudication.
- Stage III, rest pain/nocturnal pain.
- Stage IV, necrosis/gangrene.

Chronic ischaemia (see Chapter 19)

- Intermittent claudication in calf (femoral disease), thigh (iliac disease) or buttock (aorto-iliac disease).
- Cold peripheries and prolonged capillary refill time.
- Rest pain, especially at night.
- Venous guttering.
- Absent pulses.
- Arterial ulcers, especially over pressure points (heels, toes).
- Knee contractures.
- Leriche's syndrome (intermittent claudication, impotence, absent femoral pulses) indicates aortic occlusion.

Acute ischaemia (see Chapter 21)

- Pain.
- Pallor.
- Pulselessness.
- Paraesthesia and paralysis – indicate limb-threatening ischaemia that requires immediate treatment.
- 'Perishing' cold.
- 'Pistol shot' onset.
- Mottling.
- Muscle rigidity.

Investigations

Chronic ischaemia

- ABI (normal >0.9) at rest and postexercise on treadmill.
- Digital pressures (normal toe pressure >50 mmHg)
- FBC (exclude polycythaemia).
- Doppler waveform analysis.
- Digital plethysmography (in diabetes).
- Duplex ultrasound, e.g. assessing a stenosis in the femoral artery.
- Angiography (MRA, CTA or catherter angiography).

Acute ischaemia

- ECG, cardiac enzymes.
- Angiography, may be performed peroperatively.
- Find source of embolism. Holter monitoring. Echocardiograph. Ultrasound aorta for AAA.

Prognosis

Non-disabling claudication

>65% respond to conservative management. The rest require more aggressive treatment.

Disabling claudication/critical ischaemia

- Angioplasty (may be subintimal) and bypass surgery overall give good results.
- The more distal the disease the poorer the results of intervention.

Acute ischaemia

- Limb salvage 85%; mortality 10–15%.

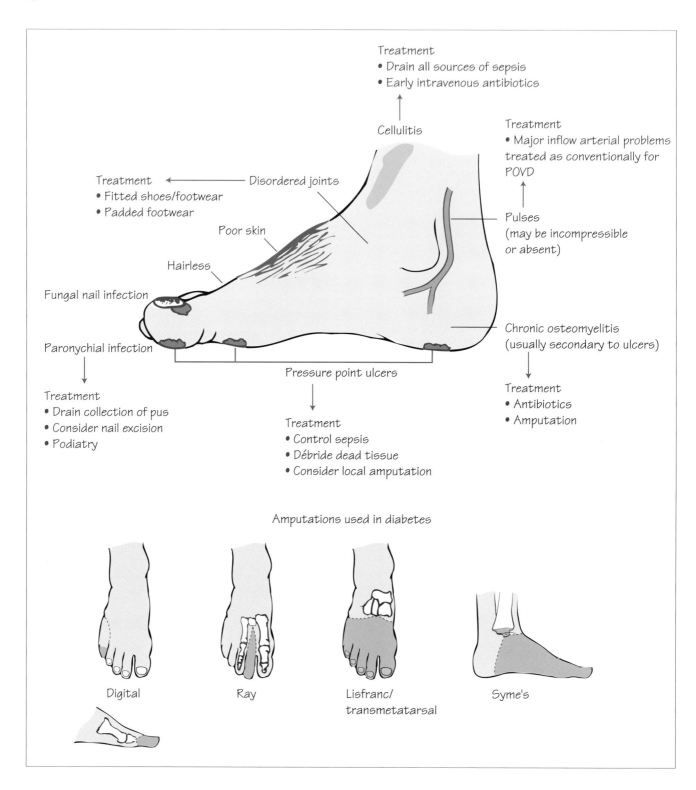

Treatment
• Drain all sources of sepsis
• Early intravenous antibiotics

Cellulitis

Treatment
• Major inflow arterial problems treated as conventionally for POVD

Treatment
• Fitted shoes/footwear
• Padded footwear

Disordered joints

Poor skin

Hairless

Pulses
(may be incompressible or absent)

Fungal nail infection

Paronychial infection

Chronic osteomyelitis
(usually secondary to ulcers)

Pressure point ulcers

Treatment
• Drain collection of pus
• Consider nail excision
• Podiatry

Treatment
• Control sepsis
• Débride dead tissue
• Consider local amputation

Treatment
• Antibiotics
• Amputation

Amputations used in diabetes

Digital

Ray

Lisfranc/
transmetatarsal

Syme's

Definition

The term *diabetic foot* refers to a spectrum of foot disorders ranging from superficial cellulitis to ulceration and gangrene occurring in people with diabetes mellitus (DM) as a result of peripheral neuropathy or ischaemia, or both.

Key points

- Prevention is all important with diabetic feet.
- All infections should be treated aggressively to reduce the risk of tissue loss.
- Osteomyelitis is frequently present in the phalanges or metatarsals.
- Treat major vessel POVD as normal – improve 'inflow' to the foot.
- Limb loss is a significant risk in patients with diabetic foot ulcers.

Pathophysiology

Three distinct processes lead to the problem of the diabetic foot:
- *Ischaemia*: macro- and microangiopathy. Higher incidence of atherosclerosis with DM.
- *Neuropathy*: sensory, motor and autonomic – multifactorial in origin.
- *Sepsis*: the glucose-saturated tissue promotes bacterial growth.

Clinical features

Neuropathic features
- Sensory disturbances – loss of vibratory and position sense.
- Trophic skin changes.
- Plantar ulceration.
- Degenerative osteoarthropathy (Charcot's joints) – occurs in 2% of DM patients.
- Pulses often present.
- Sepsis (bacterial/fungal).

Ischaemic features
- Rest pain.
- Painful ulcers over pressure areas.
- History of intermittent claudication.
- Absent pulses.
- Sepsis (bacterial/fungal).

Investigations

- FBC: leucocytosis.
- Serum glucose and gylcosylated Hb (HbA1c): diabetic control may be poor due to sepsis.
- Non-invasive vascular tests: ABI, segmental pressure, digital pressure. ABI may be falsely elevated due to medial sclerosis. Digital pressures more accurate in patients with DM.
- X-ray of foot or CT/MRI may show osteomyelitis or abscess.
- Arteriography (MRA, CTA or catheter angiography).

Essential management

Should be undertaken jointly by surgeon and physician as diabetic foot may precipitate diabetic ketoacidosis. Diabetic patients should be prescribed an antiplatelet agent and a statin.

Patient education
Do
- Carefully wash and dry feet daily.
- Inspect feet daily.
- Take meticulous care of toenails.
- Use antifungal powder.

Do not
- Walk barefoot.
- Wear ill-fitting shoes.
- Use a hot water bottle.
- Ignore any foot injury.

Neuropathic disease
- Control infection with antibiotics effective against both aerobes and anaerobes.
- Wide local excision and drainage of necrotic tissue ± skin grafting later.
- Pressure offloading: avoid weight-bearing on the wound/ulcer – special footwear, total contact casting.
- These measures usually result in healing.

Ischaemic disease
- Formal assessment of the vascular tree by angiography and reconstitution of the blood supply to the foot (either by angioplasty or bypass surgery) must be achieved before the local measures will work.
- After restoration of blood supply treat as for neuropathic disease.

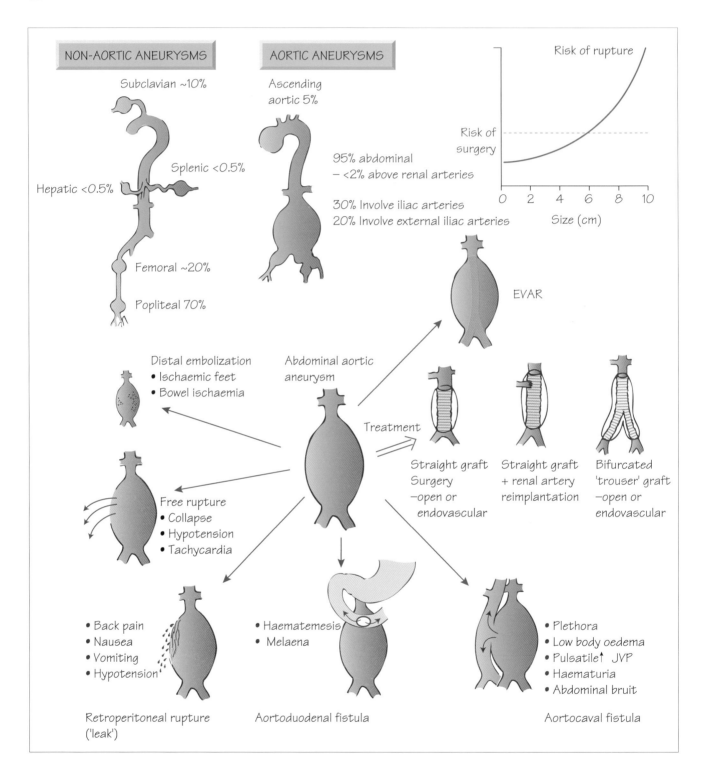

NON-AORTIC ANEURYSMS

Subclavian ~10%

Hepatic <0.5%

Splenic <0.5%

Femoral ~20%

Popliteal 70%

AORTIC ANEURYSMS

Ascending aortic 5%

95% abdominal
– <2% above renal arteries

30% Involve iliac arteries
20% Involve external iliac arteries

Risk of rupture

Risk of surgery

Size (cm)

Distal embolization
• Ischaemic feet
• Bowel ischaemia

Free rupture
• Collapse
• Hypotension
• Tachycardia

Abdominal aortic aneurysm

Treatment

EVAR

Straight graft Surgery –open or endovascular

Straight graft + renal artery reimplantation

Bifurcated 'trouser' graft –open or endovascular

• Back pain
• Nausea
• Vomiting
• Hypotension

Retroperitoneal rupture ('leak')

• Haematemesis
• Melaena

Aortoduodenal fistula

• Plethora
• Low body oedema
• Pulsatile↑ JVP
• Haematuria
• Abdominal bruit

Aortocaval fistula

Definitions

An *aneurysm* is a permanent localized dilatation of an artery to the extent that the affected artery is 1.5 times its normal diameter. A *pseudo* or *false aneurysm* is an expanding pulsating haematoma in continuity with a vessel lumen. It does not have an epithelial lining.

Key points

- Screening for AAA by ultrasound in men aged 65–79 years results in a significant reduction in mortality from AAA. No benefit from screening in women or younger men.
- All patients with other vascular disease should be examined for AAA.
- There is no medical treatment for AAA but small aneurysms may be safely managed by surveillance and regular monitoring with intervention at ≥5.5 cm.
- Mortality for elective surgery is reduced by careful patient evaluation for hidden coronary or pulmonary disease.
- Beware of the diagnosis of left renal colic in the elderly.

Sites

Abdominal aorta, iliac, femoral and popliteal arteries. Cerebral and thoracic aneurysms (TAA) are less common.

Aetiology

- Atherosclerosis.
- Familial (abnormal collagenase or elastase activity).
- Congenital (cerebral (berry) aneurysm).
- Bacterial aortitis (mycotic aneurysm).
- Syphilitic aortitis (thoracic aneurysm).

Risk factors

- Cigarette smoking.
- Hypertension.
- Hyperlipidaemia.
- Marfan syndrome and Ehlers – Danlos syndrome for TAA.
- Trauma for pseudoaneurysm, e.g. arterial puncture.

Pathology

- Aneurysms increase in size in line with the law of Laplace ($T = RP$), T = tension on the arterial wall, R = radius of artery, P = blood pressure. Increasing tension leads to rupture.
- Thrombus from within an aneurysm may be a source of peripheral emboli.
- Popliteal aneurysms may undergo complete thrombosis leading to acute leg ischaemia.
- Aneurysms may be fusiform (AAA, popliteal) or saccular (thoracic, cerebral).
- Acute *aortic dissection* (i.e. tear of the intima with blood tracking between the intima and media producing a second lumen) may occur with TAA.

Clinical features of AAA
Asymptomatic

The vast majority have no symptoms and are found incidentally. This has led to the description of an AAA as 'a U-boat in the belly' and the development of screening programmes. Most TAAs are also asymptomatic and discovered on CXR.

Symptomatic AAA

- Back pain from pressure on the vertebral column.
- Rapid expansion causes flank or back pain.
- Rupture causes collapse, back pain and an ill-defined mass.
- Erosion into IVC causes CCF, loud abdominal bruit (machinery murmur), lower limb ischaemia and gross oedema.

Symptomatic TAA

- Pain: ascending aorta – chest pain; aortic arch – neck pain; descending aorta – back pain. Pain may be chronic from pressure or acute implying impending rupture.
- Most patients are hypertensive.
- Hoarseness, SVC obstruction, dysphagia, stridor and acute aortic valve incompetence may all occur.

Investigations
Detection of AAA

- Physical examination: not accurate.
- Plain abdominal X-ray: aortic calcification.
- Ultrasonography: best way of detecting and measuring aneurysm size – many localities have effective U/S-based screening services to reduce acute presentations of rupture.
- CT or MR angiography scan: provides good information regarding relationship between AAA, renal and iliac arteries.
- Angiography: needed for anatomical detail for planning endovascular repair.

Detection of TAA

- CXR and CT or MR angiography.

Determination of fitness for surgery

- History and examination.
- ECG ± stress testing.
- Radionuclide cardiac scanning (MUGA or stress thallium scan).
- Pulmonary function tests.
- U+E and creatinine for renal assessment.

Essential management

- Endovascular or surgical repair is the treatment of choice for AAA.
- AAA or TAA of ≥5.5 cm should be repaired electively as they have a high rate of rupture. AAA <5.5 cm may be monitored with serial ultrasound or CT examinations every 6 months. Hypertension control is important in managing patients with small TAA.
- Endovascular repair of AAA with graft/stent devices is a commonly used method of repair in many patients now. 30-day mortality 2%.
- Surgical repair of AAA with inlay of a synthetic graft (open or rarely laparoscopic) may be used for those patients not suitable for endovascular repair. 30-day mortality 5%.
- TAA: ascending aorta – surgical repair ± aortic valve repair; aortic arch – open surgery; descending – open surgery or endovascular aneurysm repair (EVAR) (small risk of paraplegia).
- Ruptured AAA or TAA require immediate surgical (or endovascular) repair (perioperative mortality 50%, but 70% of patients die before they get to hospital so that overall mortality is 85%).

Prognosis

Most patients do well after AAA/TAA repair and have an excellent quality of life.

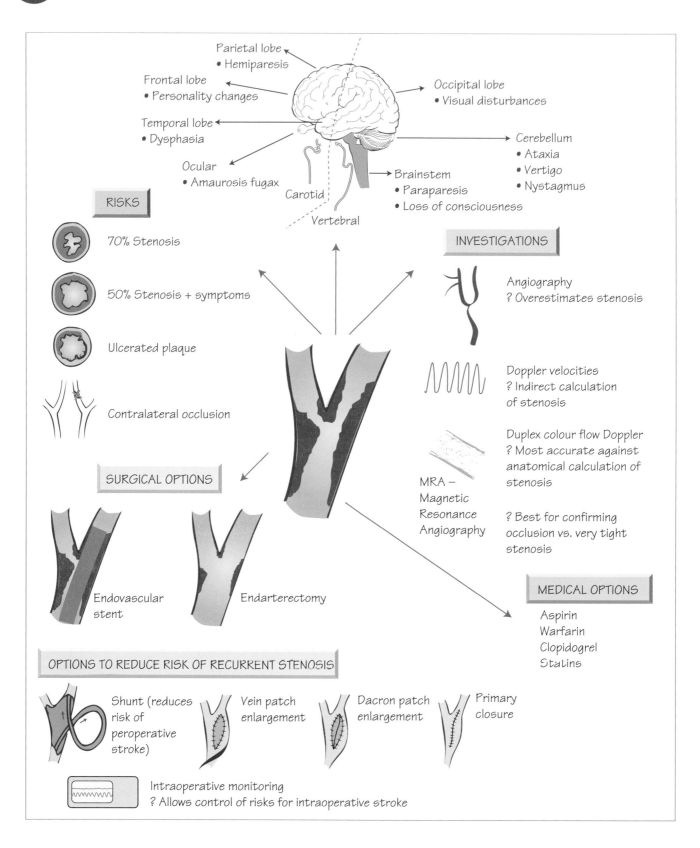

Parietal lobe
• Hemiparesis

Frontal lobe
• Personality changes

Temporal lobe
• Dysphasia

Occipital lobe
• Visual disturbances

Cerebellum
• Ataxia
• Vertigo
• Nystagmus

Ocular
• Amaurosis fugax

Carotid

Vertebral

Brainstem
• Paraparesis
• Loss of consciousness

RISKS

70% Stenosis

50% Stenosis + symptoms

Ulcerated plaque

Contralateral occlusion

INVESTIGATIONS

Angiography
? Overestimates stenosis

Doppler velocities
? Indirect calculation
of stenosis

Duplex colour flow Doppler
? Most accurate against
anatomical calculation of
stenosis

MRA –
Magnetic
Resonance
Angiography

? Best for confirming
occlusion vs. very tight
stenosis

SURGICAL OPTIONS

Endovascular
stent

Endarterectomy

MEDICAL OPTIONS

Aspirin
Warfarin
Clopidogrel
Statins

OPTIONS TO REDUCE RISK OF RECURRENT STENOSIS

Shunt (reduces
risk of
peroperative
stroke)

Vein patch
enlargement

Dacron patch
enlargement

Primary
closure

Intraoperative monitoring
? Allows control of risks for intraoperative stroke

Definition

Extracranial arterial disease is a common disorder characterized by atherosclerosis of the carotid or vertebral arteries resulting in cerebral (*stroke, TIA*), ocular (*amaurosis fugax*) or cerebellar (*vertigo, ataxia, drop attacks*) ischaemic symptoms. A *transient ischaemic attack* (TIA) is defined as: a focal neurological or ocular deficit lasting not more than 24 hours. A newer definition is: a transient episode of neurological dysfunction caused by focal brain, spinal cord, or retinal ischemia without infarction (American Heart Association, 2009). A *stroke* (*brain attack*) is a neurological deficit which lasts for more than 24 hours. New definition: an infarction of central nervous system tissue.

Key points

- All patients with transient neurological symptoms should undergo duplex ultrasound examination for carotid disease – clinical examination is not accurate.
- All patients should be treated with antiplatelet agents, statins and risk factor control.
- Carotid endarterectomy (CEA) offers optimal risk benefit for stroke prevention in well identified groups of patients.
- Carotid artery stenting (CAS) should be performed only in high-risk for CEA patients.

Epidemiology

Male > female before 65 years. Increasing risk with increasing age.

Aetiology

- Atherosclerosis and thrombosis.
- Thromboemboli.
- Fibromuscular dysplasia.

Risk factors

- Cigarette smoking.
- Hypertension.
- Cardiac disease.
- Hyperlipidaemia.
- Diabetes
- Obesity.

Pathophysiology

- The most common extracranial lesion is an atherosclerotic plaque at the carotid bifurcation. Platelet aggregation and subsequent *platelet embolization* cause ocular or cerebral symptoms.
- Symptoms due to *flow reduction* are rare in the carotid territory, but vertebrobasilar symptoms are usually flow-related. Reversed flow in the vertebral artery in the presence of ipsilateral subclavian occlusion leads to cerebral symptoms as the arm 'steals' blood from the cerebellum – subclavian steal syndrome.

Clinical features

- Cerebral symptoms (contralateral):
  motor (weakness, clumsiness or paralysis of a limb)
  sensory (numbness, paraesthesia)
  speech-related (receptive or expressive dysphasia).
- Ocular symptoms (ipsilateral): amaurosis fugax (transient loss of vision described as 'a veil coming down over the visual field').
- Cerebral (or ocular) symptoms may be transitory (TIA) or permanent (stroke).
- Vertebrobasilar symptoms: vertigo, ataxia, dizziness, syncope, bilateral paraesthesia, visual hallucinations.
- A *bruit* may be heard over a carotid artery, but it is an unreliable indicator of pathology.

Investigations

- Duplex scanning: B-mode scan and Doppler ultrasonic velocitometry: method of choice for assessing degree of carotid stenosis.
- Carotid angiography: now often performed as MRA, which is safer than standard angiography.
- CT or MRI brain scan: demonstrate the presence of a cerebral infarct.

Essential management

Medical

- Risk factor modification: smoking cessation, weight loss, blood pressure and diabetes control.
- Antiplatelet agent: inhibits platelet aggregation for the life of the platelet (aspirin or clopidogrel: 75 mg/day).
- All patients with evidence of vascular disease should be prescribed a statin.
- Anticoagulation is indicated in patients with cardiac embolic disease.

Interventional

- Carotid endarterectomy (CEA) (+ maximum medical therapy). Most benefit is achieved if carotid endarterectomy is performed within 2 weeks on onset of symptoms.
- Carotid artery stenting (CAS) should be performed only in high-risk for CEA patients, e.g. previous surgery or radiotherapy. Dual antiplatelet treatment (aspirin and clopidogrel) and carotid protection devices should be used during CAS.

Indications for carotid endarterectomy

- Symptomatic. Carotid distribution TIA or stroke with good recovery and >50% ipsilateral stenosis: CEA within 2 weeks of patient's last symptoms. Surgeon should have perioperative stroke/death rate <6%.
- Asymptomatic. >70–99% stenosis in >75-year-old men. Perioperative stroke/death rate should be <3%. CEA should only be considered in younger fit asymptomatic women as benefit significantly less than in men.

73 Venous thromboembolism

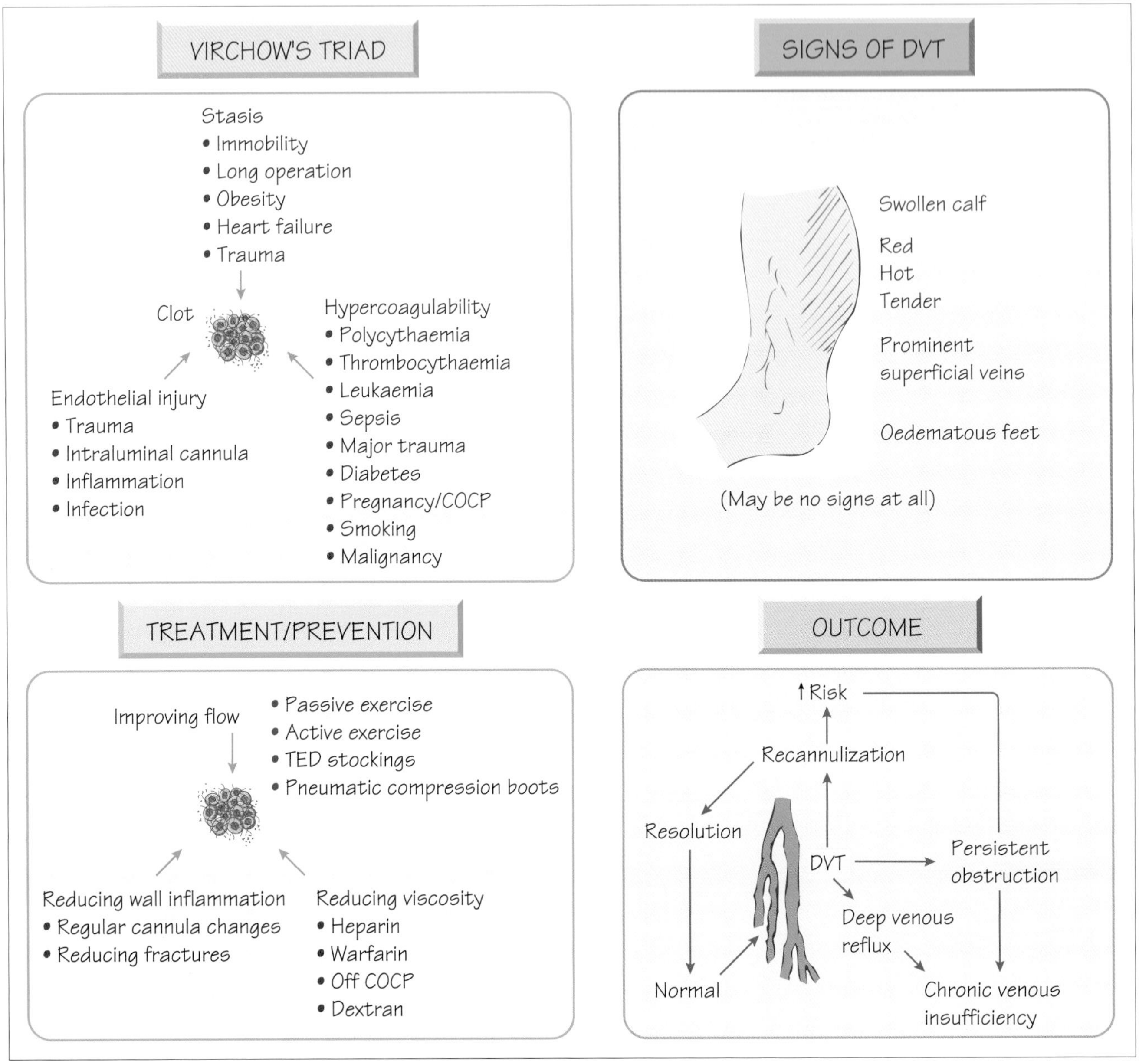
VIRCHOW'S TRIAD
Stasis
• Immobility
• Long operation
• Obesity
• Heart failure
• Trauma
Clot
Hypercoagulability
• Polycythaemia
• Thrombocythaemia
• Leukaemia
• Sepsis
• Major trauma
• Diabetes
• Pregnancy/COCP
• Smoking
• Malignancy
Endothelial injury
• Trauma
• Intraluminal cannula
• Inflammation
• Infection
SIGNS OF DVT
Swollen calf
Red
Hot
Tender
Prominent superficial veins
Oedematous feet
(May be no signs at all)
TREATMENT/PREVENTION
Improving flow
• Passive exercise
• Active exercise
• TED stockings
• Pneumatic compression boots
Reducing wall inflammation
• Regular cannula changes
• Reducing fractures
Reducing viscosity
• Heparin
• Warfarin
• Off COCP
• Dextran
OUTCOME
↑Risk
Recannulization
Resolution
DVT
Persistent obstruction
Deep venous reflux
Normal
Chronic venous insufficiency

Definitions

A *thrombus* is a solid mass of platelet, fibrin and other components of blood that forms locally in a vessel. A *deep venous thrombosis* (DVT) is a condition in which the blood in the deep veins of the legs or pelvis (rarely upper limbs) forms into a clot. Embolization of the thrombus results in a pulmonary embolus (PE) while local venous damage may lead to chronic venous insufficiency (CVI) also known as post-thrombotic or postphlebitic syndrome.

Key points

- All patients in hospital should be considered for DVT prophylaxis.
- Low probability Well's score and negative D-dimers very unlikely to have DVT.
- In clinically suspected DVT or PE, heparin should be commenced immediately.
- Recurrent DVT may lead to chronic disabling postphlebitic limb.
- DVT may be the first manifestation of an occult malignancy.

Epidemiology

DVT is extremely common among medical and surgical patients, affecting 10–30% of all general surgical patients over 40 years who undergo a major operation. PE is a common cause of sudden death in hospital patients (0.5–3.0% of patients die from PE).

Aetiology

Virchow's triad (see opposite)
Pathology

- Aggregation of platelets in venous valve cusps (area of maximum stasis or injury).
- Activation of clotting cascade producing fibrin.
- Fibrin production overwhelms the natural anticoagulant/fibrinolytic system.
- Natural history: complete resolution vs. PE vs. CVI.

Clinical features

Deep venous thrombosis
- Asymptomatic.
- Calf tenderness or aching, ankle oedema, mild pyrexia.
- Phlegmasia alba/caerulea dolens.

Pulmonary embolism
- Dyspnoea ± pleuritic chest pain.
- Tachycardia and tachypnoea.
- Cough ± haemoptysis, fever.
- Massive PE causes circulatory arrest.

Chronic venous insufficiency (see Chapter 70)
- ± History of DVT.
- Aching limb.

- Leg swelling and varicose veins.
- Venous lipodermatosclerosis (inverted bottle-shaped leg).
- Venous eczema and ulceration.

Diagnosis and investigations

Deep venous thrombosis
- D-dimers (byproduct of fibrinolysis – 95% sensitivity. A negative test excludes DVT in low to moderate risk patients (Wells' score <2)

Wells' clinical prediction score for DVT (quantifies probability of DVT).

Active cancer	+1
Post bed rest for >3 days or major surgery	+1
Entire leg swelling	+1
Pitting oedema	+1
Collateral superficial veins (non varicose)	+1
Paralysis or recent POP lower limb	+1
Tender over deep venous system	+1
Calf swelling >3 cm over other leg	+1
Previous documented DVT	+1
Alternative diagnosis more likely	−2

Probability of DVT: high ≥3, medium 1 or 2, low ≥0.

---

but a positive test does not confirm a DVT. A duplex image is required if D-dimers positive).

- Duplex imaging: compression ultrasonography gold standard for DVT diagnosis. Excellent for femoral and popliteal DVT, less accurate for calf and iliac – MRI is more accurate.
- CT venography may used if ilio-femoral DVT is suspected.

Pulmonary embolism
- ECG: tachycardia, S1, Q3, T3 or right bundle branch block, atrial fibrillation.
- WBC may be elevated.
- D-dimer testing.
- Pulse oximetry, arterial blood gases: hypoxia, hypocapnia.
- Chest X-ray: atelectasis, small pleural effusion, elevated hemi-diaphragm, infiltrates.
- Nuclear scintigraphic V/Q scanning of the lung.
- Multidetector CTA – if available, is the preferred primary diagnostic modality for PE.

Chronic venous insufficiency
- Colour duplex imaging.
- Plethysmography.
- Ascending ± descending venography.
- Ambulatory venous pressure.

Essential management

Prophylaxis against DVT
Indications
Presence of risk factors (see above).

Methods
- Mechanical compression: (TED) stockings or intermittent pneumatic compression devices.
- Pharmacological:
  low dose unfractionated heparin (LDUH) – 5000 IU s.c., b.i.d.
  low molecular weight heparin (LMWH) – dose depends on drug – better prevention but more more expensive than LDUH
  fondaparinux (Factor Xa inhibitor) – 2.5 mg/day
  warfarin and newer anticoagulants (hirudin, lepirudin).

Definitive treatment
Deep venous thrombosis
- Anticoagulation for 12 weeks:
  initial Rx: IV unfractionated heparin (check efficacy with APTT) *or* s.c. LMWH (no APTT monitoring required)
  maintenance: oral anticoagulation (warfarin) in nonpregnant patients (target INR 2.0–3.0). In pregnant use LMWH
- Compression stockings: graduated-compression below-knee elastic stockings × 2 years reduces risk of developing postphlebitic limb.

- (Thrombolysis: may be useful in selected patients with iliofemoral DVT – haemorrhage a major side-effect. Thrombectomy rarely performed.)

Pulmonary embolism
Emergency treatment:
- Fibrinolysis should be considered in all patients unless specifically contraindicated. Definite indications: haemodynamically unstable, right heart strain, likely recurrent PE.
- Prompt anticoagulation with heparin.
- Oxygen therapy.
- Pulmonary embolectomy or extracorporeal membrane oxygenation may be indicated.

Later management:
- Anticoagulation for at least 6 months.
- Look for source of embolus.
- Compression stockings.
- IVC filters for recurrent PE despite treatment, anticoagulation treatment contraindicated, 'high risk' DVTs.

Chronic venous insufficiency
- Limb elevation.
- Compression: four-layer bandaging to achieve ulcer healing. Graduated compression stockings to maintain healing.
- Varicose veins should be treated if there is an unobstructed deep venous system.
- Venous valvuoplasty or venous transposition has been used for deep venous incompetence.

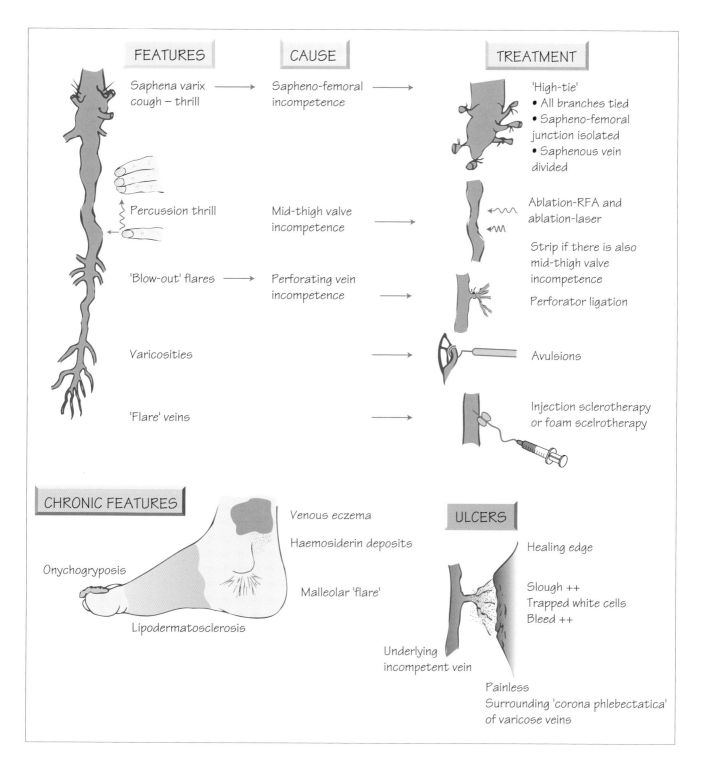

FEATURES

Saphena varix cough – thrill

Percussion thrill

'Blow-out' flares

Varicosities

'Flare' veins

CAUSE

Sapheno-femoral incompetence

Mid-thigh valve incompetence

Perforating vein incompetence

TREATMENT

'High-tie'
• All branches tied
• Sapheno-femoral junction isolated
• Saphenous vein divided

Ablation-RFA and ablation-laser

Strip if there is also mid-thigh valve incompetence

Perforator ligation

Avulsions

Injection sclerotherapy or foam scelrotherapy

CHRONIC FEATURES

Onychogryposis

Lipodermatosclerosis

Venous eczema

Haemosiderin deposits

Malleolar 'flare'

ULCERS

Healing edge

Slough ++
Trapped white cells
Bleed ++

Underlying incompetent vein

Painless
Surrounding 'corona phlebectatica' of varicose veins

Definition

Varicose veins (*VV*) are tortuous, dilated, prominent, superficial veins in the lower limbs, often in the anatomical distribution of the long and short saphenous veins.

Key points

- Pre-treatment colour duplex imaging should be considered in all patients undergoing treatment for varicose veins.
- Modern treatments include compression stockings, foam sclerotherapy, radiofrequency or laser ablation and surgery.

Epidemiology

Very common in the Western world, affecting about 50% of the adult population.

Aetiology

- Primary or familial varicose veins.
- Pregnancy (progesterone causes passive dilatation of veins).
- Secondary to postphlebitic limb (perforator failure).
- Congenital:
  Klippel–Trenaunay syndrome (port-wine stain, varicose veins, bony and soft tissue hypertrophy involving an extremity)
  Parkes–Weber syndrome (cutaneous flush with underlying multiple microarteriovenous fistulas, in association with soft tissue and skeletal hypertrophy of the affected limb).
- Iatrogenic: following formation of an arteriovenous fistula.

Pathophysiology

Venous valve failure, usually at the sapheno-femoral or sapheno-popliteal junction (and sometimes in perforating veins), results in increased venous pressure in the LSV or SSV with progressive vein dilatation and further valve disruption.

Clinical features

CEAP classification for lower extremity venous disease

- Clinical   0   No visible or palpable signs of venous disease
  1   Telangiectasia, reticular veins
  2   Varicose veins
  3   Oedema without skin changes
  4   Skin changes: (a) pigmentation, venous eczema; (b) lipodermatosclerosis
  5   Healed ulcer venous ulcer
  6   Active venous ulcer
  s   Symptomatic (ache, pain, tightness, irritation, heaviness, cramp)
  a   Asymptomatic
- Etiology: Ec (congenital), Ep (primary), Es (secondary – postthrombotic), En (no cause).
- Anatomy: As (superficial), Ap (perforator), Ad (deep), An (no venous location identified).
- Pathophysiological: Pr (reflux), Po (obstruction), Pr,o reflux + obstruction, Pn (no venous pathophysiology.)

The date of CEAP assessment should also be recorded, e.g. C4a,s, Ep, As Pr (28-7-2008).

Complications of VVs are: bleeding, superficial thrombophlebitis and venous ulceration.

Investigations

The level of investigations depends on the severity of the disease: usually history, clinical examination (Trendelenburg tests) and colour duplex scanning gives all information required.

Essential management

General

- Avoid long periods of standing or sitting.
- Weight loss and exercise.
- Elevate limbs and use skin lotions.
- Compression: wear support hosiery.

Specific

Ultrasound-guided foam sclerotherapy

- Foam prepared by mixing the sclerosing agent (polidocanol) with air is injected into the vein (under ultrasound guidance) causing chemical thrombophlebitis and occlusion. The vein must be compressed to press the walls together and prevent recanalization.
- Occlusion rates of 80%. Outpatient procedure. Minimally invasive. Cheap. Can be repeated. Extravasation of agent may cause pigmentation. Rarely foam entering the arterial circulation via a patent foramen ovale causes visual or cerebral symptoms.

Endovenous ablation

- An energy-delivering catheter (radiofrequency or laser) is placed into the vein (LSV or SSV) after infiltration of anaesthesia along its course. Ablation is achieved by heat produced by the energy source.
- Achieve occlusion rates of 80–90%. Can be performed under LA and is safe. Expensive.

Surgical ablation (standard treatment until recently)

- The LSV or SSV is surgically disconnected from the superficial femoral or popliteal vein.
- The elongated veins are 'stripped' and/ or 'avulsed' via multiple stab incisions.
- Compression stockings are worn for several weeks and exercise is encouraged.
- Standard surgery improves quality of life and is cost effective.

75 Lymphoedema

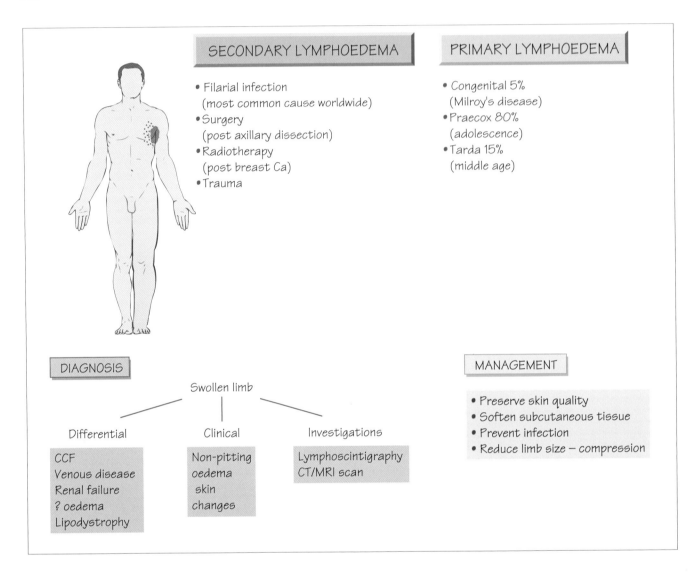

SECONDARY LYMPHOEDEMA

- Filarial infection
  (most common cause worldwide)
- Surgery
  (post axillary dissection)
- Radiotherapy
  (post breast Ca)
- Trauma

PRIMARY LYMPHOEDEMA

- Congenital 5%
  (Milroy's disease)
- Praecox 80%
  (adolescence)
- Tarda 15%
  (middle age)

DIAGNOSIS

Swollen limb

Differential

CCF
Venous disease
Renal failure
? oedema
Lipodystrophy

Clinical

Non-pitting
oedema
 skin
changes

Investigations

Lymphoscintigraphy
CT/MRI scan

MANAGEMENT

- Preserve skin quality
- Soften subcutaneous tissue
- Prevent infection
- Reduce limb size – compression

Definition

Lymphoedema is a persistent swelling of the tissues caused by the accumulation of protein-rich fluid as a result of failure of lymph transport from the tissues.

Key points

- Lymphoedema is a chronic condition that causes considerable morbidity.
- Filiariasis is the most common cause of lymphoedema worldwide.
- Up to 25% of patients post breast cancer therapy develop lymphoedema.
- Surgery is rarely indicated in the management of lymphoedema.

Classification of lymphoedema

Lymphoedema	Lymphatic defect
Primary (uncommon)	
Congenital (Milroy's disease) (rare)	Aplasia (15%)
Praecox – appears in adolescence (80% of primary lymphoedema)	Hypoplasia (70%)
Tarda – appears in middle age	Hyperplasia/varicosity (15%)
Secondary (common)	
Infection (filariasis,* TB, lymphogranuloma, actinomycosis, chronic lymphangitis	Hyperplastic/varicose
Surgery (especially after axillary dissection for breast cancer)	
Radiation therapy (especially for breast cancer)	
Trauma	

*Parasitic infestation with filarial worm *Wuchereria bancrofti*.

Clinical features

Limb swelling
- Starts distally and ascends proximally over period of months.
- Characteristic 'tree trunk' appearance to lower limb.
- Absence of pigmentation differentiates lower limb lymphoedema from venous insufficiency.

Clinical grades
- Grade 1: pitting oedema and decrease in swelling on limb elevation.
- Grade 2: non-pitting oedema and little decrease in swelling on elevation.
- Grade 3 (elephantiasis): gross swelling of the limb with skin changes.

Investigations
- Diagnosis is usually made on history and clinical examination.
- Lymphangiography – traditional lymphangiography not used anymore, but magnetic resonance lymphangiography (MRL) provides good images.
- Lymphoscintigraphy – best method of measuring lymphatic function.
- CT or MRI scanning of limb – good for imaging oedema and fibrosis.
- Duplex ultrasound to exclude venous disease.

Essential management

Lymphoedema is a chronic condition that cannot be cured but it can be managed.

Aims of management
- Preserve skin quality.
- Soften subcutaneous tissue.
- Prevent lymphangitis.
- Reduce limb size.

Complex physical therapy
- Complete decongestive therapy.
- Manual lymphatic drainage and exercise to promote lymph flow.
- Compression bandages.
- External pneumatic compression using sequential gradient pumps to decrease limb size.
- Compression sleeves and stockings to decrease limb size.
- Skin care to avoid infection and further lymphatic damage.
- Aggressive treatment of infection if it occurs.

Drug therapy
Flavonoids, antibiotics, diuretics (benzopyrones), (all have been used but usefulness unproven, benzopyrones may cause hepatic impairment).

Surgery (rarely indicated)
- Excisional debulking procedures (lymphangiectomy).
- Liposuction.
- Lymphatico-venous anastomosis.

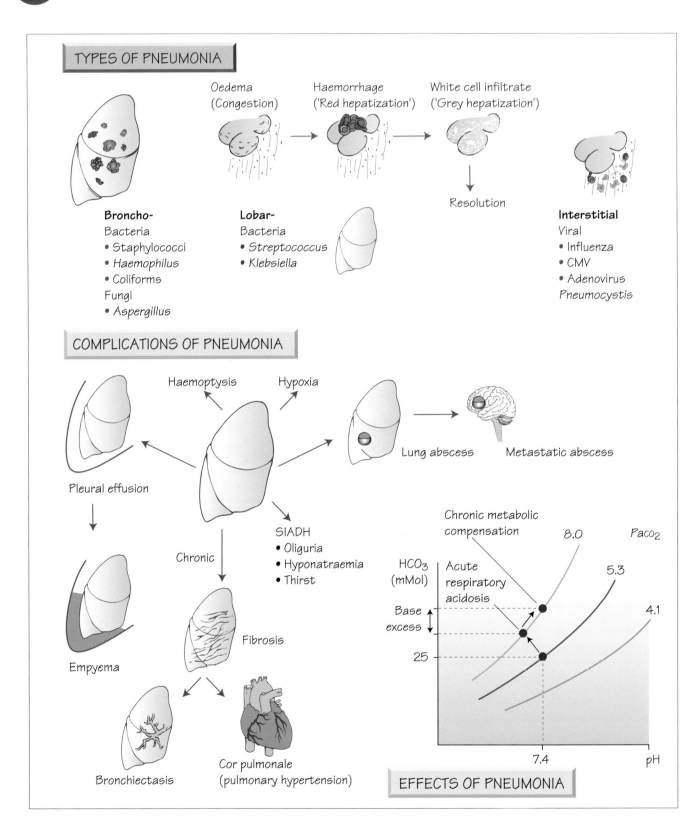

TYPES OF PNEUMONIA

Oedema (Congestion) → Haemorrhage ('Red hepatization') → White cell infiltrate ('Grey hepatization') → Resolution

Broncho-
Bacteria
• Staphylococci
• Haemophilus
• Coliforms
Fungi
• Aspergillus

Lobar-
Bacteria
• Streptococcus
• Klebsiella

Interstitial
Viral
• Influenza
• CMV
• Adenovirus
Pneumocystis

COMPLICATIONS OF PNEUMONIA

Haemoptysis   Hypoxia

Lung abscess   Metastatic abscess

Pleural effusion

SIADH
• Oliguria
• Hyponatraemia
• Thirst

Chronic

Empyema

Fibrosis

Bronchiectasis   Cor pulmonale (pulmonary hypertension)

EFFECTS OF PNEUMONIA

Chronic metabolic compensation

HCO_3 (mMol)

Acute respiratory acidosis

Base excess

25

8.0   5.3   4.1 Pa_{CO_2}

7.4   pH

Definitions

Pulmonary collapse or *atelectasis* results from alveolar hypoventilation such that the alveolar walls collapse and become de-aerated. *Pneumonia* is an infection with consolidation of the pulmonary parenchyma.

> **Key points**
>
> - Thoracic and upper abdominal incisions are at high risk of postoperative pulmonary collapse ± infection.
> - Aggressive prophylaxis is key to prevention of complications.
> - Postoperative pneumonia is often due to mixed organisms.
> - Postoperative pulmonary complications prolong hospital stay by 1–2 weeks.

Aetiology/pathophysiology

Postoperatively patients frequently develop atelectasis, which may develop into a pneumonia.

Pulmonary collapse

- Proximal bronchial obstruction.
- Trapped alveolar air absorbed.
- Common in smokers.
- Common with COPD, asthma or sleep apnoea.

Pneumonia

- Infection with micro-organisms.
- Bacterial: *Streptococcus pneumoniae, Staphylococcus, Haemophilus influenzae*.
- Viral: influenza, CMV.
- Fungal: *Candida, Aspergillus*.
- Protozoal: *Pneumocystis, Toxoplasma*.

Pulmonary embolism

See venous thromboembolism (see Chapter 73).

Predisposing factors

- Secretional airway obstruction.
- Bronchorrhoea post surgery.
- Mucus plugs block bronchi.
- Impaired ciliary action.
- Postoperative pain prevents effective coughing
- Organic airway obstruction.
- Bronchial neoplasm.

Patients prone to severe pneumonia

- The elderly.
- Alcoholics.
- Chronic lung and heart disease.
- Debilitated patients.

- Diabetes.
- Post-CVA.
- Immunodeficiency states.
- Post-splenectomy.
- Atelectasis post surgery.

Clinical features

Pulmonary collapse

- Pyrexia.
- Tachypnoea.
- Diminished air entry.
- Bronchial breathing.

Pneumonia

- Respiratory distress.
- Painful dyspnoea.
- Tachypnoea.
- Productive cough ± haemoptysis.
- Hypoxia – confusion.
- Diminished air entry.
- Consolidation.
- Pleural rub.
- Cyanosis.

Investigations

- Chest X-ray: consolidation, pleural effusion, interstitial infiltrates, air–fluid cysts.
- Sputum culture: essential for correct antibiotic treatment.
- Blood gas analysis: diagnosis of respiratory failure.

> **Essential management**
>
> **Prophylaxis**
>
> - Stop smoking – preferably for 8 weeks.
> - Pre-operative deep-breathing exercises.
> - Incentive spirometry and chest physiotherapy.
> - Nebulized bronchodilators ± ipratropium if needed.
> - Adequate analgesia postoperatively.
> - Early ambulation.
>
> **Treatment**
>
> - Pain control, epidural anaesthesia, PCA.
> - Intensive chest physiotherapy.
> - Respiratory support: humidified O_2; adequate hydration; bronchodilators
> - Specific antimicrobial therapy.
>
> **Complications**
>
> - Respiratory failure.
> - Lung abscess.

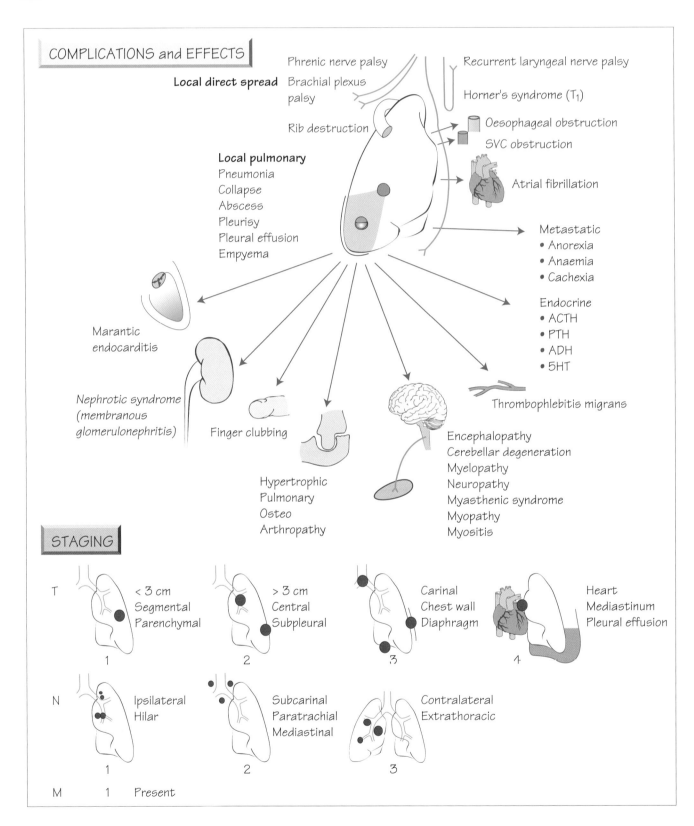

COMPLICATIONS and EFFECTS

Local direct spread

Phrenic nerve palsy
Brachial plexus palsy
Rib destruction

Recurrent laryngeal nerve palsy
Horner's syndrome (T_1)
Oesophageal obstruction
SVC obstruction
Atrial fibrillation

Local pulmonary
Pneumonia
Collapse
Abscess
Pleurisy
Pleural effusion
Empyema

Metastatic
• Anorexia
• Anaemia
• Cachexia

Endocrine
• ACTH
• PTH
• ADH
• 5HT

Marantic endocarditis

Nephrotic syndrome (membranous glomerulonephritis)

Finger clubbing

Hypertrophic Pulmonary Osteo Arthropathy

Thrombophlebitis migrans

Encephalopathy
Cerebellar degeneration
Myelopathy
Neuropathy
Myasthenic syndrome
Myopathy
Myositis

STAGING

T
< 3 cm
Segmental
Parenchymal
1

> 3 cm
Central
Subpleural
2

Carinal
Chest wall
Diaphragm
3

Heart
Mediastinum
Pleural effusion
4

N
Ipsilateral
Hilar
1

Subcarinal
Paratrachial
Mediastinal
2

Contralateral
Extrathoracic
3

M   1   Present

 Surgery at a Glance, Fifth Edition. Pierce A. Grace and Neil R. Borley. © 2013 John Wiley & Sons, Ltd. Published 2013 by John Wiley & Sons, Ltd.

Definition

Malignant lesion of the respiratory tree epithelium.

Key points

- Symptoms may be masked by coexistent lung pathology (COPD).
- Lung cancer often presents late and most are non-resectable.
- Surgically resectable tumours have a fair prognosis.
- NSCLC has a better prognosis than SCLC

Epidemiology

Male:female 5:1. Uncommon before 50 years. Most patients are in their 60s. Accounts for 40000 deaths per annum in the UK.

Aetiology

Predisposing factors:
- Cigarette smoking.
- Air pollution.
- Exposure to uranium, chromium, arsenic, haematite and asbestos.

Pathology

Non-small cell lung cancer (NSCLC) (85%)

Squamous carcinoma, large cell carcinoma, adenocarcinoma.

Small cell lung cancer (SCLC) (15%)

Also called 'oat cell'.

Spread

- Direct to pleura, recurrent laryngeal nerve, pericardium, oesophagus, brachial plexus.
- Lymphatic to mediastinal, supraclavicular and cervical nodes.
- Haematogenous to liver, bone, brain, adrenals.
- Transcoelomic pleural seedlings and effusion.

Clinical features

- History of tiredness, cough, anorexia, weight loss.
- Productive cough with purulent sputum.
- Haemoptysis.
- Finger clubbing.
- Bronchopneumonia (in lung segment distal to malignant bronchial obstruction).
- Pleuritic pain.
- Neuropathy, myopathy, hypertrophic osteoarthropathy.
- Endocrine syndromes (SCLC: ectopic secretion of ACTH (Cushing's syndrome), ADH (SIADH) or parathormone (hypercalcaemia)).
- Pancoast's tumour (apical tumour invading sympathetic trunk and brachial plexus) – Horner's syndrome, brachial neuralgia, paralysis of upper limb.
- Dysphagia and broncho-oesophageal fistula.
- Superior vena caval obstruction.

Investigations

Diagnostic

- Chest X-ray – PA and lateral (lung opacity, hilar lymphadenopathy).
- CT-guided lung biopsy.
- Sputum cytology.
- Bronchoscopy and cytology of brushings or lavage fluid.

Assess operability

- Helical CT scan of thorax/abdomen: involvement of adjacent structures, hepatic metastases, multiple primary lesions.
- Bone scan: metastases.
- Liver ultrasound: metastases.
- Mediastinoscopy: involvement of mediastinal nodes.
- Lung function test: likely patient tolerance of pulmonary resection.

Essential management

NSCLC

Curative intent
- Surgery (lobectomy or pneumonectomy) for (Stage I (T1/N0/M0 – T2/N0/M0) and Stage II (T2/N0/M0 – T2/N1/M0 – T3/N0/M0) and some Stage III (T1/N/2M0 – T4/N3/M0) when tumour is confined to one lobe or lung, no evidence of secondary deposits, carina is tumour free on bronchoscopy.
- Radiotherapy: for Stage I or II when not resectable for medical reasons, e.g. COPD.
- Neoadjuvant and adjuvant chemotherapy (cisplatin) for Stage II. (Unfortunately for most patients current treatments do not cure the cancer.)

Palliative
Radiotherapy, chemotherapy, endobronchial laser or brachytherapy: Stage III (unresectable) and Stage IV (anyT/anyN/M1) – may stop haemoptysis, relieve bone pain from secondaries, relieve SVC obstruction.

SCLC
- Limited stage disease (LD) (confined to hemithorax, mediastinum or supraclavicular nodes): chemotherapy, radiation therapy (± surgery rarely).
- Extensive stage disease (ED) (spread beyond supraclavicular area): Chemotherapy, radiotherapy.

Prognosis

Following 'curative' treatment 5-year survival rates are 30–45% for NSCLC, 14% for SCLC(LD) and 2% for SCLC(ED). Overall 5-year survival for all lung cancer is 15%.

2-week wait referral criteria for suspected lung cancer

- CXR suspicious for malignancy.
- Persistent haemoptysis in smoker or ex-smoker >40 years.
- Signs of SVC obstruction.
- Stridor.

78 Urinary tract infection

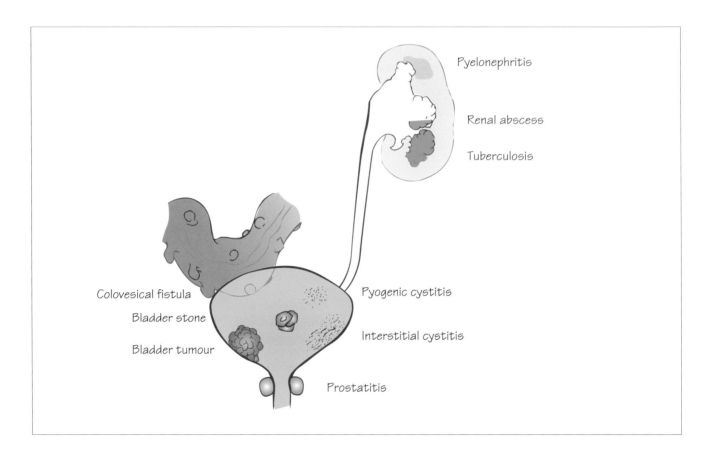

Pyelonephritis

Renal abscess

Tuberculosis

Colovesical fistula

Bladder stone

Bladder tumour

Pyogenic cystitis

Interstitial cystitis

Prostatitis

Surgery at a Glance, Fifth Edition. Pierce A. Grace and Neil R. Borley. © 2013 John Wiley & Sons, Ltd. Published 2013 by John Wiley & Sons, Ltd.

Definition

A *urinary tract infection* is a documented episode of significant bacteriuria (i.e. an infection with cfu of >100 000 single organisms per ml) which may affect the upper (*pyelonephritis*, *renal abscess*) or the lower (*cystitis*) urinary tract or both. *Colony forming units* (cfu; expressed as cfu/mL) represent the number of bacterial colonies per mL of sample.

Key points

- Lower urinary tract infection (UTI) is usually harmless and simple to treat.
- Upper UTI may be associated with renal damage and major complications. Requires prompt investigation and treatment.
- Consider an underlying cause in all recurrent or atypical infections.
- Asymptomatic bacteruria does not need to be treated (except in pregnant women).

Epidemiology

UTI is a very common condition in general practice (usually *Escherichia coli*) and accounts for 40% of hospital-acquired (*nosocomial*) infections (often *Enterobacter* or *Klebsiella*).

Risk factors

- Urinary tract obstruction.
- Instrumentation of urinary tract (e.g. indwelling catheter).
- Dysfunctional (neuropathic) bladder.
- Immunosuppression.
- Diabetes mellitus.
- Structural abnormalities (e.g. vesicoureteric reflux).
- Pregnancy.
- Dehydration.

Pathology

- Ascending infection: most UTIs caused in this way (bacteria from GI tract colonize lower urinary tract).
- Haematogenous spread: infrequent cause of UTI (seen in IV drug users, bacterial endocarditis and TB).

Clinical features
Upper urinary tract infection
- Fever, rigors/chill.
- Flank pain.
- Malaise.
- Anorexia.
- Costovertebral angle and abdominal tenderness.
- May lead to septicaemia.

Lower urinary tract infection
- Dysuria.
- Frequency and urgency.
- Suprapubic pain.
- Haematuria.
- Scrotal pain (epididymo-orchitis) or perineal pain (prostatitis).

Investigations

Gram stain and culture of a 'clean-catch' urine specimen before antibiotics have been given. Usual organisms are *E. coli*, *Enterobacter*, *Klebsiella*, *Proteus* (suggests presence of urinary calculi). >100 000 single organism cfu/ml = infection, <100 000 cfu or mixed growth suggests contamination.

Upper urinary tract infection
- FBC.
- U+E and serum creatinine: renal function.
- Renal ultrasound: pyelonephritis, stones, obstruction/hydronephrosis, secondary abscess.
- IVU: stones, structural abnormalities, obstructed collecting system.
- CT scan: abscess/tumours.
- Renal scintigraphy or isotope scanning:
  ^{99m}Tc-MAG3 ± diuretic for assessing renal blood flow/function/obstruction
  ^{99m}Tc-DMSA for renal cortical assessment, e.g. cortical scarring.

Lower urinary tract infection
- FBC.
- Cystoscopy only if haematuria – underlying neoplasm or stones.
- If obstruction is present ultrasound scan, IVU and cystoscopy may be needed.
- CT scan: colovesical fistula, prostatitis/abscess.

Essential management

Treat the infection with an appropriate antibiotic based on urine culture results and deal with any underlying cause (e.g. relieve obstruction). High fluid intake should be encouraged and potassium citrate may relieve dysuria.

Upper tract UTIs, epididymo-orchitis and prostatitis
- IV antibiotic therapy (ciprofloxacin, gentamicin, cefuroxime, co-trimoxazole).
- Relieve acute obstruction with internal (double-J stent) or external (nephrostomy) drainage (especially if acute severe sepsis).
- An abscess will require drainage either radiologically or surgically.

Cystitis and uncomplicated lower UTI
- Oral antibiotics (trimethoprim, ciprofloxacin, nitrofurantoin, cefradine).
- If there is a poor response to treatment consider unusual urinary infections: tuberculosis (sterile pyuria), candiduria, schistosomiasis, *Chlamydia trachomatis*, *Neisseria gonorrhoeae*.
- Recurrent infections should raise the possibility of underlying abnormalities requiring investigation.

Complications
- Bacteraemia and septic shock.
- Renal, perinephric and metastatic abscesses.
- Renal damage and acute/chronic renal failure.
- Chronic and xanthogranulomatous pyelonephritis.

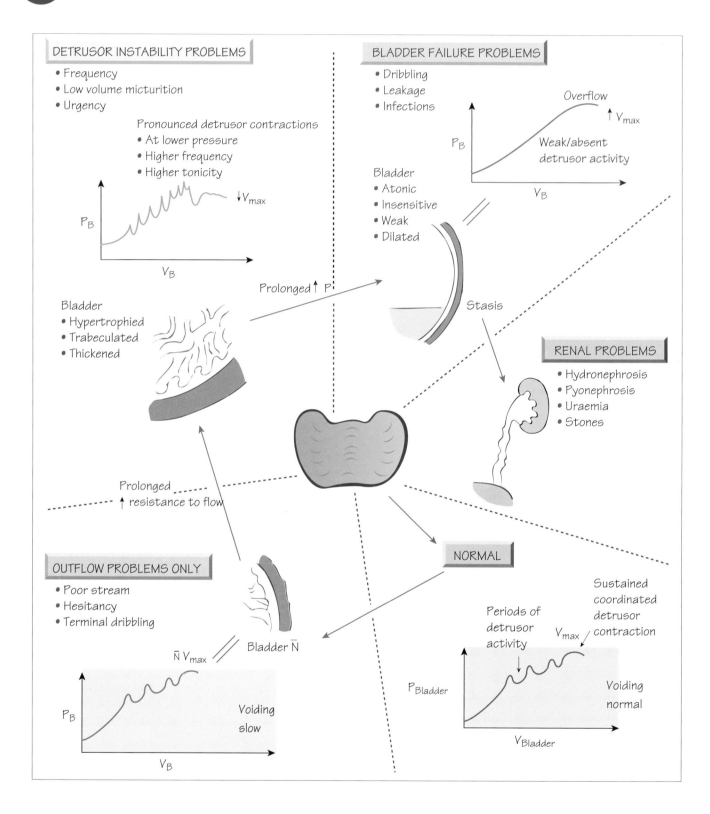

Definition

Benign prostatic hypertrophy (BPH) is a condition of unknown aetiology characterized by an increase in size of the inner zone (periurethral glands) of the prostate gland. *Lower urinary tract symptoms* (LUTS) refers to the voiding dysfunction that results from prostate gland enlargement and *bladder outlet obstruction* (BOO).

Key points

- Symptoms of BPH are initially due to obstruction-induced outflow problems, followed by bladder instability and bladder failure.
- Early treatment of symptoms prevents/reverses bladder damage and complications.
- Patients with mild LUTS can be treated with medical therapy.
- Surgical resection is safe but is associated with some significant complications.

Epidemiology

Present in 50% of 60–90-year-old men.

Pathophysiology

- Microscopic stromal nodules develop around the periurethral glands.
- Glandular hyperplasia originates around these nodules.
- As the gland increases in size, it compresses the urethra, leading to urinary tract obstruction and bladder dysfunction.

Clinical features

Initially outlet obstruction:
- Weak stream, hesitancy, intermittency, dribbling, straining to void, acute urinary retention.

  Subsequent detrusor instability:
- Frequency, urgency, nocturia, dysuria, urge incontinence.

  Finally detrusor failure and chronic retention:
- Palpable (or percussible) bladder, overflow incontinence.
- Enlarged smooth prostate on digital rectal examination.

Symptom score for BPH (International Prostate Symptom Score [IPSS]).

In past month	Never	<1 in 5 times	<50% of the time	50% of the time	>50% of the time	Almost always
Incomplete emptying	0	1	2	3	4	5
Frequency	0	1	2	3	4	5
Intermittency (stop and start)	0	1	2	3	4	5
Urgency	0	1	2	3	4	5
Weak stream	0	1	2	3	4	5
Straining	0	1	2	3	4	5
Nocturia	0	1	2	3	4	5

Total symptom score range 0–35.
0–7, mildly symptomatic; 8–19, moderately symptomatic; 20–35, severely symptomatic.

	Delighted	Mixed	Dissatisfied	Unhappy	Terrible
Bother score	0	1 2	3	4	5 6

Bother score gives an assessment of patient's perceived QoL.

Investigations

Basic investigations

- Urinalysis and urine culture for evidence of infection or haematuria.
- FBC: infection.
- U+E and serum creatinine: renal function.
- PSA: suspicion of underlying malignancy (very non-specific).

Further investigations

- Voiding diary.
- Uroflowmetry (normal maximum flow rate (Q_{max}) >15 ml/s) and post-void residual volume measurement (normal <100 ml): evidence of obstruction.
- Ultrasonography of kidneys and bladder: structural abnormalities.
- TRUS: to determine prostate size/biopsy if malignancy suspected.
- IVU: structural abnormalities.
- Cystoscopy.

Essential management

Medical

- Alter oral fluid intake, reduce caffeine intake.
- Stop anticholinergic, sympathomimetic and opioid drugs.
- α_1-Adrenergic receptor blockers (e.g. alfuzosin, doxazosin, terazosin, tamsulosin) to improve voiding.
- 5α-reductase inhibitors (e.g. finasteride) (cellular antiandrogens) to reduce prostate size.
- Consider adding anticholinergic if persistent symptoms of overactive bladder (OAB).
- Intermittent self-catheterization if detrusor failure.
- Complete obstruction requires immediate catheterization.

Surgical

Most patients are treated surgically by removing the adenomatous part of the prostate by:
- TURP with electrocautery or laser for smaller prostates and open surgery (retropublic or suprapubic approach) for larger prostates (>75 g).
- Less invasive procedures include balloon dilatation, intraurethral stents, microwave or high-intensity focused ultrasound thermotherapy, holium laser enucleation (HoLEP), electro- or radiofrequency vaporization.

Complications of surgical treatment

- Postoperative haemorrhage and clot retention.
- UTI.
- TURP syndrome: in 2% of patients absorption of irrigation fluid via venous sinuses in the prostate causes hyponatraemia, hypotension and metabolic acidosis.
- Erectile dysfunction (retrograde ejaculation, impotence) 5–35% of patients.
- Incontinence 1%.
- Urethral stricture.

Prognosis

The majority of patients have a very good QoL after prostatectomy (endoscopic or open).

80 Renal (urinary) calculi

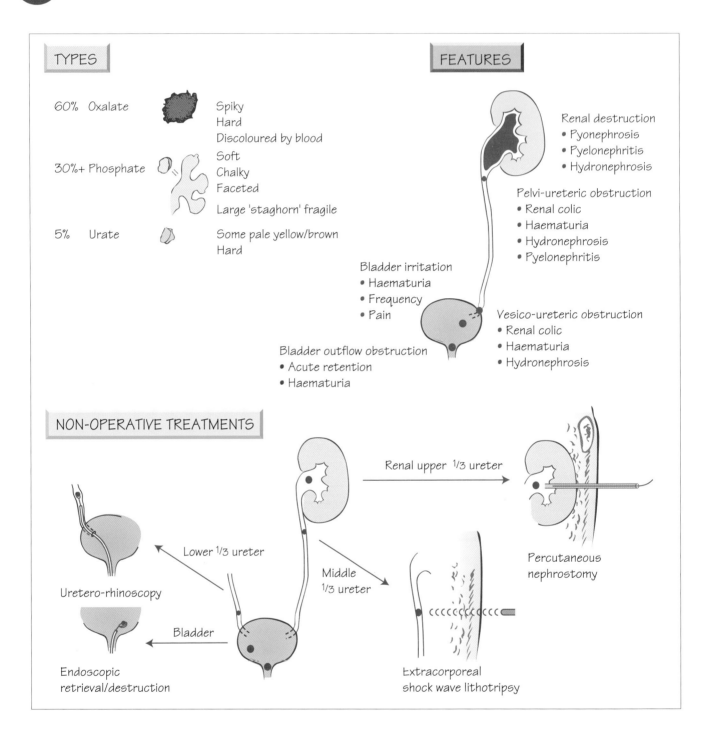

TYPES

60%	Oxalate	Spiky Hard Discoloured by blood
30%+	Phosphate	Soft Chalky Faceted Large 'staghorn' fragile
5%	Urate	Some pale yellow/brown Hard

FEATURES

Renal destruction
• Pyonephrosis
• Pyelonephritis
• Hydronephrosis

Pelvi-ureteric obstruction
• Renal colic
• Haematuria
• Hydronephrosis
• Pyelonephritis

Bladder irritation
• Haematuria
• Frequency
• Pain

Vesico-ureteric obstruction
• Renal colic
• Haematuria
• Hydronephrosis

Bladder outflow obstruction
• Acute retention
• Haematuria

NON-OPERATIVE TREATMENTS

Renal upper ⅓ ureter

Percutaneous nephrostomy

Lower ⅓ ureter

Uretero-rhinoscopy

Middle ⅓ ureter

Bladder

Endoscopic retrieval/destruction

Extracorporeal shock wave lithotripsy

Definition

Renal or *urinary* calculi are concretions formed by precipitation of various urinary solutes in the urinary tract. They contain calcium oxalate (60%), phosphate as a mixture of calcium, ammonium and magnesium phosphate – also called *struvite* – (triple phosphate stones are infective in origin) (30%), uric acid (5%) and cystine (1%).

Key points

- Calculi may develop because of or cause UTIs.
- Most stones (80–85%) pass without complication.
- Most stones are managed non-surgically.
- The pain of renal/ureteric calculi is very severe.
- Ureteric stone with obstruction and upper UTI is a urological emergency requiring immediate IV antibiotics and relief of the obstruction by ureteric stent or nephrostomy.
- Beware of the diagnosis of ureteric colic in patients >60 years – it might be a leaking AAA.

Epidemiology

Male:female 3:1. Early adult life. Among Europeans prevalence is 3%.

Pathogenesis

- Hypercalciuria: 65% of patients have idiopathic hypercalciuria.
- Nucleation theory: a crystal or foreign body acts as a nucleus for crystallization of supersaturated urine.
- Stone matrix theory: a protein matrix secreted by renal tubular cells acts as a scaffold for crystallization of supersaturated urine.
- Reduced inhibition theory: reduced urinary levels of naturally occurring inhibitors of crystallization.
- Dehydration.
- Infection: staghorn triple phosphate calculi are formed by the action of urease-producing organisms (*Proteus*, *Klebsiella*), which produce ammonia and render the urine alkaline.
- Schistosomiasis predisposes to bladder calculi (and cancer).

Pathology

- Staghorn calculi are large, fill the renal pelvis and calices, and lead to recurring pyelonephritis and renal parenchymal damage.
- Other stones are smaller, ranging in size from a few millimetres to 1–2 cm. They cause problems by obstructing the urinary tract, usually the ureter. Calyceal stones may cause haematuria and bladder stones may cause infection. Chronic bladder stones predispose to squamous carcinoma of the bladder (rare).

Clinical features

- Calyceal stones may be asymptomatic.
- Staghorn calculi present with loin pain and upper UTI.
- Ureteric colic – severe colicky pain radiating from the loin to the groin and into the testes or labia associated with gross or microscopic haematuria.
- Bladder calculi present with sudden interruption of urinary stream, perineal pain and pain at the tip of the penis.

Investigations

- FBC, U+E, serum creatinine, calcium, phosphate, urate, proteins and alkaline phosphatase.
- Urine microscopy for haematuria (present in most patients with urinary calculi) and crystals.
- Urine culture: secondary infection.
- Urine pH: <5.0 suggests uric acid stones, >7.0 suggests urea splitting organisms.
- Kidney, ureter, bladder (KUB) radiograph: 90% of renal calculi are radio-opaque.
- CT scanning: non-contrast helical CT scanning is more accurate than IVU in detecting urinary tract calculi. Gives no information about degree of obstruction or renal function.
- IVU: confirms the presence and the position of the stone in the genitourinary tract.
- An ultrasound may be indicated to exclude AAA. May show hydronephrosis or hydroureter if obstruction present.
- A renogram: may be indicated with staghorn calculi to assess renal function.
- 24-hour urine collection when patient is at home in normal environment.
- Stone analysis: origin.

Essential management

- Pain relief for ureteric colic: pethidine, diclofenac (NSAIDs as effective as opoids).
- Desmopressin (DDAVP), a vasopressin analogue given as a nasal spray, reduces the pain of acute renal colic. Usually given with diclofenac.
- High fluid intake.
- Antiemetics (metoclopramide, promethazine, prochlorperazine, hydroxyzine).
- Oral α-adrenergic blockers (e.g. tamsulosin) increase rate of spontaneous stone passage.
- 80–85% of ureteric stones pass spontaneously. Stones of <4 mm in diameter almost always pass, >6 mm almost never pass.
- Indications for intervention:
  kidney stones: symptomatic, obstruction, staghorn
  ureteric stones: failure to pass, large stone, obstruction, infection
  bladder stones: all to prevent complications
  sepsis super-added: nephrostomy.

Interventional procedures

- Obstructed infected collecting system: ureteric stents or percutaneous nephrostomy.
- Large kidney stones and staghorn calculi: percutaneous nephrolithotomy.
- Small/medium kidney stones: ESWL.
- Upper ureteric stones (above pelvic brim): ureteroscopy and manipulation of stone back into renal pelvis for ESWL or contact lithotripsy.
- Lower ureteric stones: ureteroscopy with contact lithotripsy or extraction with a Dormia basket.
- Large kidney or ureteric stones: open surgery – ureterolithotomy (rare now) or nephrolithotomy.
- Bladder stones: mechanical lithotripsy or open surgery.

Prophylaxis

Maintain high fluid intake to produce 2 L urine per day.

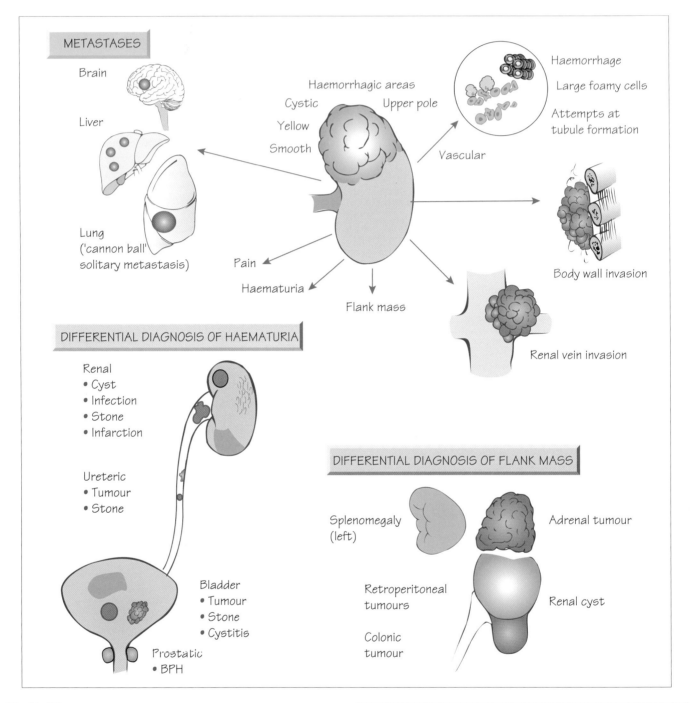

Definition

Renal cell carcinoma (RCC) (*hypernephroma* or *Grawitz' tumour*) is a malignant lesion (*adenocarcinoma*) of the kidney arising from the proximal renal tubular epithelium

Key points

- New, significant haematuria always requires investigation and may represent RCC.

- Consider RCC in unexplained anaemia, vague abdominal symptoms and recurrent UTIs. RCC is one of the great 'mimics' of medicine.
- Radical surgery offers the best hope of long-term survival. >50% of patients with early stage RCC are cured.
- Tumours are occasionally familial and a family history should be sought.

Epidemiology

Male:female 1.6:1. Uncommon before 40 years. Accounts for 2–3% of all tumours in adults and 90% of all renal tumours. (Other renal tumours: urothelial tumours, Wilms' tumour (children) and sarcomas.)

Aetiology

Predisposing factors

- Diet: high intake of fat, oil and milk.
- Toxic agents: lead, cadmium, asbestos, petroleum byproducts, large amounts of phenacetin-containing analgesics.
- Cigarette smoking doubles the risk of RCC.
- Hypertension and obesity, especially in women.
- Genetic factors: oncogene on short arm of chromosome 3, HLA antigen BW-44 and DR-8.
- Other diseases: von Hippel–Lindau (VHL) syndrome, hereditary papillary renal carcinoma, adult polycystic disease, renal dialysis patients, post-renal transplantation.

Pathology

Histology

Adenocarcinoma (cell of origin is the proximal renal tubular epithelium). Histological subtypes are: clear cell (75%), chromophilic (15%), chromophobic (5%), oncocytoma (3% – rarely metastasize) and collecting duct (2% – very aggressive).

Spread

- Direct into renal vein and perirenal tissue.
- Lymphatic to periaortic and hilar nodes.
- Haematogenous to lung (large, 'cannon-ball' metastases), bones and contralateral kidney.

Staging and prognosis

Stage	5-year survival
Stage I: T1/N0/M0 – tumour confined within renal capsule	95%
Stage II: T2/N0/M0 – tumour confined by Gerota's fascia	85%
Stage III: T1–T3/N0–1/M0 – tumour to renal vein or IVC nodes or through Gerota's fascia	59%
Stage IV: – distant metastases or invasion of adjacent organs	0–20%

Clinical features

- Triad of haematuria (40–60%), flank pain (40–50%), abdominal mass (25–45%) but all three in <10% of patients. Often late onset of symptoms.
- Hypertension (20%), polycythaemia (due to decreased blood flow to JGA → ↑ renin, ↑ erythropoietin).
- Anaemia, weight loss, PUO, night sweats, malaise.
- Paraneoplastic conditions (caused by tumour release of IL-6, erythropoietin or nitric oxide):
  hypercalcaemia, ectopic hormone production (ACTH, ADH)
  liver dysfunction (raised enzymes and prolonged PT) in the absence of metastatic disease (Stauffer's syndrome)
  polyneuropathy, myopathy, cachexia, dermatomyositis.
- Left-sided varicocele (2% of males with RCC).
- 30% present with metastatic disease (lung, soft tissues, bone, liver, skin, CNS).

Investigations

- FBC: anaemia, polycythaemia.
- ESR.
- U+E, calcium, creatinine: renal function.
- LFTs: metastases.
- Urine culture: infection.
- Abdominal ultrasound: assess renal mass and IVC.
- IVU: image renal outline.
- Contrast-enhanced CT or MRI scan: imaging modality of choice for diagnosis and staging of RCC.
- MRA and echocardiogram: assess IVC and right atrium involvement.
- Bone scan if bony symptoms and raised alkaline phosphatase.
- CXR (+ CT thorax if abnormal).

Essential management

Surgical (Stages I and II and some Stage III)

- Offers best chance of long-term survival.
- Radical (laparoscopic) nephrectomy: aim to remove kidney, renal vessels, upper ureter, (± ipsilateral adrenal gland) and Gerota's fascia.
- Partial nephrectomy: if Stage I and part of VHL presentation.
- Isolated lung/brain metastases may also be removed surgically with good results.
- Radiofrequency thermal ablation effective for small neoplasms in selected patients.

Palliative (Stage IV)

- Palliative surgery (nephrectomy) considered for pain, haemorrhage, malaise, hypercalcaemia or polycythaemia.
- Multi-kinase inhibitor treatment – targeted agents for advanced or metastatic RCC:
  VEGF inhibitor (bevacizumab) – VEGF-receptor (VEGFR) signaling blockers (sunitinib, sorafenib, and pazopanib)
  mammalian target rapamycin (mTOR) inhibitors (temsirolimus and everolimus).
- Partial response in 40% of patients with advanced disease and prolonged survival by 6–9 months. May be toxic side-effects.
- Hormone therapy (only 5% response rate) – no standard regimen.
- Immunotherapy (IL-2, interferon alpha, BCG – selected patients will respond).
- Radiotherapy for local or metastatic symptoms.
- RCC is refractory to most chemotherapeutic agents.

Prognosis

50% of early stage RCCs are cured but outcome for Stage IV is very poor. Overall survival is 40% at 5 years.

2-week wait referral criteria for suspected urological cancer

- Macroscopic haematuria in adult.
- Microscopic haematuria >50 years.
- Testicular body swelling.
- Solid renal mass on imaging.
- Increased PSA (if life expectancy >10 years).
- Increased PSA with malignant feeling prostate/bone pain.
- Suspected penile cancer.

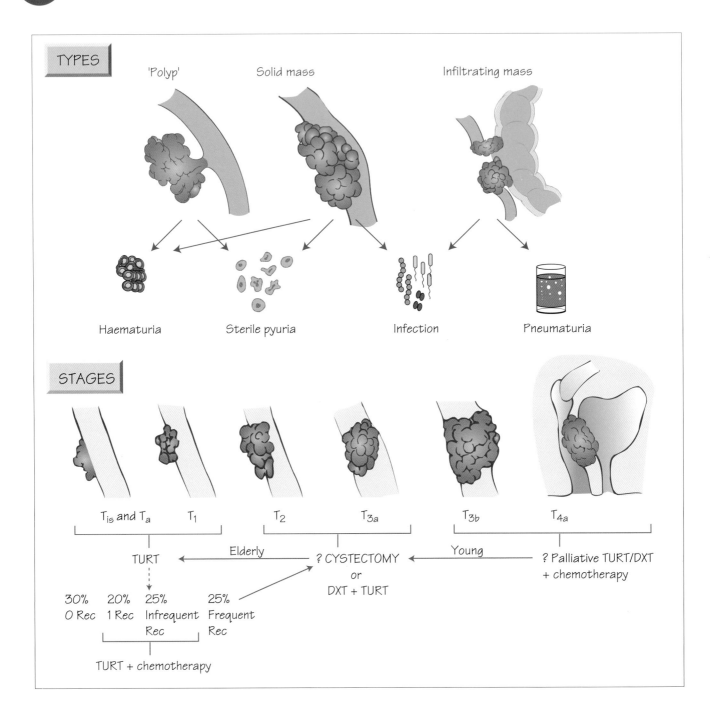

TYPES

'Polyp'　　　Solid mass　　　Infiltrating mass

Haematuria　　　Sterile pyuria　　　Infection　　　Pneumaturia

STAGES

T_{is} and T_a　　　T_1　　　T_2　　　T_{3a}　　　T_{3b}　　　T_{4a}

TURT　　←　Elderly　　? CYSTECTOMY　　←　Young　　? Palliative TURT/DXT
　　　　　　　　　　　　　　or　　　　　　　　　　+ chemotherapy
　　　　　　　　　　　　　DXT + TURT

30%　　20%　　25%　　　25%
0 Rec　1 Rec　Infrequent　Frequent
　　　　　　　Rec　　　　Rec

TURT + chemotherapy

Definition

Malignant lesion of the bladder epithelium.

Key points

- Commonly presents with gross painless haematuria.
- Ranges from 'benign'- acting recurrent bladder 'polyps' to rapidly progressive infiltrating masses.
- Transitional cell lesions are a 'field' change and often multiple.
- Local recurrence rate for non-muscle invasive TCC is high (80%).

Epidemiology

Male:female 3:1. Uncommon before 50 years. Increasing incidence of bladder cancer in recent years. Death rate is 7.6/100 000.

Aetiology

Predisposing factors:
- Smoking: associated with 50% of all bladder cancers; smokers have 2–6 times increased risk of developing bladder carcinoma. Carcinogens in smoke: 2-naphthylamine, 4-aminobiphenyl and nitrosamines.
- Exposure to aromatic amines in dyes, paints, solvents and rubber.
- Prior exposure to radiation of the pelvis or chemotherapy with cyclophosphamide (via exposure to its metabolite, acrolein).
- Bladder irritation from *Schistosomiasis*, bladder stones or long-term indwelling catheters (squamous carcinoma).
- Congenital abnormalities (extrophy of the bladder) (adenocarcinoma).
- Genetic mutations of tumour suppressor genes on chromosomes 17 (*p53*, high grade) and 9 (*p15* and *p16*, low grade) are linked to bladder cancer. Other mutations may also be involved.

Pathology
Histology
- Transitional cell carcinoma (TCC) or urothelial carcinoma (90%).
- Squamous cell carcinoma (5%). (In developing world SCC is common because of association with *Schistosomiasis*.)
- Adenocarcinoma (2%).

Staging and prognosis for TCC

Stage	5-year survival
Non muscle invasive (70%)	
Stage 0: T1s/N0/M0 – Tumour confined to urothelium	80–100%
Stage I: T1/N0/M0 – Lamina propria involved	85%
Muscle invasive tumours (25%)	
Stage II: T2/N0/M0 – Muscularis propria invasion	75%
Stage III: T3/N0/M0 – Perivesical tissue invaded	50%
Advanced disease (5%)	
Stage IV: anyT/anyN/M1 – Invasion of adjacent pelvic organs	10%
Grade: Low (grades 1 and 2), high (grade 3)	

Spread

- Direct into pelvic viscera (prostate, uterus, vagina, colon, rectum).
- Lymphatic to periaortic nodes.
- Haematogenous to liver and lung.

Clinical features
- Painless intermittent gross haematuria (95%).
- Dysuria, urgency or frequency (10%).

Investigations
- Urine analysis and microscopy.
- Urine cytology (significant false negative rate).
- FBC: anaemia.
- U+E creatinine: renal function.
- CT urography or IVU: occult upper tract tumours.
- Ultrasound: obstruction.
- CT scan: local invasion, distant metastases.
- Cystourethroscopy and biopsy.

Essential management

Non-muscle invasive tumours (Stages 0 and I)
- TURT of bladder and surveillance cystoscopy.
- Intravesical immunotherapy with BCG ± interferon α or interferon-γ. Patients with recurrence of T_{CIS} after BCG should be considered for radical cystectomy as most (80%) will progress to muscle invasive bladder cancer.
- Intravesical chemotherapy may be useful in patients refractory to intravesical immunotherapy.

Invasive tumours (Stages II and III)
- Radical cystectomy + pelvic lymphadenectomy + urinary diversion (e.g. ileal conduit) (± neoadjuvant chemotherapy). 90% 5-year survival if tumour confined to bladder.
- External beam radiation therapy has been used but results not as good as radical surgery – 20–40% 5-year survival if tumour confined to bladder.

Advanced disease (Stage IV)
- Chemotherapy: (MVAC) methotrexate, vinblastine, doxorubicin (adriamycin), cisplatin or (GC) gemcitabine and cisplatin, (CMV) cisplatin, methotrexate, vinblastine. Most patients will die within 2 years in spite of Rx.

2-week wait referral criteria for suspected urological cancer

- Macroscopic haematuria in adult.
- Microscopic haematuria >50 years.
- Testicular body swelling.
- Solid renal mass on imaging.
- Increased PSA (if life expectancy >10 years).
- Increased PSA with malignant feeling prostate/bone pain.
- Suspected penile cancer.

83 Carcinoma of the prostate

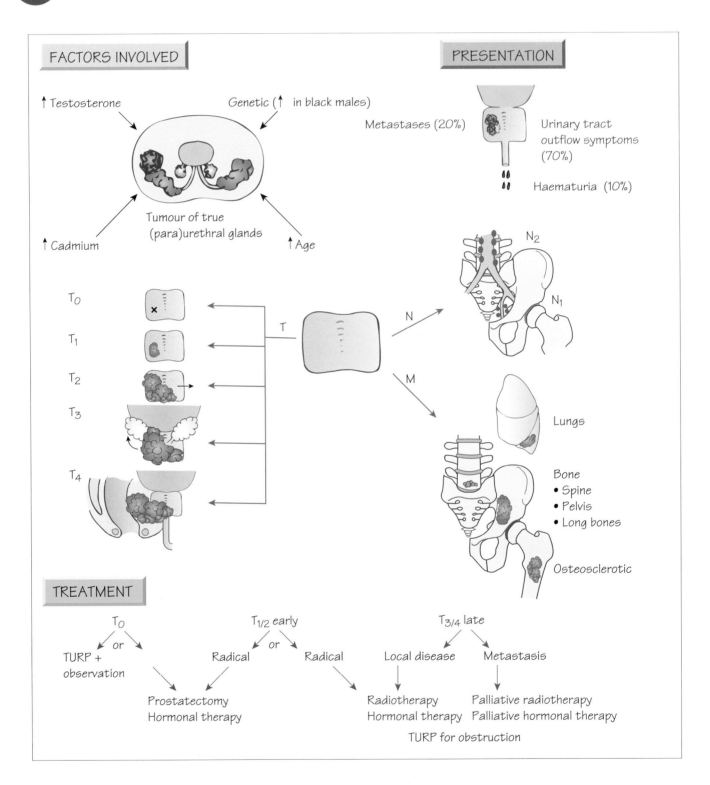

FACTORS INVOLVED

↑Testosterone   Genetic (↑ in black males)

Tumour of true
(para)urethral glands

↑Cadmium   ↑Age

T_0
T_1
T_2
T_3
T_4

T

N

M

PRESENTATION

Metastases (20%)   Urinary tract
outflow symptoms
(70%)

Haematuria (10%)

N_2
N_1

Lungs

Bone
• Spine
• Pelvis
• Long bones

Osteosclerotic

TREATMENT

T_0
or
TURP +
observation

$T_{1/2}$ early
or
Radical   Radical

Prostatectomy
Hormonal therapy

$T_{3/4}$ late
Local disease   Metastasis

Radiotherapy   Palliative radiotherapy
Hormonal therapy   Palliative hormonal therapy

TURP for obstruction

Definition
Malignant lesion of the prostate gland.

Key points

- Prostate cancer is commonly found in older men. Variable clinical course.
- Increasingly found (asymptomatic) by screening using PSA and digital rectal examination. Screening may detect non-lethal tumours. Need prostatic biopsy to make diagnosis.
- Non-metastatic disease has good 5-year survival with radical local therapy.
- Metastatic disease is best managed medically and has a poor outlook.

Epidemiology
Uncommon before 60 years. 80% of prostate cancers are clinically undetected (latent carcinoma) and are only discovered on autopsy. The true incidence of this disease is considerably higher than the clinical experience would indicate.

Aetiology
- Increasing age.
- More common in black men.
- Hormonal factors: growth enhanced by testosterone and inhibited by oestrogens or antiandrogens.

Pathology
- Prostatic tumours are often multicentric and located in the periphery of the gland.
- Adenocarcinoma arising from glandular epithelium.
- Gleason grading (1–5) is used to grade differentiation. The most common and second most common pattern are each graded 1–5; the sum of these gives the Gleason score (2–10).
- Staging: TNM, PSA levels and Gleason grading are all used to calculate 'stage'.

Spread
- Direct into remainder of gland and seminal vesicles.
- Lymphatic to iliac and periaortic nodes.
- Haematogenous to bone (usually osteosclerotic lesions), liver, lung.

Clinical features
- Bladder outflow obstruction (poor stream, hesitancy, nocturia).
- New onset erectile dysfunction.
- Symptoms of advanced disease (ureteric obstruction and hydronephrosis or bone pain from metastases, classically worse at night).
- Nodule or irregular firm mass detected on rectal examination.

Investigations
- FBC: anaemia.
- U+E, creatinine: renal function.
- Specific markers: PSA, PSA velocity (3 measurements over 2 years), free:total PSA ratio.
  PSA: >10 ng/ml (carcinoma unlikely to be organ confined) – prostatic bx.
  PSA: 4–10 ng/ml (carcinoma may be organ confined) – prostatic bx.
  PSA: <4 ng/ml (only 20% will have cancer) – ± prostatic bx.
- Transrectal U/S and MRI: local staging.
- Transrectal U/S guided needle biopsy of the prostate: tissue diagnosis.
- Bone scan: metastases.

Essential management

Localized prostate cancer (Stages I–III)

Risk	PSA (ng/mL)		Gleason		Clinical	Rx
Low (Stage I)	<10	+	≤6	+	T1–T2a	Active surveillance or radical Rx
Intermediate (Stage II)	10–20	or	7	or	T2b–T2c	Radical Rx
High (Stage III)	>20	or	8–10	or	T3–T4	Radical Rx (EBRT + androgen deprivation therapy (ADT) or RP + adjuvant RT)

Active surveillance: observed for biochemical, histological or clinical progression. If progression occurs patients should be offered radical Rx.
  Radical Rx: radical prostatectomy (RP) or radiotherapy (RT) (external beam (EBRT) or interstitial brachytherapy).

Metastatic prostate cancer (Stage IV)
- Primary hormonal Rx: Androgen deprivation therapy: orchidectomy ± gonadotropin releasing (also known as 'luteinizing') hormone (GnLH or LHRH) agonist – may be 'tumour flare' for first 2 weeks of Rx with GnLH, which is controlled by simultaneous administration of antiandrogens; oestrogens not used very much because of CVS side effects.
- Secondary hormonal Rx: antiandrogens, cytochrome P450 enzyme inhibitor, corticosteroids.
- Hormone resistance: miotoxanone or docetaxel + steroid; immunotherapy (sipuleucel-T).
- Painful bone metastases: local EBRT or bone-targeted radioisotopes: samarium-153 or strontium-89.

Prognosis
- Localized tumours: 90% 5-year survival.
- Local spread: 70% 5-year survival.
- Metastases: 30% 5-year survival.

2-week wait referral criteria for suspected urological cancer

- Macroscopic haematuria in adult.
- Microscopic haematuria >50 years.
- Testicular body swelling.
- Solid renal mass on imaging.
- Increased PSA (if life expectancy >10 years).
- Increased PSA with malignant feeling prostate/bone pain.
- Suspected penile cancer.

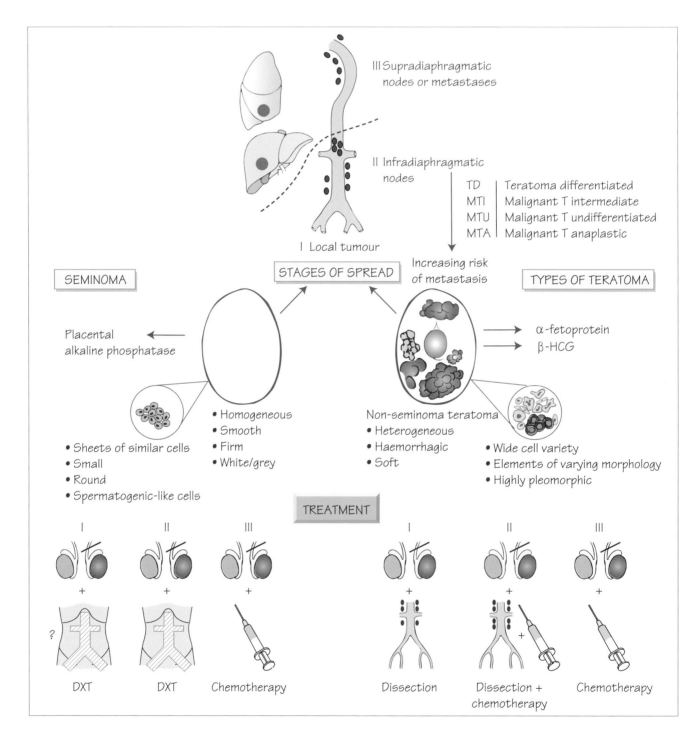

Definition
Malignant lesion of the testis.

- Early tumours have an excellent prognosis with surgery alone.
- Late tumours have a good prognosis with surgery and medical therapy.
- Orchidectomy for tumour should be via a groin incision.
- Prognosis is generally good but depends on stage and histology.

Epidemiology

Age 20–35 years. Most common solid tumours in young males. The incidence of testicular cancer seems to be increasing.

Aetiology

• Crypto-orchidism – 40 to 50-fold increase in risk of developing testicular germ cell cancer. Risk is unaffected by orchidopexy.
• Exposure to high prenatal oestrogen levels, chemical carcinogens, trauma, orchitis.
• Higher incidence in white men.

Pathology

Classification of testicular tumours

• Germ-cell tumours (95%) (secrete AFP and β-HCG):
seminoma (SGCT) (40%)
non-seminoma (NSGCT) – embryonal carcinoma (25%), teratoma/teratocarcinoma (30%), choriocarcinoma (1%), yolk sac tumour (rare).
• Non-germ-cell tumours (stromal tumours) (5%):
Leydig cell
Sertoli cell
granulosa cell.
Non-germ-cell tumours are rare and only 10% of them are malignant.
• Metastatic tumours.

Staging

• Stage I: confined to scrotum.
• Stage II: spread to retroperitoneal lymph nodes below the diaphragm.
• Stage III: distant metastases.

Spread

• Germ-cell tumours to para-aortic nodes, lung and brain.
• Stromal tumours rarely metastasize.

Clinical features

• Painless, hard swelling of the testis, often discovered incidentally or after trauma.
• Vague testicular discomfort common, bleeding into tumour may mimic acute torsion.
• Rarely evidence of metastatic disease or gynaecomastia (5%).
• Examination: hard, irregular, non-tender testicular mass.

Investigations

• Blood for tumour markers, i.e. AFP, β-HCG and LDH. Very useful in following success of treatment.
• AFP is elevated in 75% of embryonal and 65% of teratocarcinoma.
• AFP is not elevated in pure seminoma or choriocarcinoma. If an AFP elevation is noted in a pathologically diagnosed seminoma, the diagnosis should be changed to NSGCT.
• β-HCG is elevated in 100% choriocarcinoma, 60% embryonal carcinoma, 60% teratocarcinoma and 10% pure seminoma.
• Scrotal ultrasound: diagnosis is made by seeing a mass in the testis usually confined by the tunica albuginea.
• Chest X-ray to assess lungs and mediastinum: metastases.

• CT scan of chest and abdomen and pelvis: to detect lymph nodes and stage disease.
• Consider sperm banking for future fertility options.

Essential management

Radical orchidectomy (via groin incision) and histological diagnosis. Further treatment depends on histology and staging.

Seminoma

• Stage I: radical orchidectomy + active surveillance ± radiotherapy to retroperitoneal nodes or carboplatin chemotherapy.
• Stage II: radical orchidectomy + radiotherapy to retroperitoneal nodes or cisplatin chemotherapy.
• Stage III: radical orchidectomy + chemotherapy (bleomycin, etoposide, cisplatin (BEP)).

Non-seminoma germ cell

• Stage I: orchidectomy + active surveillance or RPLND or adjuvant BEP.
• Stage II: orchidectomy + RPLND ± BEP.
• Stage III: primary chemotherapy (+ RPLND if good response).

Testicular cancers can also can be subdivided into good, intermediate and poor risk, depending on levels of tumour markers, size of mediastinal nodes, presence of cervical nodes and number of mediastinal metastases. (RPLND (open or laparoscopic) may be complicated by lack of antegarde ejaculation.)

Prognosis

• Overall cure rates for testicular cancer are over 90% and node-negative disease has almost 100% 5-year survival.
• SGCT: Stages I and II, 98–100% 5-year survival; Stage III, 86–90% 5-year survival.
• NSGCT: Stage I, 98% 5-year survival; Stage II, 92% 5-year survival; Stage III, good risk 92%, intermediate risk 80% and poor risk 48% 5-year survival.
• Survivors of testicular cancer are at a risk of developing secondary cancers because of young age and exposure to radiotherapy ± chemotherapy.

2-week wait referral criteria for suspected urological cancer

• Macroscopic haematuria in adult.
• Microscopic haematuria >50 years.
• Testicular body swelling.
• Solid renal mass on imaging.
• Increased PSA (if life expectancy >10 years).
• Increased PSA with malignant feeling prostate/bone pain.
• Suspected penile cancer.

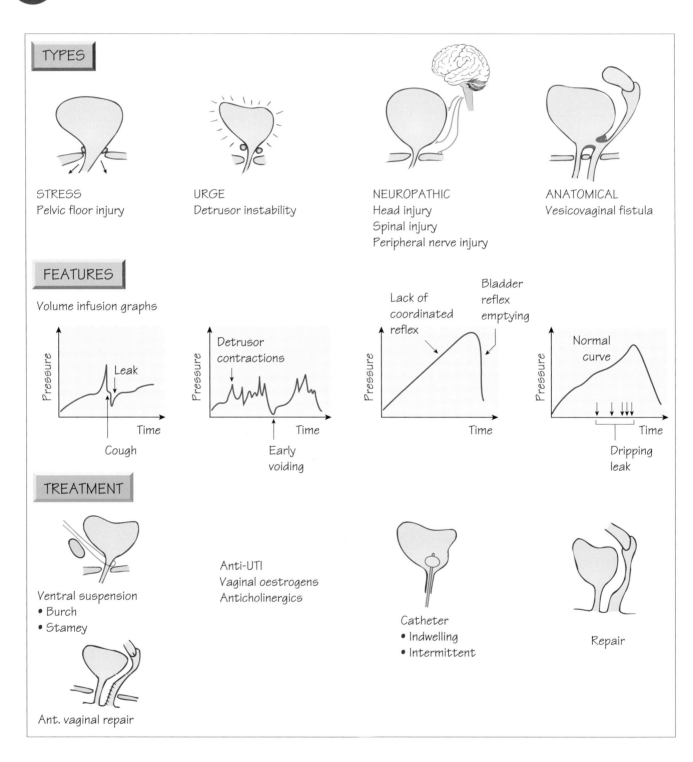

TYPES

STRESS
Pelvic floor injury

URGE
Detrusor instability

NEUROPATHIC
Head injury
Spinal injury
Peripheral nerve injury

ANATOMICAL
Vesicovaginal fistula

FEATURES

Volume infusion graphs

Leak
Cough

Detrusor contractions
Early voiding

Lack of coordinated reflex
Bladder reflex emptying

Normal curve
Dripping leak

TREATMENT

Ventral suspension
• Burch
• Stamey

Ant. vaginal repair

Anti-UTI
Vaginal oestrogens
Anticholinergics

Catheter
• Indwelling
• Intermittent

Repair

Definition

Urinary incontinence (UI) is defined as the involuntary loss of urine that can be demonstrated objectively.

> ## Key points
>
> - A common and socially disabling condition, often undetected and undertreated.
> - Full assessment and investigation is required to elicit precise cause and tailor treatment.

Epidemiology

UI affects 15–30% of the general population. More common in females (male:female 1:3) and in the elderly. UI rarely causes death but is a huge source of morbidity (perineal irritation and sepsis, frequency and nocturia, social isolation and embarrassment).

Classification

Urethral incontinence

- Urethral abnormalities: obesity, multiparity, difficult delivery, pelvic fractures, post-prostatectomy.
- Bladder abnormalities: neuropathic or non-neuropathic detrusor abnormalities, infection, interstitial cystitis, bladder stones and tumours.
- Non-urinary abnormalities: impaired mobility or mental function.

Non-urethral incontinence

- Urinary fistula: vesicovaginal.
- Ureteral ectopia: ureter drains into urethra (usually a duplex ureter).

Pathophysiology

- *Stress incontinence*: urine leakage when infra-abdominal pressure exceeds urethral pressure (e.g. coughing, laughing, straining or lifting). Urethral incompetence often develops as a result of impaired urethral support due to pelvic floor muscle weakness.
- *Urge incontinence*: uninhibited bladder contraction from detrusor hyperactivity causes a rise in intravesical pressure and urine leakage. May be caused by loss of cortical control (e.g. stroke) or bladder inflammation from stone, infection or neoplasm. Characterized by an overactive bladder: urgency, frequency and nocturia.
- *Mixed incontinence* is a combination of stress and urge incontinence.
- *Overflow incontinence (incomplete bladder emptying)*: damage to the efferent fibres of the sacral reflex causes bladder atonia. The bladder fills with urine and becomes grossly distended with constant dribbling of urine. May result from bladder outlet obstruction (e.g. BPH), spinal cord injury or congenital defect (e.g. spina bifida) or neuropathy (e.g. diabetes).

Clinical features

- Stress incontinence: loss of urine during coughing, straining, etc. These symptoms are quite specific for stress incontinence.
- Urge incontinence: inability to maintain urine continence in the presence of frequent and insistent urges to void.
- Nocturnal enuresis: 10% of 5-year-olds and 5% of 10-year-olds are incontinent during sleep. Bed-wetting in older children is abnormal and may indicate bladder instability.

- May be symptoms of an underlying cause: infection (frequency, dysuria, nocturia); obstruction (poor stream, dribbling); trauma (including surgery, e.g. abdominoperineal resection); fistula (continuous dribbling); neurological disease (sexual or bowel dysfunction) or systemic disease (e.g. diabetes).
- Assessment of impact on QoL should be made (e.g. *CONTILIFE* questionnaire).

Investigations

- Voiding (or bladder) diary: useful to establish baseline and assess efficacy of treatment.
- Urine culture: to exclude infection.
- IVU: to assess upper tracts and obstruction or fistula.
- Urodynamics – essential in determining type of incontinence accurately:
    uroflowmetry: measures flow rate
    cystometry: demonstrates detrusor contractures
    video cystometry: shows leakage of urine on straining in patients with stress incontinence
    urethral pressure flowmetry: measures urethral and bladder pressure at rest and during voiding
    postvoid residual volume is measured by ultrasound or passing a catheter and draining the bladder 5 minutes after micturition.
- Cystoscopy: if bladder stone or neoplasm is suspected.
- Vaginal speculum examination ± cystogram if vesicovaginal fistula suspected.
- MRI to visualize pelvic floor defects.

> ## Essential management
>
> ### Urge incontinence
>
> - Medical treatment: modify fluid intake, avoid caffeine and alcohol, treat any underlying cause (infection, tumour, stone); bladder training; pelvic floor exercises (Kegel exercises); anticholinergic drugs with antimuscarinic effects (oxybutynin, tolterodine).
> - Surgical treatment (uncommon): cystoscopy and bladder distension, augmentation cystoplasty.
>
> ### Stress incontinence
>
> - Medical treatment: lose weight, pelvic floor exercises, topical oestrogens for atrophic vaginitis, vaginal pessary.
> - Surgical treatment (common): retropubic or endoscopic urethropexy, vaginal repair, artificial sphincter, periurethral bulking injections, implantation of artificial sphincter (rare).
>
> ### Overflow incontinence
>
> - Avoid medicines that cause detrusor hypoactivity: anticholinergics, calcium-channel blockers.
> - If obstruction present: treat cause of obstruction, e.g. TURP.
> - If no obstruction: short period of catheter drainage to allow detrusor muscle to recover from over-stretching, then short course of detrusor muscle stimulants (bethanechol; distigmine).
> - Clean intermittent self-catheterization is a very effective way to manage neurogenic overflow incontinence.
>
> ### Urinary fistula
>
> - Always requires surgical treatment.

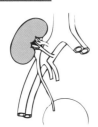

RENAL

Typical outcomes
1 yr graft survival 90%
5 yr graft survival 65%

- Typical indications
  - Diabetic nephropathy
  - Glomerulopathies
  - Renal cystic disease
  - Renal arterial disease
  - Metabolic diseases
- Technical notes
  - Donor sources (cadaveric, LRD, LURD)
  - Graft placed in iliac fossa
  - Blood supply from external iliac vessels
  - Ureter implanted into bladder
- Typical complications
  - Acute rejection
  - Chronic rejection
  - Urine leak ('urinoma')
  - Vascular thrombosis
  - Lymphatic leak ('lymphocoele')

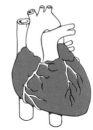

CARDIAC

Typical outcomes
1 yr graft survival 80%
5 yr graft survival 65%

- Typical indications
  - Cardiomyopathies
  - Ischaemic heart disease
  - Congenital heart disease
- Technical notes
  - Donor sources (cadaveric)
  - Fully anatomical transplantation
- Typical complications
  - Acute rejection
  - Chronic rejection
  - Recurrent coronary artery disease

HEPATIC

Typical outcomes
1 yr graft survival 80%
5 yr graft survival 55%

- Typical indications
  - Alcoholic disease
  - Viral hepatitis
  - Toxin induced liver failure
  - Autoimmune hepatic/biliary diseases
  - Metabolic diseases
  - Congenital disorders
  - Budd–Chiari syndrome
- Technical notes
  - Donor sources (cadaveric, LRD, LURD)
  - May be part of a liver or complete liver
- Typical complications
  - Primary acute non-function
  - Bile leak
  - Recurrent coronary artery disease
  - Vascular thrombosis
  - Biliary stricture

PANCREATIC

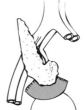

Typical outcomes
1 yr graft survival 75%

- Typical indications
  - Diabetes
- Technical notes
  - Pancreas and duodenum implanted into iliac fossa
  - Often with simultaneous kindey transplant
- Typical complications
  - Pancreatitis
  - Acute rejection
  - Vascular thrombosis

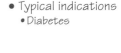

SMALL BOWEL

Typical outcomes
1 yr graft survival 60%

- Typical indications
  - Short bowel due to resection/ vascular accident
  - Congenital atresia
- Typical complications
  - Acute rejection
  - GVHD

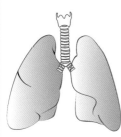

LUNG

Typical outcomes
1 yr graft survival 70%
5 yr graft survival 55%

- Typical indications
  - COPD
  - Cystic fibrosis
  - Fibrosing alveolitis
  - Pulmonary hypertension
- Technical notes
  - Donor sources (cadaveric, LURD ('domino'))
  - May be part combined heart–lung, double lung or single lung
- Typical complications
  - Pulmonary infection

Definitions

Transplantation is the procedure whereby cells, tissues or organs are moved from one site to another to provide structure and/or function. A *graft* is the organ or tissue transplanted. *Autografting* is transplantation from one part of a patient's body to another e.g. toe to replace thumb. *Allografting* (also known as *homografting*) is transplantation between organisms of the same species (i.e. human to human). *Xenografting* is transplantation between organisms of different species (e.g. pig to human). Grafts may be placed in the 'correct' anatomical location (*orthotopic* transplantation; e.g. heart transplant) or in a non-anatomical location (*heterotopic* transplantation; e.g. kidney transplant). The graft comes from a *donor* and is implanted into a *recipient (host)*. Donors may be *cadaveric* (usually brainstem death victims), *living related* (LRD) (family members sharing large genetic elements with the recipient) or *living unrelated* (LURD) (altruistic individuals donating one of a pair of organs). *Natural or innate immunity* refers to the non-specific immune response (macrophages, neutrophils, natural killer cells, cytokines). *Adaptive immunity*, refers to the response to a specific antigen (T-cells and B-cells).

Key points

- All but identical twin transplants require immunosuppression.
- Graft rejection can be hyperacute, acute or chronic.
- Long-term immunosuppression causes disease in its own right.
- Kidney, pancreas, liver, heart and lung transplantation are well established with high success rates. Small bowel transplantation is being progressively developed.

Immunology of transplantation

- Pre-existing cell surface antigens (e.g. ABO and related blood groups) stimulate pre-existing humoral immunity in the form of antibodies. All grafts must be ABO-matched or hyperacute rejection will occur.
- Class 1 MHC antigens (e.g. HLA-A, HLA-B, HLA-C) exist on nucleated cell surfaces and stimulate activation of recipient CD8 positive (cytotoxic) T lymphocytes. Optimizing Class 1 matching reduces the risk of acute rejection episodes.
- Class 2 MHC antigens (e.g. DR, DP, DQ) are found on cells such as macrophages, monocytes and B lymphocytes and stimulate CD4 positive (helper) T lymphocytes. Optimizing Class 2 matching reduces the risk of mixed humoral/cell-mediated rejection.
- Mechanism of rejection: sensitization stage (pro-inflammatory mediators and T cells), allo-recognition (direct and indirect pathways), effector stage (macrophage infiltration, NK cells), apoptosis.

Graft rejection

- Hyperacute rejection – occurs shortly after graft enters host circulation. Caused by preformed antibody recognition of cell surface antigens. Prevented by crossmatching between recipient serum and donor cells.
- Acute rejection – can occur at any time in the life of a graft but is most common in the first months after transplantation. Caused by

cell-mediated immunity against HLA antigens. May be reduced or prevented by immunosuppression. Single episodes of acute rejection are easy to treat and rarely lead to organ failure.

- Chronic rejection – occurs after months and years. Causes may be multifaoctorial including low grade cell-mediated attack due to HLA mismatching, chronic infection, underlying organ disease. Leading cause of organ transplant failure.
- Flu-like symptoms and evidence of failing function of the transplanted organ indicate rejection. Diagnosis confirmed by biopsy.

Immunosuppression

- All immunosuppressives result in non-specific suppression of immune defence and increase the life time risk of infection (CMV, herpes group viruses, *Pneumocystis*, *Candida*, *Aspergilla*, *Cryptococcus*) and malignancy (BCC skin, SCC skin, B-cell lymphomas) for the recipient.

Drug group	Effect	Side-effects
Corticosteroids	Suppress all inflammatory elements of the immune response	'Cushingoid' effects
Anti-proliferatives (methotrexate, azathioprine, mycophenolate)	Prevent cell-mediated cell mitosis and amplification of response	Renal and hepatic dysfunction, marrow suppression
Calcineurin blockade (ciclosporin, tacrolimus)	Suppress T cells and inhibit IL-2 release	Nephrotoxicity
mTOR inhibitors (sirolimus/ rapamycin, everolimus)	Prevents T- and B-cell activation in response to IL-2	Interstitial pneumonitis
Biological effectors (monoclonal anti-IL-2 receptor antibody (Basiliximab) and anti CD20 antibody (Rituximab); polyclonal anti T-cell antibodies)	Block specific parts of the immune responses	May induce severe reactions, e.g. cytokine release syndrome

Graft-versus-host disease

- Caused by donor immune cells present in the graft mounting immunological attack on recipient (host) tissues. Mediated mostly by T-cells. Most often follows bone marrow, liver and small bowel TxP.
- Causes fever, skin rash, rapidly developing multisystem failure. 75% mortality.
- May be reduced by perfusing the graft thoroughly prior to implantation to 'wash-out' donor lymphocytes.

Paediatric 'general' surgery/1

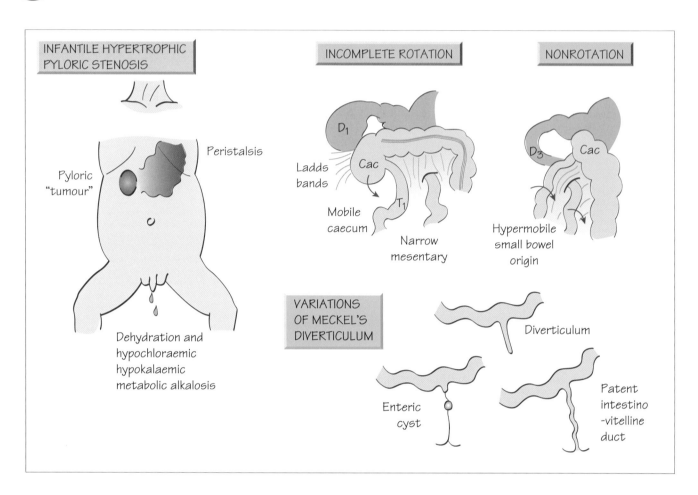

Infantile hypertrophic pyloric stenosis

Definition
This is a condition characterized by hypertrophy of the circular muscle of the gastric pylorus that obstructs gastric outflow.

Aetiology
The aetiology is unknown but it affects 1 in 450 children; 85% male, often firstborn; 20% have family history.

Clinical features
- Non-bile-stained, projectile vomiting (after feeds) beginning at 2–6 weeks. May be bloodstained.
- Baby is hungry, constipated and dehydrated. Loss of H^+ and Cl^- from stomach and K^+ from kidney causes hypochloraemic, hypokalaemic metabolic alkalosis.
- Palpable pyloric 'tumour' during a test feed or after vomiting.
- Gastric peristalsis may be seen. Ultrasound confirms the diagnosis.

Management
- Correct dehydration and electrolyte imbalance with **0.9% NaCl with added K^+** (20 mmol/L) (contains 170 mmol Cl^-/L) or **0.45% NaCl in dextrose 5% with added K^+** (20 mmol/L)(contains 95 mmol Cl^-/L). May take 24–48 hours to become normal.
- Ramstedt's pyloromyotomy via transverse RUQ or per umbilical incision or laparoscopically. Normal feeding can commence within 24 hours.

Malrotation of the gut

Definition and aetiology
'Malrotation' is often used to describe a number of conditions (1 in 500 live births) that are caused by failure of the intestine to rotate into the correct anatomical position during embryological development. Most common types are incomplete rotation and non-rotation.

Complications that can result include:
- Volvulus (leading to risk of bowel necrosis); usually small bowel ± caecum/proximal colon.
- Internal herniation (via abnormally large paraduodenal recesses and paracolic spaces).
- Duodenal obstruction (usually incomplete and intermittent); often said to be due to Ladd's bands (peritoneal tissue related to incomplete rotation) but probably due to rotation of a narrow small bowel mesenteric origin.

Clinical features
Bile-stained vomiting in the newborn period is the most common presentation but older children may present with recurrent abdominal pain, abdominal distension and vomiting.

Management
- If diagnosed prior to acute presentation: surgery to 'complete' the non-rotation; placing the colon in the left abdomen and small bowel to the right (widening the mesenertic attachment with fixation).
- Acute presentations: release the obstructions, resect non-viable bowel ± fixation of the bowel in normal anatomical position.

Meckel's diverticulum

Definition
Meckel's diverticulum is the remnant of the vitello-intestinal duct forming a blind-ending pouch on the antimesenteric border of the terminal ileum and is present in 2% of the population.

Clinical features
Most are asymptomatic.
   May present with:
- Rectal bleeding (often due to ulceration of the normal ileal mucosa opposite the diverticulum due to acid secreting (gastric antral type) epithelium within the diverticulum – detectable by technetium pertechnate scan in 70% of cases.
- 'Appendicitis' (Meckel's diverticulitis).
- Acute ileoileal intussusception.
- Volvulus (due to intestine-vitelline band/duct with small bowel rotation around it).

Management
Surgical excision, even if found incidentally.

Paediatric 'general' surgery/2

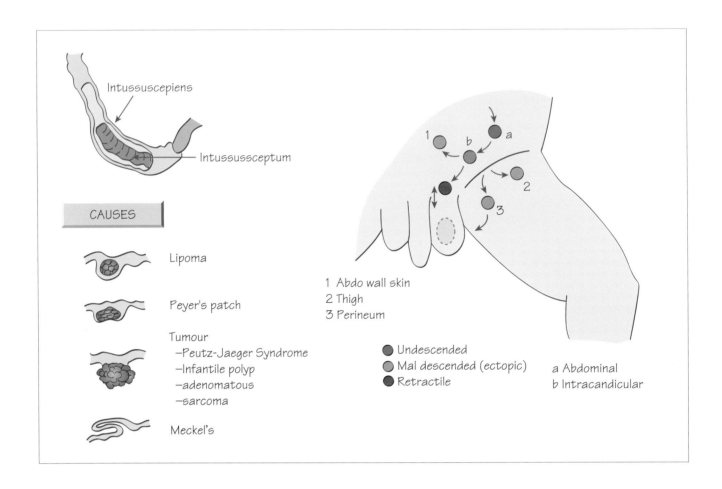

Intussuscepiens

Intussussceptum

CAUSES

Lipoma

Peyer's patch

Tumour
  —Peutz-Jaeger Syndrome
  —Infantile polyp
  —adenomatous
  —sarcoma

Meckel's

1 Abdo wall skin
2 Thigh
3 Perineum

● Undescended
● Mal descended (ectopic)
● Retractile

a Abdominal
b Intracandicular

Gastro-oesophageal reflux
Definition
This is a common condition characterized by incompetence of the LOS, resulting in retrograde passage of gastric contents into the oesophagus, leading to vomiting.

Aetiology
Transient LOS relaxation caused by:
- Increased volume of feed overwhelming gastric capacity.
- 'Slumped' seating position.

Clinical features
- Vomiting, usually bile-stained, not related to feeds, may contain blood (indicates oesophagitis) and rarely is projectile.
- Respiratory symptoms are frequently present of often caused by microaspiration of gastric content.
- Apnoea, stridor, wheezing, chronic (nocturnal) cough and failure to thrive may all be present.

Investigations
Most cases require no investigations and the diagnosis and treatment can be based on clinical features. If oesophagitis, stricture, anaemia or aspiration is suspected, a barium swallow, gastric scintigraphy (good for diagnosis of pulmonary aspiration), oesophagoscopy and biopsy, 24-hour pH monitoring and oesophageal manometry are indicated.

Treatment
As there is a natural tendency towards spontaneous improvement with age (most have resolved by age 18 months), a conservative approach is adopted initially: smaller, thicker feeds, positioning infant in 30° head-up prone position after feeds, antacids, H_2 receptor blockers, proton pump inhibitors ± prokinetic agents.

Surgery (laparoscopic Nissen fundoplication) is reserved for failure for respond to conservative treatment with oesophageal stricture or severe pulmonary aspiration.

Intussusception
Definitions
Intussusception is the invagination of one segment of bowel into an adjacent distal segment. The segment that invaginates is called the *intussusceptum* and the segment into which it invaginates the *intussuscepiens*. The tip of the intussusceptum is called the *apex* or *lead point*.

Aetiology

• 90% are idiopathic.
• Viral infection can lead to hyperplasia of Peyer's patches which become the apex of an intussusception.
• Other lead points include Meckel's diverticulum, a polyp or a duplication cyst.

Clinical features

• Most common cause of intestinal obstruction in infants 3–12 months. Males > females.
• Presents with pain (attacks of colicky pain every 15–20 minutes, lasting 2–3 minutes with screaming and drawing up of legs), pallor, vomiting and lethargy between attacks.
• Sausage-shaped mass in RUQ, empty RIF (sign de Dance).
• Passage of blood and mucus ('redcurrant jelly' stool).
• Tachycardia and dehydration.

Diagnosis

• Plain X-ray may show intestinal obstruction and sometimes the outline of the intussusception.
• Ultrasonography investigation of choice: 'target sign', 'pseudo-kidney'.
• Definite diagnosis by air or (less common) barium enema.

Management

• IV fluids to resuscitate infant (shock is frequent because of fluid sequesteration in the bowel).
• Air reduction of intussusception if no peritonitis (success in 75%–90% of cases).
• Remainder require surgical reduction.

Inguinoscrotal conditions
Acute scrotum
Definition

The *acute scrotum* is a red, swollen, painful scrotum caused by torsion of the hydatid of Morgagni (60%), torsion of the testis (30%), epididymo-orchitis (10%) and idiopathic scrotal oedema (10%).

Management

• All cases of 'acute scrotum' should be explored.
• If true testicular torsion, treatment is bilateral orchidopexy (orchidectomy of affected testis if gangrenous).
• If torsion is hydatid of Morgagni, treatment is removal of hydatid on affected side only.

Inguinal hernia and hydrocele
Definitions and aetiology

During the seventh month of gestation the testis descends from the posterior abdominal wall into the scrotum through a peritoneal diverticulum called the *processus vaginalis*, which obliterates just before birth. An *inguinal hernia* in an infant is a swelling in the inguinal area due to failure of obliteration of the processus vaginalis, allowing bowel or omentum to descend within the hernial sac below the external inguinal ring. A *hydrocele* is a collection of fluid around the testis that has trickled down from the peritoneal cavity via a narrow, but patent, processus vaginalis.

Diagnosis

• Diagnosis of a hydrocele is usually obvious: the scrotum contains fluid and transilluminates brilliantly.
• Diagnosis of a hernia may be entirely on the mother's given history or a lump may be obvious.
• Strangulation is a serious complication as it may compromise bowel and/or the blood supply to the testis.

Management

• Hernia should be treated by early operation to obliterate the patent processus vaginalis.
• Hydroceles often close during the first two years. Should be repaired if persist after that.

Undescended testis
Definitions and aetiology

A *congenital undescended testis* (UDT) is one that has not reached the bottom of the scrotum at 3 months post-term. A *retractile testis* is one that can be manipulated to the bottom of the scrotum. An *ectopic testis* is one that has strayed from the normal path of descent.

Diagnosis

Most UDTs are found at the superficial inguinal pouch and associated with hypoplastic hemi-scrotum and inguinal hernia.

Management

• Treatment is by orchidopexy and should be performed at 6–12 months.
• UDTs are at increased risk of developing malignancy, even after orchidopexy and require long-term surveillance.

Index